EDITION

2

Sports Nutrition

A Guide for the Professional Working With Active People

Dan Benardot, PhD, RD

Editor-in-Chief

Sports and Cardiovascular Nutritionists (SCAN)
A Practice Group of The American Dietetic Association

The American Dietetic Association

SCAN is a practice group composed of sports and cardiovascular nutritionists who are members of The American Dietetic Association. The objectives of SCAN are threefold:

▶ to promote the integration of nutrition, exercise, and respiratory fitness necessary for the achievement and maintenance of optimal health;

▶ to help prevent or control cardiovascular disease; and

▶ to utilize nutrition and fitness to enhance the quality of life for all people.

Library of Congress Cataloging-in-Publication Data
Sports nutrition : a guide for the professional working with active people / Dan Benardot, editor-in-chief ; Sports and Cardiovascular Nutritionists, a practice group of The American Dietetic Association. — 2nd ed.
    p.   cm.
   includes bibliographical references and index.
   ISBN 0-88091-106-9
   1. Athletes—Nutrition. 2. Exercise—Physiological aspects. I. Benardot, Dan, 1949– . II. American Dietetic Association. Sports and Cardiovascular Nutritionists.
   [DNLM: 1. Exercise—physiology. 2. Nutrition. 3. Sports. QT260 S7632]
RC1235.S6637 1992
613.2′08′8796—dc20
DNLM/DLC
for Library of Congress   92-49945
                                                      CIP

The views expressed in this publication are those of the authors and do not necessarily reflect policies and/or official positions of The American Dietetic Association. Mention of product names in this publication does not constitute endorsement by the authors or The American Dietetic Association. The American Dietetic Association disclaims responsibility for the application of the information contained herein.

First edition published 1986.

Cover photo credits: *Tennis scene* ©1992, Terje Rakke/The Image Bank. *Orange* ©1992, Chicago Photographic Company

Contributors

EDITOR-IN-CHIEF
Dan Benardot, PhD, RD

ASSOCIATE EDITORS
Section 1, Ann Marie Hedquist, PhD, RD
Section 2, Melinda Manore, PhD, RD
Section 3, June Alberici, MS
Section 4, Mitchell Kanter, PhD
Section 5, Susan M. Kleiner, PhD, RD

CONTRIBUTING WRITERS
Dan Benardot, PhD, RD; Jacqueline Berning, MS, RD; Sharon Bortz, MS, RD;
Barbara A. Bowman, PhD; Joan Buchbinder, MS, RD; Nancy Clark, MS, RD;
Mildred Cody, PhD, RD; Julane Contursi, MS, RD; Lisa Dorfman, RD;
Marie Dunford, PhD, RD; Steven Fike, MEd, RD; Ann Grediagin, MS, RD;
Karen Hare, RD; Charlene Harkins, MEd, RD; Sara Hinkle, MS, RD; Mitchell Kanter, PhD;
Jane Kerstetter, PhD, RD; Susan M. Kleiner, PhD, RD; Susan Kosharek, MS, RD;
Page Love, MS, RD; Melinda Manore, PhD, RD; Elizabeth Markley, PhD, RD;
Gerald D. McKibben, PhD, RD; Jill Mielcarek, RD; Meg Binnie Molloy, MPH, RD;
Connie Mueller, MS, RD; Peggy H. Paul, RD; Kathy Quinn, MS, RD; Sheri L. Riel, MS;
Monique Ryan, RD; Josephine Connolly Schoonen, MS, RD; Ann Snyder, PhD;
Patti Tveit, MS, RD

RESOURCE CONTRIBUTORS
Susan M. Kleiner, PhD, RD; Penny Kris-Etherton, PhD, RD; James T. Ledford Jr;
Page Love, MS, RD; Jill Mielcarek, RD; Robin Shearn, MS, RD; Patti Tveit, MS, RD

REVIEWERS
Jacqueline Berning MS, RD; Kristine Larson Clark, PhD, RD;
Karen Reznik Dolins, MS, RD; Lori Valencic, MEd, RD

SCAN FUNCTIONAL COORDINATORS FOR PUBLICATIONS
Lori Valencic, MEd, RD; Joanne Milkereit, MHSA, RD; Nikki Salmons Zeidner, RD

Contents

Preface

This second edition of *Sports Nutrition* enlarges on the scope of the first edition, while maintaining the goal of providing a guide for the nutrition professional in meeting the objectives of the Sports and Cardiovascular Nutritionists dietetic practice group. This manual is intended for registered dietitians and other health professionals who provide clients with up-to-date and reliable information through individual nutrition and exercise counseling, group programs in sports medicine clinics, wellness programs, cardiac rehabilitation counseling, corporate fitness programs, and counseling professional and amateur sports teams.

The manual is organized in sections to help the reader obtain needed information quickly. Material that is applicable to more than one population or condition is repeated for the reader's convenience. In addition, the manual has an extensive index. These strategies help make *Sports Nutrition* comprehensive, as one would expect of a text, and easy to reference, as one would expect of a manual.

As scientific fields go, sports nutrition is still in its relative infancy. In spite of this, enough has been learned over the past two decades to confirm that sports nutrition is, indeed, a science, and this requires that established rules of scientific evidence be applied to the collection and distribution of information. This means that we can learn by carefully collecting data from those who have achieved the best in sports performance or who have shown improvement by following a particular protocol. However, the generalization of this information to others— given nutritional, psychological, physiological, anatomical, and motivational differences—is not easy to do. Therefore, while global generalizations on how to achieve optimal performance or health can be made, even to relatively homogeneous groups or sports teams, our strength lies in understanding and focusing on the individual.

There is still much to learn in the area of sports nutrition, and we will all require more time to understand fully what we think we already know. The information base is increasing so rapidly that existing paradigms are constantly being questioned and reevaluated. It would be comforting to think that an increase in activity is associated with a concomitant increase in food intake, so that the increased nutrient demands of activity are automatically met. After all, doesn't regular activity help to influence appetite so that physiological needs are met? In reality, however, some nutrients are used or lost at a rate faster than can easily be replaced by typical food intakes, and many athletes suffer from eating disorders that put them at frank nutritional risk. Most people who work in the area of sports nutrition have learned about gastric emptying and intestinal absorption rates, especially as these concepts relate to optimal rehydration. Yet, the individual differences in how fluids and foods leave the stomach and become absorbed are so great that we may be putting undue limitations in the recommendations we make. These are just a few of the many issues that should encourage you to place a great deal of emphasis on understanding the individual. To make the best possible nutritional recommendations, it is critical that we understand how and what our clients eat, their food tolerances and intolerances, how often and with what intensity they train, their physical condition, their family concerns, and their motivation to excel. We hope that this book will assist you in understanding the issues so that the best information can be provided as you work to optimize health and sports performance.

▶ **ACKNOWLEDGMENTS**

For this edition of *Sports Nutrition*, nutrient analyses were computed using data from the USDA Nutrient Database for Standard Reference, full version, release 9 (Oct 1992). At the time of publication, this is the latest USDA computer database release.

Many people contributed in various ways to this manual. I have attempted to identify those whose significant efforts, through writing and contributing resources, merit mention and praise. Their names appear throughout the body of the manual in the sections they worked on. But many other people contributed to the manual through their encouragement, energy, ideas, and comments. Among these are members of the SCAN executive board, and the Publications Division of The American Dietetic Association. Those who worked on the first edition must also be thanked, for without them our job on this second edition would have been interminably longer and more difficult. My colleagues at Georgia State University have been terrific at keeping an open eye for new developments in sports nutrition. I've lost track of the number of times they placed key new articles on my desk for review. The Sports and Cardiovascular Nutritionists dietetic practice group gratefully acknowledges the financial support of the Gatorade Sports Science Institute. Finally, a special thanks goes to my family and the families of all the SCAN members who contributed time to this project. Their understanding and encouragement made this manual a reality.

Dan Benardot, PhD, RD
Department of Nutrition and Dietetics
College of Health Sciences
Georgia State University
Atlanta

Metabolic Needs of Exercise

Ann Marie Hedquist, Editor

The relationship between nutrition and exercise is clear, straightforward, and well known. Reduced to its essential elements, this relationship focuses on two major factors:

▶ Exercise increases the rate of utilization of energy substrate and certain nutrients, with a concomitant rise in heat production.

▶ The increase in heat production results in a greater loss of body water (and associated minerals) via sweat, in the body's attempt to maintain normal body temperature.

Thus, the essential goal of the qualified nutritionist or registered dietitian is to help the athlete obtain energy, fluid, and associated nutrients in the right amounts and at the right times. While this may seem a relatively easy task, it is not. The specifics of individual requirements vary by sport, body size, gender, exercise intensity and duration, age, ambient temperature and humidity, conditioned level of the athlete, altitude, muscle-type predominance, body composition, and individual genetic variability. Further, since sports nutrition is a relatively young science, there is still much to learn about the individual nutrient requirements associated with exercise of different intensity and duration. This section presents an overview of our current knowledge about energy metabolism and exercise physiology and their implications on various activities.

Physiology of Anaerobic and Aerobic Exercise

Sharon Bortz, Josephine Connolly Schoonen, Mitchell Kanter, Susan Kosharek, and Dan Benardot

▶ MUSCLE FIBER-TYPE PREDOMINANCE

There are three types of muscle tissue in the human body:

- ▶ smooth
- ▶ cardiac
- ▶ skeletal

It is important to understand the functions of skeletal muscle when considering the energy demands of physical activity. Skeletal muscle constitutes approximately 40% of body weight, and it has three major functions: motion, heat production, and posture (body support).[1] Distinct types of muscle fibers make up skeletal muscle (see *Table 1.1*). Although there are individual differences in the distribution of each of these different muscle fibers, their relative proportion remains constant throughout life. It is these individual differences in fiber-type distribution that may be at least partially responsible for producing elite marathon runners who could never compete at the same level as sprinters, or elite gymnasts who could never be competitive as long-distance swimmers. These muscle fibers follow[2,3]:

- ▶ Type I (slow twitch)–oxidative endurance; also classified as "red" fibers due to their high myoglobin content
- ▶ Type IIA (fast twitch)–oxidative, glycolytic
- ▶ Type IIB (pure fast twitch)–glycolytic; may also be called white fibers

The proportion of muscle fiber types is largely determined by genetics. Aerobic training will enhance the oxidative capacities of the type IIA muscle

TABLE 1.1 Muscle Fiber Types and Their Characteristics

Muscle Fiber	Type I	Type IIA	Type IIB
Glycolytic capacity	Low	Moderate	High
Oxidative capacity	High	Moderate	Low
Contraction speed	Slow	Fast	Fast
Glycogen storage	Moderate-high	Moderate-high	Moderate-high
Triglyceride storage	High	Moderate	Low
Capillary supply	Good	Moderate	Poor

Adapted with permission from Saltin B, Henriksson J, Nygaard E, et al. Muscle fiber types and their characteristics. *Ann NY Acad Sci.* 1979;301:3-29.

fibers and may bring about a relative change in size. Training will not change the overall composition of the muscle fibers.

Muscular contraction and relaxation involve actin and myosin filaments in the muscle fibers. In order for either process to proceed, adenosine triphosphate (ATP) must be present. ATP provides the fuel for muscle contraction, active transport of nutrients, and biosynthesis within the body.[4]

► ENERGY SYSTEMS: ANAEROBIC METABOLISM (PHOSPHOCREATINE-ATP SYSTEM)

There are three major metabolic pathways by which ATP can be produced during exercise (see *Table 1.2*):

- ► the phosphagen system
- ► anaerobic glycolysis
- ► aerobic metabolism

The phosphagen system involves stored energy in the form of high-energy phosphate bonds of ATP and creatine phosphate (CP) molecules. ATP molecules are the first to lose their high-energy phosphate molecules and provide energy for muscle contraction.

Muscle cells can store only about 3 mol of ATP, which is capable of providing energy for only a few seconds of high-intensity exercise. To allow muscle contraction to continue, the ATP molecules are continuously resynthesized. For immediate resynthesis, CP serves as the phosphate donor. However, the amount of CP stored in the muscle fiber is only about five times as great as the ATP stores. The combined energy stores in the form of ATP and CP is, therefore, able to fuel muscle contractions for only a short time (less than 1 minute). To continue ATP resynthesis and to allow further exercise, energy must be derived from stored substrates by means of the anaerobic, glycolytic, and aerobic pathways (see *Figure 1.1*).

When the demand for energy persists and the ATP and CP stores are depleted, the accumulation of the byproducts of ATP breakdown initiates anaerobic glycolysis. This process, which is a series of reactions that converts

TABLE 1.2 General Characteristics of the Three Systems by Which ATP Is Formed

System	Food or Chemical Fuel	O_2 Required	Speed	Relative ATP Production
Anaerobic ATP-PC system (phosphagen system)	Phosphocreatine	No	Fastest	Little; limited
Lactic acid system (anaerobic glycolysis)	Glycogen (glucose)	No	Fast	Little; limited
Aerobic oxygen system (aerobic metabolism)	Glycogen, fats, proteins	Yes	Slow	Much; unlimited

Adapted from Fox EL, Mathews D. *The Physiological Basis of Physical Education and Athletics.* 3rd ed. New York, NY: Saunders College Publishing; 1981. Reprinted with permission.

FIGURE 1.1   Derivation of energy from the metabolism of the three basic foodstuffs.

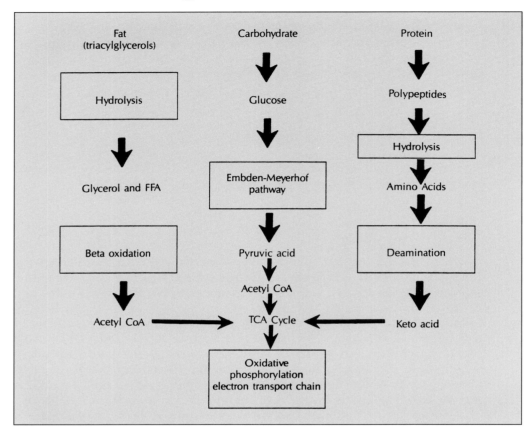

Adapted from deVries HA. *Physiology of Exercise for Physical Education and Athletics.* 3rd ed. Dubuque, Iowa: Wm C Brown Publishers; 1980. Reprinted with permission.

glucose to lactic acid, can fuel exercise for several minutes without oxygen.[5,6]

Once glycogen is used, the muscle cell can no longer contract at high intensity, and muscle fatigue sets in. In anaerobic glycolysis, the major energy metabolic process in high-intensity, near-maximum-effort exercise, glycogen is used at a rate that is 18 times faster than during oxidative phosphorylation for the same ATP yield. Much of the lactic acid that accumulates as a byproduct of anaerobic metabolism diffuses from the muscle and into the blood. This increase in blood lactate concentration, which happens quickly during intense exercise, inhibits lipolysis and enhances carbohydrate utilization, further increases lactic acid, and eventually contributes to muscle fatigue during prolonged aerobic exercise. This is done by the inhibition of glycolysis as a result of a decrease in pH in the intracellular compartment of the working cell.

At the initiation of any activity, more energy is derived from anaerobic metabolism than aerobic metabolism.[7] As activity continues, however, the proportion of energy derived from anaerobic metabolism decreases and the proportion of energy derived from aerobic metabolism increases. The aerobic system is far more efficient than the anaerobic system with respect to ATP production. The amount of ATP that can be synthesized from stored muscle glycogen is approximately 50 times more than that supplied by all the anaerobic systems combined.[8]

▶ ENERGY SYSTEMS: ANAEROBIC GLYCOLYSIS (LACTACID SYSTEM)

Many physiological adaptations occur in response to training. One way to examine the differences between trained and untrained individuals is to examine the metabolic responses to a bout of exercise. In fact, exercise is often described in terms of the metabolic response it elicits. Comparison of the metabolic response during exercise with the resting metabolic rate or with the maximal metabolic rate describes the absolute (as well as the relative) intensity of an exercise bout.

As the intensity of exercise increases, oxygen consumption ($\dot{V}O_2$max) increases linearly and the level of blood lactic acid remains relatively unchanged until exercise intensity approaches 60% to 80% of $\dot{V}O_2$max. At the point that the rate of lactic acid production exceeds the rate of lactic acid removal there is an exponential rise in the concentration of lactic acid in the blood. This inflection has mistakenly been called the "anaerobic threshold," but may best be described as the lactate threshold (Tlac). In trained individuals, Tlac is reached at approximately 70% to 85% of $\dot{V}O_2$max, whereas in untrained subjects the Tlac may occur at a lower intensity of exercise, 50% to 60% of $\dot{V}O_2$max. The rise in Tlac as a result of endurance training apparently occurs as a result of an increase in the rate of lactate removal in trained individuals.

In addition to bringing about changes in the clearance rate of lactic acid, endurance training also results in changes in the maximal amount of blood that can be pumped by the heart every minute (cardiac output, or CO). The increase in CO enables the trained individual to supply more oxygen to exercising muscle. Concomitant to the increase in CO, endurance training also increases the mitochondrial content in skeletal muscle, enlarging the quantity of oxidative enzymes. The increase in oxidative enzymes, along with the increase in oxygen delivery, enables the aerobically trained individual to metabolize fat at a greater rate than an untrained individual.

▶ ENERGY SYSTEMS: AEROBIC METABOLISM

The second phase of the ATP-generating energy system is called aerobic metabolism (*Figure 1.2*). As the name implies, this pathway ultimately requires the presence of oxygen. It is through this energy system that most of the ATP (energy) is produced. Aerobic metabolism can be divided into two stages:

Stage 1:   Oxidative metabolism
a. Pyruvate–acetyl CoA
b. Krebs cycle (also known as tricarboxylic acid cycle or citric acid cycle)
Stage 2:   Electron transport chain (also known as oxidative phosphorylation or the respiratory chain)

Once pyruvate is formed from glycolysis, it is transferred from the cytoplasm to the mitochondria of the cell, where the enzymes for mediating the reactions of aerobic metabolism are localized. A series of reactions are necessary to convert pyruvate into acetyl CoA, after which acetyl CoA enters the Krebs cycle. The purpose of the Krebs cycle is to produce coenzymes that are ultimately used for the electron transport chain.

Two important coenzymes involved in aerobic metabolism are flavin-adenine dinucleotide (FAD) and nicotinamide-adenine dinucleotide (NAD), since it is through these coenzymes that all of the ATP is produced. For each pyruvate-to-acetyl CoA reaction, a hydrogen atom is removed and transferred

FIGURE 1.2   Anaerobic and aerobic energy systems.

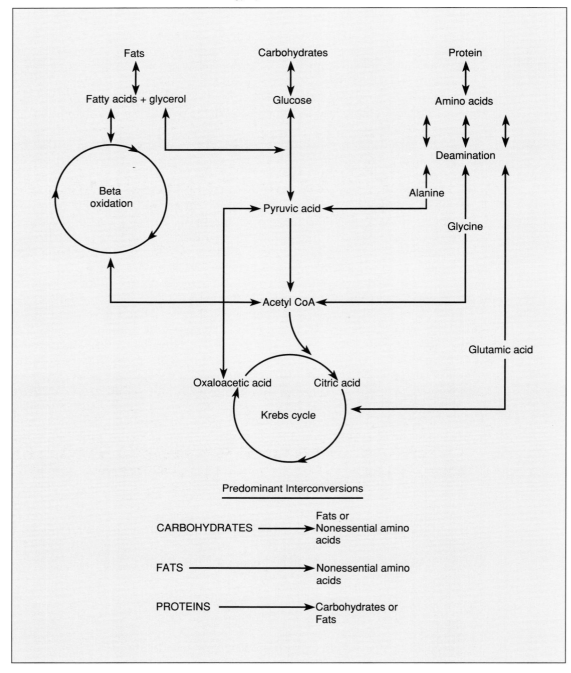

to one NAD. For each cycle of Krebs, 3 NAD and 1 FAD are used similarly. These coenzymes are then shuttled to the electron transport chain, which involves a chain of reactions for transporting the hydrogen electrons from the coenzymes. This series of reactions is driven by oxygen, and the ultimate products produced are water and ATP.

Carbohydrate, fat, and protein break down to forms that can enter anaerobic and aerobic metabolism. The carbohydrate breakdown product is glucose, which is the starting point for glycolysis and eventually follows the pathway to the Krebs cycle and the electron transport chain. The primary fat molecule, triglyceride, breaks down to form glycerol and three fatty acids. Glycerol reacts to form one of the components of glycolysis, from which point it can proceed through glycolysis and the Krebs cycle, or it can reform glucose (gluconeogenesis). The fatty acids have carbon units taken off two at a time (a process called beta oxidation), with each two-carbon unit producing acetyl CoA. The protein breakdown product, amino acids, can go one of two ways for producing ATP. Through the process of deamination, they form keto acids, which enter the Krebs cycle at various sites depending on the amino acid. Similarly, through transamination the amino group of an amino acid is transferred to a keto acid. Depending on the amino acid, it enters at either glycolysis or the Krebs cycle.

Glucose, fatty acids, and amino acids are all important sources of energy during exercise. Glucose and fatty acids provide for the majority of energy needs. Because the potential amount of energy produced from these substrates is related to carbon skeleton length and metabolic factors, the amount of energy derived from the metabolism of one molecule of these substrates varies widely.

There is some evidence that exercise results in an increased hepatic gluconeogenesis. Although it is not clear whether the amino acid alanine is formed from glucose or other amino acids, studies have demonstrated an increased release of alanine from exercising muscle. This alanine could be used to form additional glucose (via the glucose-alanine cycle), but it is still unclear whether this represents a net increase in available glucose, because the carbon skeleton of alanine may be derived from glucose.[9,10]

The amount and type of fuel used and the proportion of aerobic to anaerobic metabolism called into play depend on three main factors: intensity and duration of the exercise, condition of the athlete, and diet.[8] Environmental conditions can also affect fuel usage, with more muscle glycogen breakdown at higher temperatures.[11] See *Table 1.3* for a summary of major sports and their predominant energy systems.

Carbohydrates are preferable as the anaerobic fuel source because the ATP produced from their catabolism is immediate, due to the direct pathway from the working muscle. Muscle glycogen is the preferred carbohydrate fuel source for activities with an intensity greater than 65% $\dot{V}O_2$max.[12] Glycogen supply is limited, though, providing energy for roughly 2 hours of exercise.[13] When this fuel source is depleted, fatigue sets in.

Carbohydrates are also used by the marathon runner. The amount used depends on the runner's speed (the faster the speed, the more carbohydrates used) and his or her diet. If the runner previously consumed a high-carbohydrate diet, more stored carbohydrate in the form of glycogen will be available as a fuel source, thus delaying the onset of fatigue. Also, consuming high-carbohydrate drinks during the run allows the runner to use blood glucose instead of glycogen stores for immediate energy.

As the exercise intensity decreases and the duration of the activity increases, fat as a fuel source becomes more important (*Figure 1.3*). Fats are mobilized from muscle and adipose tissue. During exercise, trained endurance athletes experience increased fat utilization for the following reasons:

1. Aerobically trained muscles have an improved ability to utilize fat.
2. Lipoprotein-lipase activity is higher in trained muscle.
3. Taking points 1 and 2 together, there is an increased potential for the utilization of intramuscular triglycerides.

Fats make up the largest depot of fuel in the body, with enough fuel for 6.5 days of running.[14] The more fat can substitute for glucose and its precursor, glycogen, as a fuel source, the more the body can spare these limited fuel sources, thereby prolonging the activity.

TABLE 1.3 Major Sports and Their Predominant Energy Systems

Sport or Sport Activity	Emphasis According to Energy Systems		
	ATP-PC and LA*	LA-O_2†	O_2‡
Baseball	80	20	–
Basketball	85	15	–
Fencing	90	10	–
Field hockey	60	20	20
Football	90	10	–
Golf	95	5	–
Gymnastics			
Ice hockey			
forwards, defense	80	20	–
goalie	95	5	–
Lacrosse			
goalie defense, attack men	80	20	–
midfielders, man-down	60	20	20
Rowing	20	30	50
Skiing			
slalom, jumping, downhill	80	20	–
cross-country	–	5	95
pleasure skiing	34	33	33
Soccer			
goalie, wings, strikers	80	20	–
halfbacks or link men	60	20	20
Swimming and diving			
50 yd diving	98	2	–
100 yd	80	15	5
200 yd	30	65	5
400-500 yd	20	40	40
1500-1650 yd	10	20	70
Tennis	70	20	10
Track and field			
100-200 yd	98	2	–
field events	90	10	–
440 yd	80	15	5
880 yd	30	65	5
1 mile	20	55	25
2 miles	20	40	40
3 miles	10	20	70
6 miles (cross-country)	5	15	80
marathon	–	5	95
Volleyball	90	10	–

Adapted from Fox EL, Mathews D. *The Physiological Basis of Physical Education and Athletics.* 3rd ed. New York, NY: Saunders College Publishing; 1981. Reprinted with permission.

  *Anaerobic (phosphagen system)

  †Combination (lactic acid-oxygen)

  ‡Aerobic (oxygen)

It is important to realize that during all types of exercise, anaerobic and aerobic metabolism work together (Table 1.3). During the first several minutes of any activity, anaerobic metabolism provides most of the energy. As the time of activity increases, but intensity remains low to moderate, the contribution of aerobic metabolism increases (see Figure 1.3). This process can be summarized as follows:

▶ High exercise intensity (high $\dot{V}O_2$max) relies more heavily on glucose as a fuel.

▶ Low exercise intensity (low $\dot{V}O_2$max), with adequate oxygen and oxidative enzymes, relies on a mixture of fat and carbohydrate as a fuel.

FIGURE 1.3 The anaerobic/aerobic combination.

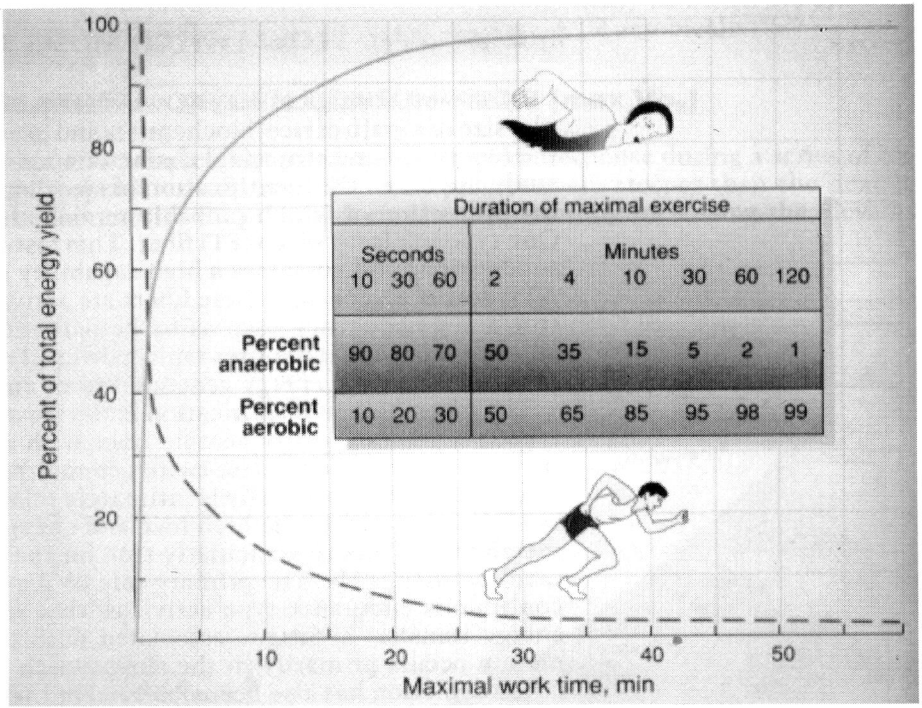

Percent of total energy yield
100
80
60
40
20
Maximal work time, min
10
20
30
40
50
Duration of maximal exercise
Seconds
10 30 60
Minutes
2 4 10 30 60 120
Percent anaerobic
90 80 70 50 35 15 5 2 1
Percent aerobic
10 20 30 50 65 85 95 98 99

Relative contribution of aerobic and anaerobic energy during maximal physical activity of various durations. It should be noted that 1.5 to 2 minutes of maximal effort requires 50% of the energy from aerobic and anaerobic processes. Adapted from Åstrand PO, Rodahl K. *Textbook of Work Physiology.* New York, NY: McGraw-Hill Book Co; 1977. Used with permission of McGraw-Hill Book Co.

REFERENCES

1. McArdle WD, Katch F, Katch V. *Exercise Physiology, Energy, Nutrition and Human Performance.* Philadelphia, Pa: Lea & Febiger; 1986.
2. Fox EL. *Sports Physiology.* 2nd ed. Philadelphia, Pa: Saunders College Publishing; 1984.
3. Wright DE, Paige DM. Physical exercise and energy requirements. *J Clin Nutr.* 1988;7:9-17.
4. Katch F, McArdle WD. *Nutrition Weight Control and Exercise.* 2nd ed. Philadelphia, Pa: Lea & Febiger; 1983.
5. Guyton AC. *The Textbook of Medical Physiology.* 6th ed. Philadelphia, Pa: WB Saunders Co; 1981.
6. Murray RK, Granner DK, Mayes PA, Rodwell VW. *Harper's Biochemistry.* 21st ed. Norwalk, Conn: Appleton and Lange; 1988.
7. deVries H. *Physiology of Exercise.* 3rd ed. Dubuque, Iowa: WC Brown Co; 1980.
8. Fox E, Matthews D. *The Physiological Basis of Physical Education and Athletics.* 3rd ed. New York, NY: Saunders College Publishing; 1981.
9. Felig P, Wahren J. Amino acid metabolism in exercising man. *J Clin Invest.* 1971;50:2703.
10. Goldstein L, Newsholme EA. The formation of alanine from amino acids in diaphragm muscle of the rat. *Biochem J.* 1976;154:555.
11. Fink WJ, Costill DL, Van Handel PJ. Leg metabolism during exercise in the heat and cold. *Eur J Appl Physio.* 1975;34:183-190.
12. Saltin B, Karlsson J. Muscle glycogen utilization during work of different intensities. In: Pernow B, Saltin B, eds. *Muscle Metabolism During Exercise.* New York, NY: Plenum Press; 1971:289-300.

13. Lamb DR, Murray R. *Perspectives in Exercise Science and Sports Medicine.* Vol 1, *Prolonged Exercise.* Indianapolis, Ind: Benchmark Press; 1988.
14. Lemon PWR, Yarasheski KE, Dolony DG. The importance of protein for athletes. *Sports Med.* 1984;1:474-484.

Fuel Supplies for Exercise

Jacqueline Berning, Gerald McKibben, Dan Benardot, and Steven Fike

▶ CARBOHYDRATES

Carbohydrates can be categorized as either *simple* or *complex*. Simple carbohydrates include the common monosaccharides and disaccharides: glucose, fructose, sucrose, and galactose. Whereas simple carbohydrates are commonly associated with sweets and candy, they also occur naturally in fruits and vegetables. Complex carbohydrates include the digestible and indigestible polysaccharides, and are associated with starches (pasta, bread, cereal, legumes, starchy vegetables) and other fruits and vegetables.

Carbohydrates and Muscle Glycogen Storage

Both simple and complex carbohydrates are important components of an athlete's diet. It has been recommended that athletes derive 60% to 70% of total calories from carbohydrates, with 45% to 50% from complex carbohydrates and 8% to 12% from simple carbohydrates.[1] Several studies have evaluated the relative effects of different carbohydrates as fuels for exercise. Costill and colleagues compared the effects of simple and complex carbohydrate consumption during a 48-hour period after glycogen-depleting exercise.[2] During the first 24 hours, no statistically significant differences were found in muscle glycogen synthesis between the simple and complex carbohydrates (75 mmol/kg for complex; 70 mmol/kg for simple). At 48 hours, however, the complex-carbohydrate diet resulted in significantly greater muscle glycogen synthesis than the simple-carbohydrate diet (22 mmol/kg for complex; 8 mmol/kg for simple). It was hypothesized that complex carbohydrates sustained a higher level of insulin than simple carbohydrates, and this was responsible for the enhanced muscle glycogen storage during the second 24-hour period. In a similar comparison, the effects of simple and complex carbohydrates on skeletal muscle glycogen content were compared.[3] It was found that significant increases in muscle glycogen content could be achieved with the provision of either simple or complex carbohydrates.

It should be considered that, especially in the long run, complex carbohydrates have an advantage over simple carbohydrates because they tend to be more nutrient-dense. Complex carbohydrates provide more B vitamins necessary for energy metabolism, and they may also provide more fiber and iron. Because consumption of complex carbohydrates contributes to a more nutritionally balanced diet, athletes should be encouraged to consume diets higher in complex carbohydrates and lower in simple carbohydrates.

Glycogen

Glycogen, an intracellular polysaccharide, is the body's predominant storage form of carbohydrate. It is the primary source of fuel in endurance events, such as marathon running, cross-country skiing, distance cycling, and swimming. Liver and muscle cells store the body's limited glycogen supply. When this supply is lowered or depleted, muscle fibers lack the fuel needed for contraction, and fatigue results. Any method that either delays glycogen depletion or maximizes glycogen storage capability is important to endurance athletes, or to athletes who train daily.

In the late 1960s, Scandinavian researchers popularized a training and diet regimen now known as carbohydrate loading or glycogen loading.[4,5] This technique allows an athlete to store two to three times the normal amount of muscle glycogen. Usual muscle glycogen stores represent about 1500 kcal of carbohydrate.[6] Liver glycogen stores contribute an additional 320 kcal, and a smaller amount is in blood. For the endurance athlete, the combined glycogen-glucose pool can last about 2 hours.

The glycogen-loading technique is useful in delaying glycogen depletion and premature exhaustion in athletes exercising continuously for greater than 1 hour. The classical carbohydrate depletion and loading technique is presented here to compare the process with current theories.

Glycogen Loading

Depletion. The first phase (depletion of glycogen stores) begins 1 week prior to the event. A long and hard training session helps to deplete existing muscle glycogen stores. For the next 3 days, moderate exercise further reduces muscle glycogen stores, and muscles become "hungry" for carbohydrates. The diet during this phase is low in carbohydrates (100 g per day) and high in fat and protein.

Loading. In the 3 days before the competition little exercise is done, to give muscles a rest and to limit glycogen utilization. High-carbohydrate meals are consumed to supersaturate muscles with glycogen stores. These precompetition meals provide 60% to 70% of total calories in starchy carbohydrates (250 to 600 g carbohydrate per day). The high-carbohydrate meals contain a moderate amount of protein and a low amount of fat. This regimen is theorized to "load" the muscles with glycogen and enhance athletic performance.

After the competition, high-carbohydrate meals are once again consumed to replace the glycogen used during the competition. This early and classical carbohydrate-loading regimen is controversial because it often causes physiological side effects that may physically or psychologically impair performance for some athletes. The first phase of heavy workouts, without carbohydrate repletion, leaves athletes feeling weak, sore, dizzy, and tired. During the subsequent loading phase, the athlete may feel bloated, heavy, and uncomfortable. Three to five grams of water are retained per gram of glycogen stored.[7] The retained water yields a typical 2-lb to 7-lb weight gain that may leave the athlete feeling fat and sluggish. In addition, the athlete must also reduce activity; thus, his or her regular training pattern is disrupted. Younger athletes, people with diabetes, people at high risk of cardiovascular disease, and survivors of a myocardial infarction should completely refrain from this regimen because of the dietary manipulations involved. Because of the potential for negative side effects, this classical approach to glycogen loading is *not* recommended.

Research indicates that carbohydrate deprivation during the depletion phase is not necessary and has numerous detriments.[8] Endurance training itself stimulates increased glycogen synthetase activity, which encourages glycogen synthesis and storage.[9] Therefore, enforced dietary carbohydrate depletion is unnecessary.

Safe Glycogen Loading

To obtain maximal muscle glycogen stores *safely*, athletes should consume a high-carbohydrate diet as a standard part of their regular conditioning program. Meals during this conditioning program should supply at least 50% (preferably 60% to 70%) of total calories in carbohydrates.[10] At 50% of total calories for a person who consumes 3000 kcal per day, this represents a minimum of 375 g of carbohydrates per day. Three days prior to an endurance event, physical training should taper to allow muscles to rest. Dietary carbohydrates should gradually be increased and culminate in precompetition meals that contain 60% to 70% of total calories from carbohydrates. This represents a minimum of 450 g of carbohydrates per day for a 3000-kcal intake. The combination of rest and increased carbohydrate intake encourages glycogen storage that is comparable to the traditional carbohydrate-loading regimen, but is not associated with any of the potentially negative side effects.[11]

Although carbohydrate loading does not help an athlete run faster, the regimen might help the athlete perform longer before tiring. Because inadequate muscle and liver glycogen are associated with reduced performance, athletes (especially those involved in endurance events) should assure adequate glycogen stores by consuming a high proportion of total calories from carbohydrates.

The carbohydrates in an athlete's diet should come primarily from complex carbohydrate sources (fruits, vegetables, legumes, juices, breads, cereals, and pastas). Simple sugars have limited nutritional value and should be used sparingly by the training athlete when carbohydrate loading. More healthful food choices contribute energy plus needed vitamins and minerals.

With carbohydrate loading, the total daily calories should not increase; rather, the athlete should increase the percentage of carbohydrate calories. Some high-carbohydrate foods, such as pizza, ice cream, and pastas with rich sauces, are also high in fat and, thus, calorically dense. However, because these are the foods athletes eat, consider offering athletes suggestions on how to make these foods more acceptable. Encourage them, for example, to choose vegetable pizza with a thick crust, pasta with marinara sauce, and frozen yogurt. (See appendix 1 for a list of foods commonly consumed and the distribution of carbohydrate, fat, and protein as percentages of total calories.)

▶ FATS

Dietary fat serves several major functions:

> ▶ It is an energy source.
> ▶ It provides an essential fatty acid (linoleic acid).
> ▶ It aids in the absorption and transport of fat-soluble vitamins.

Fats commonly contribute 35% to 45% of the calories in the typical American diet, a level far higher than that necessary to maintain optimal health.[12] Fats are a natural component of some foods, such as whole milk, meat, nuts, and cheese, and they are often added in food processing to make, for example, potato chips and desserts.

Dietary fat is hydrolyzed primarily by pancreatic lipase in the small intestine after the fats have been emulsified by bile salts. The end products are monoglycerides, fatty acids, and glycerol. After being transported into the intestinal cell walls, the fatty acids and glycerol combine to form triacylglycerols, which are then absorbed into the lymph as chylomicrons, and eventually transported into the blood. The major storage site of fat is adipose tissue, although the muscles and other tissues may also serve as minor storage deposits.

The contribution of fat as an energy source decreases as the intensity of the exercise increases. Fatty acids cannot generate ATP anaerobically, and, as the exercise intensity increases, fat assumes a lesser role in total energy metabolism. In addition, fatty acid metabolism requires more oxygen than the metabolism of carbohydrates.

Fat is a concentrated source of energy, providing more than twice the potential energy of protein or carbohydrate (9 kcal/g v 4 kcal/g). Aside from the extremely small amounts (3 to 6 g per day) of fat needed as a carrier of the fat-soluble vitamins and the essential fatty acid (linoleic acid), dietary fat is not necessary. The body is fully capable of manufacturing storage fat from extra (beyond that needed for total energy requirement) dietary protein and carbohydrate. Also, most people already have sufficient stores of fat, so increasing fat intake as a means of providing energy is not necessary. Typically, it is not fat that is a limiting factor in performance at low work loads, but related substrates that are necessary for the metabolism of fat. For instance, low blood glucose and liver glycogen levels may be responsible for shortening endurance even in the presence of large amounts of free fatty acids. Consuming a high-fat diet may result in a slightly larger proportion of fats used during exercise. However, because this type of diet limits the amount of carbohydrates stored, and because carbohydrates are necessary for the complete oxidation of fats, the ultimate effect is to reduce endurance.[13]

The average 150-lb person with 10% to 20% body fat stores has between 63 000 and 126 000 potential calories as fat. However, this same person would only have 1800 to 2000 potential calories stored as carbohydrate. Therefore, even the leanest athletes have adequate fat storage to meet the metabolic demands of endurance activity.

Triglycerides

Triglycerides are the primary storage form of fat in the body, but triglycerides are not used directly as fuel. Much like glycogen is a storage form for glucose, triglycerides are a storage form for metabolizable fatty acids and glycerol. Triglycerides can be stored in fat cells around the body, and also within muscle cells. The triglycerides stored within muscle cells are available for immediate muscular work, while those stored in adipose cells must be transported to the tissues where they are needed. Of the three potential body sources of fat (stored triglycerides, blood triglycerides, and free fatty acids), stored triglycerides in adipose tissue and in muscle are the only practical energy sources during exercise.[14] Free fatty acids in the blood total approximately 0.75 g (<7 kcal), and blood triglycerides total approximately 8 g (72 kcal).

Fat stored in adipose tissues (as triglyceride) is mobilized by lipolysis. The resulting free fatty acids are the energy form usable by muscle cells. In addition to the free fatty acids that are generated by the hydrolysis of triglycerides in adipose tissue, a portion of the lipids oxidized during prolonged exercise are derived from plasma and intramuscular triglyceride hydrolysis.[15] This contribution of plasma triglyceride is relatively small during exercise. However, intramuscular lipid stores have been reported to decrease 30% to 50% during 30 and 100 km races.[15] Training increases the capacity of skeletal muscle to utilize fat. A highly trained marathon athlete running at a pace that is 70% $\dot{V}O_2$max for 1 hour can derive up to 75% of the total energy requirement through fat metabolism.[12]

Fats and Exercise

At the initiation of exercise, muscles are provided with more oxygen and free fatty acids in preparation for fuel needs. The degree to which lipids are used as fuel during exercise is determined by five variables[16]:

▶ exercise intensity
▶ exercise duration
▶ diet
▶ endurance training history
▶ altered metabolic state

Exercise of <50% $\dot{V}O_2$max (low-intensity) mainly involves use of type I (slow-twitch) muscle fibers. These may rely extensively on free fatty acids for fuel. As exercise intensity increases, type IIA and type IIB fibers are gradually recruited, leading to a greater requirement for glucose as a fuel.

Endurance (aerobic) training has the effect of increasing the number of mitochondria per cell and adding enzymes involved in fatty-acid oxidation. This training effect causes an increase in endurance capacity by enhancing the athlete's ability to burn fat as an energy substrate. This increased ability to burn fat as a fuel is demonstrated in four distinct ways[17]:

1. Lower respiratory ratio at the same exercise intensity (representing a more efficient use of oxygen)
2. Lower respiratory quotient (representing more oxygen able to be used at a given work load)
3. Decreased rate of glycogen utilization (representing more fat used to meet energy needs)
4. Lower lactate production (representing more complete oxidation–improved oxygen utilization–of energy substrates)

Because fatty acids do not provide a significant proportion of the energy used by type II (fast-twitch) muscle fibers, the rate at which lipids are used for fuel declines in proportion to exercise intensity. However, training does increase the rate of fat utilization by these muscles by changing their oxidative potential.

▶ PROTEINS AND AMINO ACIDS

Protein has long been a nutrient of interest for athletes and a controversial issue for nutritionists. Many athletes believe large quantities of protein are necessary to build muscle tissue, add strength, and provide extra energy. Protein and amino acids are among the most popular supplements taken by athletes involved in weight training. Amino acids (see *Table 1.4*), the building blocks of protein, are commonly believed to be absorbed and assimilated into muscle tissue more efficiently than protein. Other athletes believe amino acids will stimulate the release of growth hormone, causing rapid muscle and strength gains. The role of protein and amino acids in athletic performance is a complex issue, one that is not yet completely understood. The Food and Nutrition Board of the National Research Council has stated that protein requirements do not increase for individuals engaged in strenuous activity.[18] However, a growing

TABLE 1.4 Essential and Nonessential Amino Acids

Essential Amino Acids	Nonessential Amino Acids
Histidine	Alanine
Isoleucine	Arginine
Leucine	Asparagine
Lysine	Aspartic acid
Methionine	Cysteine
Phenylalanine	Glutamic acid
Threonine	Glutamine
Tryptophan	Glycine
Valine	Proline
	Serine
	Tyrosine

body of scientific evidence shows that protein needs of athletes may be greater than those of nonathletes.

Functions

Second to water, protein makes up the largest percentage of material in the human body–around 45%.[19] The requirement for protein is actually a requirement for amino acids. Protein is like a chain-link fence, with amino acids as the links. Protein is a component of many hormones, including growth hormone and insulin. It supplies antibodies for the body's immune system, and it is part of every enzyme in the body. Other body proteins that have a role in athletic performance include hemoglobin and myoglobin, which are involved in oxygen transport to muscles. A lesser role of protein is to supply energy, as amino acids, during starvation or intense exercise. In aerobic sports, amino acids may supply up to 15% of the total energy used. It is easy to see that an inadequate supply of protein will quickly harm one's health and performance.

Factors Affecting Protein Requirements

An individual's protein requirement is dependent on the following factors[20]:

1. Energy intake
2. Degree of training
3. Intensity of training

The most important factor affecting protein requirement is calorie intake. At any given protein intake, increasing energy intake will improve protein utilization.[21] Conversely, when energy intake is below the requirement, protein breakdown and loss increases.[22]

The second factor affecting a person's protein requirement is degree of training or conditioning. The effect of training on protein needs appears to be transient. Initially, protein losses increase with training, but they return to normal after an adaptation period of 5 to 14 days.[23] In fact, training may actually increase the efficiency of protein utilization.[24] The implication is that well-trained individuals need less protein than those beginning an exercise program.

The third factor affecting protein requirement is training intensity. There is some discrepancy in data regarding the effect of intensity on protein requirement.[20] Some data show that protein losses increase with a heavy training bout,[25,26] while other researchers have found the opposite.[27] This discrepancy may be due to timing of the study, actual intensity, and poor dietary controls. It does appear that, as intensity increases to the anaerobic level, protein breakdown (from increased amino acid use) increases.[28] The rate of amino acid use appears to be dependent on glycogen stores. One study found an increased rate of amino acid utilization during exercise in individuals with depleted glycogen stores.[29] Adequate muscle glycogen stores may, therefore, have a protein-sparing effect.

Protein Needs of Endurance Athletes

Contrary to conventional wisdom, it appears that endurance athletes have greater protein needs than strength-training athletes.[25,30] Although the reasons for this are not entirely clear, they include increased utilization of branched-chain amino acids and increased breakdown of protein (similar to what happens during starvation).[13] Recent studies have indicated that, to maintain nitrogen balance, a protein intake of 0.94 to 1.37 g/kg per day is necessary for endurance athletes.[26,30] Athletes in this category might include distance runners, swimmers, soccer players, cross-country skiers, triathletes, and road cyclists.

Protein Needs of Strength Athletes

Weight training may actually improve the efficiency of protein utilization.[24] A recent study found that the protein needs of weight-training athletes were actually closer to those of inactive individuals than to those of endurance athletes.[30] Again, the time when the training starts is important in determining needs. Early reports from Eastern Europe recommending protein intakes in excess of 2 g/kg per day lacked adequate diet controls.[31,32] More recent reports have suggested that adequate protein stores and muscle growth can be obtained on an intake of 0.8 to 1.2 g/kg per day.[24]

Determining Requirements

Contrary to popular belief, muscle tissue is not mostly protein; rather, it is approximately 70% water. It is not known how much muscle tissue can be assimilated in a given time period. In a best-case scenario, an adult in weight training may be able to add 1 kg of muscle in a week. Since muscle is approximately 20% protein, the following formula can be used to calculate the amount of protein needed above minimal requirements to add this extra kilogram of muscle. One kilogram of muscle $\times$ 20% = 0.2 kg. Thus, 200 extra grams of protein per week would be needed to add 1 kg of muscle (200 g/7 = 28 g protein per day). This would amount to an extra 4 oz of meat per day. Of course, this scenario assumes that all extra protein is converted into lean tissue.

Actual Intake

Diet studies performed on athletes indicate that both strength and endurance athletes generally consume well in excess of the Recommended Dietary Allowance (RDA) of protein.[32-34] Football players have been reported to consume 1.8 to 2 g of protein per kilogram of body weight.[34,35] Bodybuilders may consume even more.[36] Reports on triathletes indicate intakes around 2 g/kg of body weight.[32,33] It appears that those athletes who generally consume supplemental protein and amino acids (bodybuilders and strength-training athletes) are actually the ones who need them the least. On the other hand, athletes (such as gymnasts) who may need extra protein (due to their low calorie intake and increased requirements for growth) seldom consume supplemental protein.

▶ PROBLEMS WITH ALCOHOL AS AN ENERGY SUBSTRATE

In the early 1900s, marathoners sometimes received brandy during a race. Like strychnine, which marathoners also received, alcohol was thought to enhance performance in endurance events.[37] Alcohol is one of the most abused drugs in the United States. Although it is a concentrated source of calories, it has limited food value. While alcohol has a high caloric yield (7 kcal/g), it is not a significant energy supplier during exercise. Once metabolized, most of the alcohol's energy yield is released as heat; hence, alcohol is not stored for future use as body fuel. *Table 1.5* provides the energy content of typical alcoholic beverages.

In moderate amounts (one to two drinks), alcohol does not appear to affect performance negatively, provided it is not ingested the day of the competition. If one drink (12 oz of beer, 4 oz of wine, or 1 oz of 80 proof [40% alcohol] liquor) is consumed before a workout or event, the alcohol will have a direct effect on the nervous system. Alcohol acts on the brain by depressing its ability to reason and make judgments. Information-related processes are slowed; fine motor skills are decreased; reaction time is reduced; coordination, balance, and visual perception are altered; and muscular reflexes are impaired. Athletes involved in sports like tennis and racquetball, which demand the athlete's rapid reflex response, are most affected.

Alcohol can weaken the heart's pumping force[38] and diminish sprinting, middle-distance[39] and endurance performance.[40] One of the most harmful effects of alcohol in an athletic event is evident in prolonged endurance contests. The liver is the primary organ for the detoxification of alcohol. Once alcohol is present in the blood, the metabolism of alcohol takes priority over other liver functions. During prolonged exercise, when the body needs the extra glucose that can be formed by the liver, an elevated level of blood alcohol may block this biochemical pathway. A drop in blood glucose during an endurance event could lead to early fatigue.

Alcohol is absorbed into the bloodstream via the stomach and small intestine. Peak concentration in the blood occurs within 1 hour of consumption, depending on whether food is in the stomach. The absorbed alcohol is distributed within the water compartments of cells. This can disturb the water balance in muscle cells and consequently alter the cellular enzymatic activity that produces ATP, the substrate that provides fuel for muscle contraction, active transport, and biosynthesis within the body.

Body size and composition will alter dose/response rates to alcohol. A small, lean athlete whose body has a high percentage of body water is likely to experience fatigue from the effects of alcohol sooner than would a larger person with more body fat.

Research indicates that moderate levels of alcohol are associated with elevated levels of high-density lipoprotein cholesterol (HDL-C). Levels of HDL-C are also increased as a result of exercise, and are associated with a reduced risk of heart disease. However, two distinct subfractions of HDL have been

TABLE 1.5 Energy Content of Typical Alcoholic Beverages

Beverage	Amount, oz	CHO, g	CHO, kcal	Alcohol, g	Alcohol, kcal	Total kcal
Beer	12	14	56	13	91	147
Wine, table	4	4	16	12	84	100
Liquor (80 proof)	1.5	0	0	14	98	98

Adapted from Adams C. *Nutritive Value of American Foods in Common Units.* Washington, DC: Agriculture Research Service; 1975. US Dept of Agriculture handbook 456.

identified. The HDL$_3$-C is increased with moderate alcohol consumption; the HDL$_2$-C fraction is increased as a result of exercise. It is the HDL$_2$-C fraction that is believed to be protective against coronary heart disease.[41]

Drinking alcohol provides relaxation and can calm precompetition nervousness, and its vasodilation effect enhances blood flow to the muscles. However, drinking before training or before a competition may not improve work capacity and may lead to decreased performance levels. It is also important to remember that alcohol abuse is a major cause of automobile and other serious accidents, and that prolonged overconsumption can damage the liver, heart, muscles, and brain. Alcohol use should be discouraged.

REFERENCES

1. *US Dietary Goals*. Washington, DC: US Select Committee on Nutrition and Human Needs; 1978. US Dept of Health and Human Services and US Dept of Agriculture.
2. Costill DL, Sherman WM, Fink WJ, Witten MW, Miller JM. The role of dietary carbohydrates in muscle glycogen resynthesis after strenuous running. *Am J Clin Nutr*. 1981;34:1831-1836.
3. Roberts KM, Noble EG, Hayden DB, Taylor AW. Simple and complex carbohydrate rich diets and muscle glycogen content of marathon runners. *Eur J Appl Physiol*. 1988;57:70-74.
4. Bergstrom J, Hermansen L, Saltin B. Diet, muscle glycogen and physical performance. *Acta Physiol Scand*. 1967;71:140-150.
5. Ahlborg B, Bergstrom J, Brohult J, Ekelund L, Hultman E, Maschio G. Human muscle glycogen content and capacity for prolonged exercise after different diets. *Foersvarsmedicin*. 1967;3:85-99.
6. National Dairy Council. *Food Power*. 1984.
7. Olsson KE, Saltin B. Variations in total body water with muscle glycogen changes in man. *Biochem Exerc Med Sports*. 1969;5:159-162.
8. Sherman WM, Costill DL, Fink WJ, Miller JM. The effects of exercise and diet manipulation on muscle glycogen and its subsequent use during performance. *Int J Sports Med*. 1981;2:114-118.
9. Kochan RG, Lamb DR, Lutz SA, Perrill CV, Reimann EM, Schtender KK. Glycogen synthase activation in human skeletal muscle: effects of diet and exercise. *Am J Physiol*. 1979;236:E660-E666.
10. Williams M. *Nutrition for Fitness and Sport*. 3rd ed. Dubuque, Iowa: Wm C Brown Co; 1992.
11. Ivy J, Costill D. Influence of caffeine and carbohydrate feedings on endurance performance. *Med Sci Sports Exerc*. 1979;11:6.
12. Mattson FH. In: Hegstead DM et al, eds. *Present Knowledge in Nutrition*. 4th ed. New York, NY: Nutrition Foundation, Inc; 1976.
13. Lemon PWR, Nagle FJ. Effects of exercise on protein and amino acid metabolism. *Med Sci Sports Exerc*. 1981;13:141-149.
14. Williams MH. The role of fat in physical activity. In: *Nutritional Aspects of Human Physical and Athletic Performance*. Springfield, Ill: Charles C Thomas Publisher; 1985.
15. Connor E, Connor L. The dietary prevention and treatment of coronary heart disease. In: Connor WE, Briston JD, eds. *Coronary Heart Disease: Prevention, Complications, and Treatment*. Philadelphia, Pa: JB Lippincott; 1985.
16. Wright ED, Paige DM. Lipid metabolism and exercise. *J Clin Nutr*. 1988;7:28-32.
17. Gollnick PD. Metabolism of substrates: energy substrate metabolism during and as modified by training. *Fed Proc*. 1985;44:353-7.
18. National Research Council, Food and Nutrition Board. *Recommended Dietary Allowances*. 10th ed. Washington, DC: National Academy Press; 1989.
19. Munro HN, Crim MC. The proteins and amino acids. In: Goodhart RS, Shils ME, eds. *Modern Nutrition in Health and Disease*. 6th ed. Philadelphia, Pa: Lea & Febiger; 1980.
20. Butterfield GE. Whole-body protein utilization in humans. *Med Sci Sports Exerc*. 1987;19:S157-S167.

21. Butterfield GE, Calloway DH. Physical activity improves protein utilization in young men. *Br J Nutr*. 1984;51:171-184.

22. Todd DS, Butterfield GE, Calloway DH. Nitrogen balance in men with adequate and deficient energy intake at three levels of work. *J Nutr*. 1984;114:2107-2118.

23. Gontzea I, Sutzescu R, Dumitrach S. The influence of adaptation to physical effort on nitrogen balance in man. *Nutr Reports Intl*. 1975;11:231-236.

24. Marable NL, Hickson JF, et al. Urinary nitrogen excretion as influenced by a muscle-building exercise program and protein intake variation. *Nutr Reports Intl*. 1979;19:795-805.

25. Meredith CN, Zackin MJ, Frontera WR, Evans WJ. Dietary protein requirements and body protein metabolism in endurance-trained men. *J Appl Physiol*. 1989;66:2850-2856.

26. Dohm GL, Williams RT, Kasperek GJ, Van Rij AM. Increased excretion of urea and N-methylhistidine by rats and humans after a bout of exercise. *J Appl Physiol*. 1982;52:27-33.

27. Horswill CA, et al. Excretion of 3-methylhistidine and hydroxyproline following acute weight-training exercise. *Int J Sports Med*. 1988;9:245-248.

28. Millward DJ, et al. Effect of exercise on protein metabolism in humans as explored with stable isotopes. *Fed Proc*. 1982;41:2686-2691.

29. Lemon PWR, Mullin JP. Effect of initial muscle glycogen levels on protein catabolism during exercise. *J Appl Physiol*. 1980;48:624-629.

30. Tarnopolsky M, MacDougall D, Atkinson S. Influence of protein intake and training status on nitrogen balance and lean body mass. *J Appl Physiol*. 1988;64:187-193.

31. Celejowa I, Homa M. Food intake, nitrogen and energy balance in Polish weight lifters during a training camp. *Nutr Metabol*. 1970;12:259-274.

32. Laritcheva KA, Yalovaya NI, Shubin VI, Smirnov PV. Study of energy expenditure and protein needs of top weight lifters. In: Parizkova J, Rogozkin VA, eds. *Nutrition, Physical Fitness and Health*. Baltimore, Md: University Park; 1978:155.

33. Burke L, Read R. Diet patterns of elite Australian male triathletes. *Phys Sports Med*. 1987;15:140-145.

34. Short SH, Short WR. Four-year study of university athletes' dietary intake. *J Am Diet Assoc*. 1983;82:632.

35. Hickson JF, et al. Nutritional profile of football athletes eating from a training table. *Nutr Res*. 1987;7:27.

36. Hickson JF, Wolinsky I. Human protein intake and metabolism in exercise and sport. In: Hickson JF, Wolinsky I, eds. *Nutrition in Exercise and Sport*. Boca Raton, Fla: CRC Press; 1989.

37. Eichner ER. Ergolytic drugs. *Sports Sci Exchange*. 1989;2(15).

38. Lange RM, Borow KM, Neumann A, Feldman T. Adverse cardiac effects of alcohol ingesting in young adults. *Ann Intern Med*. 1985;102:742-747.

39. McNaughton L, Preece D. Alcohol and its effects on spring and middle distance running. *Br J Sports Med*. 1986;20:56-59.

40. Houmard JA, Langenfeld ME, Wiley RL, Seifert J. Effects of the acute ingestion of small amounts of alcohol on 5-mile run times. *J Sports Med*. 1987;27:2533-257.

41. Lieber C. To drink (moderately) or not to drink? *N Engl J Med*. 1984;310:846.

Predicting Energy Expenditure

Peggy H. Paul and Ann Snyder

▶ ENDURANCE SPORTS

Athletes who train regularly and compete for 1 or more hours per day have nutritional needs that go beyond those of a recreational athlete. Such training schedules demand efficient carbohydrate and fat metabolism and a diet that provides sufficient energy and nutrients. There are many examples of finely tuned athletes who appear to push the human system to its maximum metabolic potential. The 22-day Tour de France cycling race is one highly strenuous endurance event in which competitors require an estimated average of more than 6000 kcal per day. It is easy to see why this energy requirement is so high. Consider that a 160-lb bicyclist traveling at an average speed of 15 mph for 6 hours has an energy demand for the activity alone of about 4000 kcal.

Relative contribution of carbohydrate, protein, and fat for cyclists has been shown to be 62%, 15% and 23%, respectively, with close to 50% of those calories being consumed during the race.[1] Unfortunately, among elite athletes, such a fine example of energy expenditure paralleled with energy intake does not always occur. A recent study explored the nutritional habits of elite German athletes who trained 1 to 2 hours daily, and who competed at an international level.[2] Results were surprising, particularly regarding total calorie intake and carbohydrate content of the diet. Mean energy intake varied from 2900 to 5900 kcal per day for men and 1625 to 3100 kcal per day for women, indicating a marginal energy intake for many athletes, especially those training upward of 90 minutes per day. Contribution of carbohydrate to total intake varied from 40% to 63% of calories, an insufficient intake for most groups.[2]

The dietary focus for most endurance athletes often stresses adequacy of carbohydrate to offset depleted muscle glycogen stores, which can ultimately impair performance. While carbohydrates provide the fuel of choice for most athletes, of equal importance for endurance athletes is the ability to burn body fat as fuel. Physiologically, body fat spares muscle glycogen and can delay the onset of fatigue. With endurance training, such a physiological adaptation occurs. The highly trained body of a distance athlete can mobilize fat from adipose tissue and oxidize it in exercising muscles more efficiently than that of a less-trained athlete. Studies confirm the higher lipolytic activity and greater utilization of free fatty acids in endurance-trained persons.[3] Endurance training not only increases the amount and activity of norepinephrine (fat-mobilizing enzyme), but it also increases the size and number of fat-burning mitochondria.[4] An athlete's fat-burning capacity is critical for overall performance, especially in endurance and ultraendurance events.

Endurance athletes burn a large number of calories simply because of the time they spend in training. They do, however, burn this energy more efficiently, or more economically, than less-trained athletes. Efficiency of human movement, or the efficiency of energy burned, refers to the quantity of energy required to perform a particular task in relation to the actual work accomplished.[5] A common way to assess the economy, or efficiency, of physical effort is to evaluate the oxygen consumed while exercising. For example, at a submaximal speed of running, cycling, or swimming, an individual with greater economy of movement requires less oxygen to perform the task. The ability to use less oxygen is critical for endurance athletes when success depends on one's aerobic capacity and capabilities. An effective endurance-training program typically enhances both the economy of movement and the aerobic capacity to perform. For example, well-trained marathon runners generally run at 5% to 10% greater economy than middle-distance runners.[5] The longer and more effectively an athlete trains, the more efficient the body becomes at burning calories and using oxygen.

Despite all that is known regarding the energy and nutrient needs of endurance athletes, much remains to be discovered. Extrapolation from other population groups suggests that endurance athletes have generally elevated risks for nutrient and energy deficiencies[6] leading to chronic fatigue, weight loss, and impaired physical performance. Further research is greatly needed to determine appropriate feeding schedules for endurance events as well as the specific nutrient needs of elite athletes.

▶ NONENDURANCE SPORTS

Activities that are classified as nonendurance sports usually last less than 2 or 3 minutes, and include such activities as the sprint events in swimming and track; power events, such as high jumps, weight lifting, and throwing; and daily-living events, such as carrying bags of groceries or heavy luggage. The fuel of these activities, which require intense muscular contractions, is provided anaerobically by the stored phosphagens (ATP/CP) and glycolysis. With very intense activity, CP stores are the initial energy source to replenish ATP, but CP stores fall to low levels and remain low until the activity stops. Anaerobic glycolysis also contributes to the replenishment of ATP during high-intensity activity. The rate of glycogen utilization has been shown to increase nearly three times (from 3.4 to 10 mmol glucose units per kilogram of wet muscle per minute) for activities performed at 150% of aerobic capacity ($\dot{V}O_2$max) when compared with activities performed at 100% of aerobic capacity. Due to the great increase in the rate of anaerobic glycolysis, levels of lactic acid in the blood as high as 20 times the resting levels have been observed following high-intensity exercise. Thus, for high-intensity, nonendurance activities the major causes of fatigue would seem to be the depletion of creatine phosphate and the accumulation of lactic acid. Although normal levels of muscle glycogen are sufficient for single bouts of high-intensity exercise, repeat bouts of high-intensity activity may also be limited by the depletion of muscle glycogen.

When estimating a person's energy requirement, a number of factors must be taken into account. Metabolic rate and calorie expenditure are influenced by basal metabolism, physical activity, and the specific dynamic action of foods (dietary-induced thermogenesis). There is a known relationship between height, weight, body surface area, and energy utilization. This relationship is expressed in *Figure 1.4* as a nomogram. *Table 1.6* summarizes median energy consumption and requirements for elite male athletes in different sports.

FIGURE 1.4   Nomogram relating height and weight to surface area and calorie requirement.

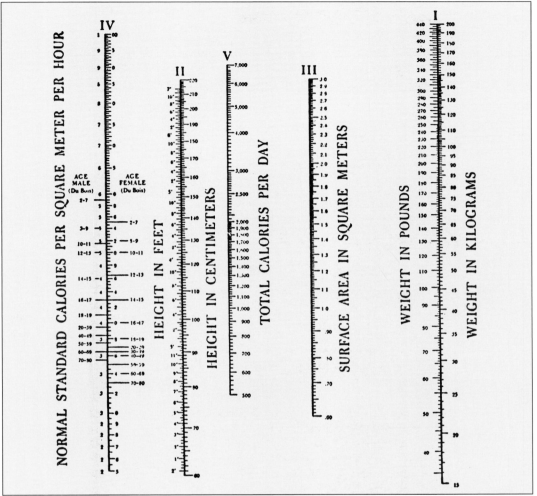

Place the chart on a flat, smooth table. Use only a ruler with a true straight edge. Do not draw lines on the chart but merely indicate their positions by the straight edge of the ruler. Locate the various points by means of needles (pin stuck through the eraser of a lead pencil). Locate the patient's normal weight on scale I and his or her height on scale II. The ruler joining these two points intersects scale III at the patient's surface area. Locate the age and sex of the patient on scale IV. A ruler joining this point with the patient's surface area on scale III crosses scale V at the *basal* energy requirement. To convert Calories (kcal) to k, multiply by 4.184. Adapted from Mayo Clinic by permission of Mayo Foundation.

TABLE 1.6   Median Energy Consumption and Corresponding Daily Food Requirements of Groups of Elite Male Athletes

Selected Sports Category 1	Expenditure of Energy per kg of Body Weight per Day (kcal) 2	Average Body Weight (kg) 3	Normative Daily Net Needs Based on Computed Energy Requirements (column 2 × column 3) (kcal) 4	Optimal Daily Gross Requirements With 10% Added for SDA Effect (kcal) 5
Group A				
Cross-country skiing	82.14	67.5	5550	6105
Crew racing	69.21	80.0	5550	6105
Canoe racing	72.72	75.0	5450	5995
Swimming	69.87	76.0	5300	5830
Bicycle racing	80.39	68.0	5450	5995
Marathon racing	79.07	68.0	5400	5940
Average values (men)			5450	5995

Rounded-off norm: 6000 kcal

Also belonging to sports of group A are skiing; Norwegian combination; middle-distance racing; walking; ice racing; modern pentathlon; equine sports; military; and touring (alpine climbing).

(continued)

TABLE 1.6 Median Energy Consumption and Corresponding Daily Food Requirements of Groups of Elite Male Athletes (continued)

Selected Sports Category	Expenditure of Energy per kg of Body Weight per Day (kcal)	Average Body Weight (kg)	Normative Daily Net Needs Based on Computed Energy Requirements (column 2 × column 3) (kcal)	Optimal Daily Gross Requirements With 10% Added for SDA Effect (kcal)
1	2	3	4	5
Group B				
Soccer	72.28	74.0	5350	5885
Handball	68.06	75.0	5100	5610
Basketball	67.93	75.0	5100	5610
Field hockey	69.18	75.0	5200	5720
Ice hockey	71.87	68.0	4900	5390
Average values (men)			5130	5643

Rounded-off norm: 5600 kcal

Also belonging to group B are rugby; water polo; volleyball; tennis; polo; and bicycle polo.

Group C				
Canoe slalom	67.16	68.0	4550	5005
Shooting	62.71	72.5	4550	5005
Table tennis	59.96	74.0	4450	4895
Bowling	62.69	75.0	4700	5170
Sailing	63.77	74.0	4700	5170
Average values (men)			4590	5049

Rounded-off norm: 5000 kcal

Also belonging to group C are circuit cycle racing (1000-4000 meters); fencing; ice sailing; and gliding.

Group D				
Sprinting	61.77	69.0	4250	4675
Running: short to middle distances	65.62	65.0	4250	4675
Pole vault	57.83	73.0	4200	4620
Diving	69.24	61.0	4200	4620
Boxing (middle- and welterweight to 63.5 kg)	67.25	63.0	4250	4675
Average values (men)			4230	4653

Rounded-off norm: 4600 kcal

Also belonging to group D are hurdle races; broad and high jump; hop-skip-and-jump; ballet swimming; figure skating; figure roller skating; and skiing; ski jump; bobsled; and tobogganing.

Group E1				
Judo (lightweight)	72.92	62.5	4550	5005
Weight lifting (lightweight)	69.15	67.5	4650	5115
Javelin	56.95	76.0	4350	4785
Gymnastics with apparatus	67.14	65.0	4350	4785
Steeplechase	63.96	68.0	4350	4785
Ski: Alpine competition	71.29	67.5	4800	5280
Average values (men)			4508	4959

Rounded-off norm: 5000 kcal

Group E2				
Hammerthrow	62.46	102.0	6350	6985
Shot put and discus	62.47	102.0	6350	6985

Rounded-off norm: 7000 kcal

Also belonging to group E1 are wrestling; automobile rallies; motor racing; gymnastics; acrobatics; parachute jumping; equine sports shows; decathlon; and bicycle gymnastics.

Adapted from W. McArdle, F. Katch, V. Katch: *Exercise Physiology: Energy, Nutrition, and Human Performance,* 2nd ed. Philadelphia, Lea & Febiger, 1981. Reprinted with permission.

REFERENCES

1. Saris WH, Van Erp Baart MA, Brouns F, Westerterp KR, Ten Hoor F. Study on food intake and energy expenditure during extreme sustained exercise: the Tour de France. *Int J Sports Med.* May 1989;10(supl 1).
2. Van Erp Baart MA, Saris WH, Binkhourst RA, Vos JA, Elvers JW. Nationwide survey on nutritional habits in elite athletes. Part 1: Energy, carbohydrate, protein, and fat intake. *Int J Sports Med.* May 1989; 10(suppl 1).
3. Friedmann B, Kindermann W. Energy metabolism and regulatory hormones in women and men during endurance exercise. *Eur J Appl Physiol.* September 1989;59(1/2):1-9.
4. Coleman E. Fat mobilization in endurance training. *Sports Medicine Digest.* 1988.
5. McArdle WD, Katch FI, Katch VL. *Exercise Physiology–Energy, Nutrition, and Human Performance.* 2nd ed. Philadelphia, Penn: Lea & Febiger; 1986.
6. McArdle WD, Katch FI, Katch VL. Substrate utilization, body composition, and nutrient requirements in endurance athletes. *Ann Sports Med.* 1987;3:104-108.

Vitamins, Minerals, and Athletic Performance

Mitchell Kanter and Dan Benardot

Vitamins are complex organic compounds that exist in tiny quantities in foods. They are essential for optimal functioning of many physiological processes. Vitamins play active roles in the action of the several hundred enzymes that serve as catalysts to normal body functions, including digestion, muscular contraction, and energy release from body stores.

It is hard to understand clearly the relationship between vitamins, minerals, and athletic performance because it is difficult to design research protocols that adequately address this relationship. For instance, it is an arduous task to isolate the independent effects of training, motivation, and belief (ie, the placebo effect) from the actual effect of individual dietary components. Nevertheless, we do have a good understanding of the metabolic functions of most vitamins and minerals, and this understanding helps us to make reasonable judgments about the potential effects of these substances on athletic performance. Where studies have been executed to evaluate the effectiveness of high-level mineral or vitamin dosing on athletic performance, the findings generally lead to the conclusion that providing an amount in high therapeutic doses is not useful and does not improve athletic performance.[1] Therefore, the focus should be on making certain that the increased caloric intake of most athletes is of sufficient quality that the vitamins and minerals necessary for optimal functioning of energy metabolic processes are present. The RDA is an excellent beginning point for establishing nutrient requirements for athletes.

▶ B-COMPLEX VITAMINS

The B-complex vitamins, including thiamin (B_1), riboflavin (B_2), niacin, pyridoxine (pyridoxal, pyridoxamine, B_6), folacin, cyanocobalamin (B_{12}), pantothenic acid, and biotin, work together to aid in muscle contraction and relaxation, energy metabolism, and healthy digestion and absorption of nutrients. Because of the well-established role of B vitamins in energy metabolism and muscle function, they are frequently taken as supplements by athletes.[2] Since the B vitamins are soluble in water, they do not have a separate storage depot. Therefore, once tissue levels reach saturation, excess levels are excreted. However, megadoses of some B vitamins can be potentially harmful, with unpleasant and harmful side effects. Any level of these vitamins that exceeds tissue saturation is not useful, so the aim should be to provide sufficient but not excessive amounts. It is safe to say that in the absence of a known deficiency, supplemental intake of these vitamins does not improve either anaerobic or aerobic potential, and does not positively affect strength, speed, or endurance.

A brief description of the exercise-related functions of the B-complex vitamins, plus the typical signs of deficiencies, the symptoms associated with overdoses, and selected food sources, are shown in *Table 1.7*.

Thiamin (Vitamin B$_1$)

The major function of thiamin is related to the metabolism of carbohydrates, but it also functions in the metabolism of proteins and fats and the formation of hemoglobin.[3] Its major energy-related coenzyme is thiamin pyrophosphate (TPP). Because of thiamin's relationship to energy metabolism, the thiamin requirement increases in relative proportion to energy utilization (approximately 0.5 mg/1000 kcal).[4] On a diet of reasonable quality that contains complex carbohydrates, this dietary requirement can be easily met.

Because carbohydrate is a primary fuel in all forms of activity, thiamin plays an important role in assuring optimal athletic performance through carbohydrate metabolism. High-level endurance activities do elevate thiamin requirements, but studies conducted to evaluate the effect of B vitamins on performance fail to support the use of thiamin supplements.[3,5-7]

It was demonstrated that individuals who ingested large amounts of sucrose had compromised thiamin status, as measured by erythrocyte transketolase.[8] The studied subjects reported numerous symptoms, including chest pains,

TABLE 1.7 The B-Complex Vitamins

Vitamin B	Exercise-related Functions	Symptoms of Deficiency	Symptoms of Overdose	Food Sources
Thiamin (B$_1$)	Carbohydrate metabolism, normal nervous system function.	Fatigue, muscle weakness. Paresthesia, uncoordinated gait	Relatively nontoxic	Liver, pork, lean meats, wheat germ, and whole grains, enriched breads, and cereals.
Riboflavin (B$_2$)	Cellular energy release and respiration.	Fatigue	Relatively nontoxic	Milk and milk products, liver, enriched breads, and cereals.
Niacin	Cellular energy processes and respiration. Carbohydrate metabolism and fat synthesis.	Fatigue, lassitude	Flushing, itchy skin, headaches, nausea, liver damage, irregular heartbeat.	Liver, poultry, fish, peanut butter.
Pyridoxine (B$_6$)	Amino acid and protein metabolism. Normal RBC formation.	Weakness, difficulty in walking. Anemia	Nerve damage, liver damage	Liver, herring and salmon, wheat germ and whole grains, lean meats.
Folacin (Folic acid)	Regulation of tissue processes. Normal RBC formation.	Reduced endurance. Anemia	Masks certain anemias	Liver, wheat bran and whole grains, spinach and other leafy greens, legumes, orange juice.
Vitamin B$_{12}$	Normal RBC development. Maintenance of nerve tissue.	Anemia. Muscular incoordination	Liver damage	Foods of animal origin, specially prepared fermented yeasts and fortified soy products.
Biotin	Synthesis of fat, glycogen; amino acid metabolism. Maintenance of nervous tissue.	Lethargy, muscular aches. Extreme sensitivity to touch or pain	Depressed secretion of gastric HCl	Egg yolk, liver, legumes
Pantothenic acid	Energy and tissue metabolism.	Fatigue, muscle cramping, impaired motor coordination	Diarrhea	Eggs, liver, wheat bran, peanuts, legumes, lean meats, spinach, and other vegetables.

Adapted with permission from Krause MV, Mahan LK. *Food Nutrition and Diet Therapy.* 6th ed. Philadelphia, Pa: WB Saunders; 1979.

sleeplessness, depression, anorexia, peripheral neuropathy, and elevated temperature. All subjects improved with thiamin supplementation. Based on these results, it has been suggested that the potential depletion of vitamins and minerals that might result from a combination of exercise and poor diet must be considered.[9]

Riboflavin (Vitamin B$_2$)

Riboflavin has an important role in the release of energy via two riboflavin-containing coenzymes: flavin mononucleotide (FMN) and flavin-adenine dinucleotide (FAD).

Compromised riboflavin status, as measured by erythrocyte glutathione reductase activity, was demonstrated in a study of exercising college females.[10] It was suggested by the authors that exercise increases the requirement for riboflavin. Although not adequately tested, it can be assumed based on our understanding of riboflavin function that poor riboflavin status may negatively affect energy metabolism and athletic performance. As with thiamin, the requirement for riboflavin is based on the amount of energy metabolized: 0.6 mg/1000 kcal.[4] It was the view of the National Research Council (1989) that riboflavin requirement does not change with increases in muscle activity. It is clear from these divergent findings that additional research is needed.

Niacin

Niacin plays an important role in energy metabolism and fat synthesis through two niacin-related coenzymes[3]: nicotinamide adenine dinucleotide (NAD) and nicotinamide adenine dinucleotide phosphate (NADP).

Niacin is currently being used as an effective hypocholesterolemic agent. However, when taken in therapeutic doses niacin has caused hepatitis, dermatitis, and uremia.[3] There is conflicting evidence on whether niacin supplementation is useful for enhancing athletic performance. It is theorized that an improvement in anaerobic threshold would occur through an inhibition of free fatty acid mobilization, thereby increasing glycogen utilization.[5] However, it is also theorized that the inhibition of free fatty acid transfer could negatively affect endurance performance by increasing the reliance on muscle glycogen as an energy substrate.[11] Several studies have found that niacin supplementation apparently does not benefit either anaerobic or aerobic capacity.[12,13]

Pyridoxine, Pyridoxal, Pyridoxamine (Vitamin B$_6$)

The coenzyme of vitamin B$_6$, pyridoxal phosphate (PLP), is an important vitamin in the metabolism of proteins, carbohydrates, and fats. It is also involved in the synthesis of amino acids, regulation of nitrogen, regulation of glycogen metabolism (as a component of phosphorylase), and formation of hemoglobin, myoglobin, and cytochromes.[3,5,14] Its relationship to energy metabolism has led to theories that associate vitamin B$_6$ with the enhancement of aerobic potential. However, studies investigating vitamin B$_6$ supplementation have not demonstrated that it improves aerobic performance.[15,16]

It is important to note that toxicity with high, continuous doses of this vitamin have been reported in the literature. A dependency to B$_6$ may be induced with a daily supplement of 200 mg of pyridoxine for 1 month.[14] Other reported problems associated with vitamin B$_6$ toxicity include numbness of the feet and hands with supplements of 2000 mg per day.[17]

Cyanocobalamin (Vitamin B$_{12}$)

The major roles of vitamin B$_{12}$ are the synthesis of red blood cells and the metabolism of carbohydrates and fats.[3] It is the latter function that encourages numerous athletes to receive intramuscular injections of vitamin B$_{12}$ in the belief that exercise endurance will be increased.[5] In spite of this common practice, studies have not found an improvement in endurance with B$_{12}$ supplementation.[18]

It should be noted that vitamin B$_{12}$ is derived from foods of animal origin *only*. Because of the low rate of usage and relatively high tissue storage level of the vitamin, it may take several years for signs of vitamin B$_{12}$ deficiency to occur with a strict vegetarian intake. Therefore, athletes who practice strict vegetarianism should consider, on the advice of their physician or other licensed health professional, taking an occasional supplement of vitamin B$_{12}$.[19]

Folacin (Folic Acid, Pteroylglutamic Acid)

Folate is an integral part of a coenzyme involved in the formation of new cells. Most commonly it is known for its involvement in red blood cell and DNA synthesis. As its name suggests (derived from *folium*, or "leaf"), it is abundant in green leafy vegetables, but it is also found in legumes, seeds, and animal liver. Because both vitamin B$_{12}$ deficiency and folacin deficiency cause a megaloblastic anemia, high levels of folacin may temporarily mask a deficiency of vitamin B$_{12}$.

As with any anemia, the megaloblastic anemia of folacin causes a lowering of oxygen-carrying capacity, which would negatively affect endurance activity. It has been confirmed from nationwide dietary surveys that folate intake may be marginal for large portions of the US population; therefore, isolated deficiencies may occur.[3] Studies to evaluate the folacin status of athletes and the efficacy of folate supplements on athletic performance have not been performed.

Biotin

Biotin is part of a coenzyme (for carboxylases) necessary for energy metabolism, fat synthesis, and glycogen synthesis.[3] These functions suggest that it is an important vitamin for endurance activities. However, because no studies have researched the relationship between biotin and endurance, it is impossible to conclude that athletic activity increases biotin requirement.

Biotin deficiency, which is extremely rare in humans, may result in an abnormal heart beat, loss of appetite, muscle pain and weakness, and early fatigue. Toxicity symptoms from high intake of this vitamin have not been reported.

Pantothenic Acid

This vitamin, which is an integral part of acetyl coenzyme A (CoA), is sufficiently widespread in the food supply to make deficiency unlikely. Acetyl CoA is a central actor in energy metabolism, involved in both pyruvate formation and fatty acid synthesis. It has been suggested that exercise may increase the requirement for pantothenic acid.[1] However, additional work must be done before this relationship is well established.

Pantothenic acid deficiency may be associated with intestinal distress (vomiting, diarrhea), fatigue, postural hypotension, and irascibility.[14] High-dose intakes may lead to occasional diarrhea.

► ASCORBIC ACID (VITAMIN C)

Vitamin C is involved in the synthesis of the connective tissue protein, collagen. It is also involved in synthesis of thyroxine (a metabolism-controlling hormone), metabolism of amino acids, absorption of iron, and resistance to infection. Although most Americans have more than adequate intakes of vitamin C, studies on athletes have been contradictory.[1] Some studies indicate that marginal vitamin C status may impair work capacity, but other studies report that high-dose intakes of the vitamin are not useful in enhancing performance.[20-22]

Symptoms of vitamin C deficiency include microcytic anemia, purpura, easy hemorrhaging, depression, and frequent infections. Symptoms of toxicity (which are rare) include red-cell breakage, nausea, frequent urination, abdominal cramps, and diarrhea.[3]

► FAT-SOLUBLE VITAMINS (VITAMINS A, D, E, AND K)

Unlike water-soluble vitamins, which do not have specific storage depots in the body and are excreted when tissue saturation levels are reached, fat-soluble vitamins are stored in specific lipid-containing cells (usually in the liver) where they can be called upon when needed. Because humans have this storage capacity (ie, backup system), it is difficult to study the effect of these vitamins on athletic performance.[1,3]

Although there has been almost no viable research on the relationship between fat-soluble vitamins and athletic performance, it has been theorized that there may be such a relationship with vitamin A. One of the functions of vitamin A is the synthesis of glycogen, and another of its functions is the synthesis of protein (muscle). In theory, it could be concluded that a deficiency of vitamin A might negatively affect both strength and endurance, but no study has adequately explored this theory.[1]

Because an excessive intake of fat-soluble vitamins may easily induce toxic symptoms, supplementation with these vitamins should only take place under the strict supervision of an appropriately licensed health professional.

► MINERALS

Calcium

Bones consist of "live" cells that are constantly changing. This change enables them to adapt, with the availability of the right nutrients in the right amounts, to the physiological stressors introduced by each person. One of the minerals responsible for this variation in bone makeup is calcium. The major functions of calcium include[3]:

► Bone formation and bone strength
► Assists in nerve impulse transmission across cell membranes
► Muscle contraction
► Blood clotting
► Helps to maintain viability of tissues

While all of these functions are critical to life, it should be clear to the reader that several of these functions are critical to athletic performance. Nevertheless, there is evidence that many athletes may have an intake of calcium that is far below the 1989 RDA of 800 to 1200 mg per day.[23,24]

Because exercise almost always increases the stress on bones, bones in healthy individuals adapt by becoming more dense in those areas of stress. However, many athletes develop fractures (commonly referred to as stress fractures) because the level of stress placed on the bones exceeds the strength of the affected bones. When bones are not sufficiently strong to control the stress placed on them, it may be the result of inadequate calcium intake, inadequate estrogen production, or both. (See *Tables 1.8* and *1.9* for dietary calcium equivalents and forms of elemental calcium; also see appendix 2 for the calcium content of common foods.) The amenorrhea commonly seen in young female athletes appears to be closely associated with lower bone mineral density.[24] While amenorrhea may result from a single factor or a combination of factors (including low body-fat percentage, inadequate calorie intake, low estrogen, high cortisol, and emotional stress), its effect on bone density has been well documented.

Because many young female athletes have a combination of low estrogen levels and low calcium intakes, they are at high risk for poor bone development and later bone disease. Estrogen assists in maintaining bone density by increasing intestinal calcium absorption and decreasing bone and kidney losses of calcium. Low estrogen levels and a low calcium intake increase the risk of inadequate supply of calcium to bone. Recent research indicates that amenorrheic athletes may reduce the risk of stress fractures by consuming >120% of the RDA.[24-26]

TABLE 1.8   Calcium Equivalents*

Buttermilk	1 cup
Cheddar cheese	1½ oz
Cottage cheese	2 cups
Yogurt	1 cup
Processed cheese	1½ slices
Ice cream	1½ cups
Ice milk	1½ cups
Tofu	8 oz
Broccoli	2 cups
Collard, turnip greens	1 cup
Kale, mustard greens	1½ cups
Oysters	1½ cups (about 16 medium)
Salmon	4 oz
Sardines	2½ oz

*Foods that contain approximately the same amount of calcium as an 8 oz cup of milk (297 mg).

Data from Adams C. *Nutritive Value of American Foods in Common Units.* Washington, DC: Agriculture Research Service; 1975. US Dept of Agriculture handbook 456.

TABLE 1.9   Elemental Calcium in Different Forms

Calcium Salt	Theoretical Tablet Size, mg	Percent Calcium	Content of Elemental Calcium, mg
Calcium gluconate	1200	9	108
Calcium lactate	1200	13	156
Calcium carbonate	1200	40	480

Adapted from Avioli VL. *Ann Rev Nutr.* 1984;4:571 with permission from the Annual Review of Nutrition, vol 4, ©1984 by Annual Reviews Inc.

Iron

Because iron is involved in the transfer of oxygen, a deficiency of iron may be associated with reduced athletic performance, even if the deficiency is only marginal.[27,28] It appears that athletes might be at increased risk for iron deficiency because of the following[29]:

▶ Inadequate iron intake
▶ Poor iron absorption
▶ Loss of iron via sweat
▶ Gastrointestinal blood loss
▶ Red cell hemolysis with hematuria

A condition referred to as sports anemia (hypochromic monocytic transient anemia) has been reported in athletes. This condition appears to be most associated with increased red blood cell destruction and decreased hemoglobin concentration at the beginning of a strenuous exercise conditioning program.[25] It has also been hypothesized that "sports anemia" may be caused by an inadequate protein intake in the early stages of training. In early training, the demand to form additional muscle tissue may compete with the demand to form additional hemoglobin, thus causing the anemia.[25] Sports anemia appears to be a transient condition, disappearing once the body has sufficient time to adapt to the training regimen.

Several studies have evaluated the rate of iron deficiency in athletes, and have found a higher prevalence in female athletes than male athletes.[30,31] It appears that the risk of iron deficiency is greatest in the following groups:

Female athletes. Regular menstrual losses increase the iron needs of females. An additional risk is imposed when these same women are also in a negative calorie balance. Typically, low calorie intakes are also inadequate in iron. The iron concentration of the typical American diet requires an intake of approximately 3000 kcal to obtain the RDA amount.[25,32]

Vegetarian athletes. Limiting or eliminating meat eliminates some of the best, most biologically available sources of iron (see appendix 3). Iron from fruit, vegetable, and cereal sources is not as well absorbed as that from animal sources.

Endurance athletes. Losses of iron from intestinal bleeding,[33] sweat,[34] urine, and feces may contribute to the need for additional dietary iron.

Growing athletes. The RDA of iron for the adolescent male and female is 18 mg due, at least in part, to fast growth and the enlargement of blood volume. Because of this growth, there is an increased need for iron for the synthesis of hemoglobin.[4]

The average rate of iron absorption from food is approximately 10%, and the RDA is set at a level that reflects this absorption level.[4] The following recommendations are aimed at enhancing iron absorption and reducing the risk of developing iron deficiency or anemia.

▶ Lean cuts of red meats and dark poultry meat should be consumed three to four times per week.
▶ Enriched or fortified breads, cereals, and pastas should be eaten regularly.

▶ Vitamin C enhances iron absorption, so vitamin C-containing foods should be consumed with iron-containing foods. This is especially important when consuming nonheme (fruit and vegetable) sources of iron.

▶ Certain foods contain substances that inhibit iron absorption, and these substances should be consumed in moderation. They include tannic acid (in tea), phytic acid (in bran), and polyphenol (in coffee).

▶ On the advice of a physician or other appropriately licensed health professional, it may be prudent for certain women of childbearing age to take iron supplements regularly.

Zinc

Zinc is intimately involved in energy metabolism, and is present in more than 70 enzymes involved in energy metabolic processes. Zinc also plays a part in[3]:

▶ Growth and development
▶ Sexual maturation
▶ Normal appetite and taste sensitivity
▶ Thyroid function and metabolic rate
▶ Immune response
▶ Sight
▶ Gastrointestinal functioning

The best sources of zinc are animal protein foods. In diets that are low in animal protein and high in high-fiber grains and cereals, there is an increased chance for zinc deficiency because of reduced absorption of available dietary zinc. This reduced absorption is caused by phytic acid, which has a high binding affinity for zinc (and other bivalent minerals) and, when bound, makes zinc unavailable for absorption.

It was found that many runners who participated in a 20-day road race in Hawaii showed signs of compromised zinc status, even though they appeared to be healthy and had no obvious signs of zinc deficiency.[35] It was suggested that this marginal zinc deficiency might be due to the following factors:

▶ Low dietary intake of zinc
▶ Increased loss of zinc via urine
▶ Increased loss of zinc via sweat
▶ Redistribution of zinc into muscle and liver, and out of the blood

It has been found that the greater the daily running distance, the lower the serum zinc concentration.[30,36] However, this finding conflicts with that of Lukaski and colleagues[37], who found no difference in plasma zinc values between athletes and control subjects. These conflicting findings suggest a need for a great deal more work in understanding the relationship between zinc and exercise.

Sodium

Sodium makes up 40% of common table salt; chloride makes up the other 60%. Sodium is an essential mineral needed by the body to regulate water balance in the cells, to maintain blood volume, and to maintain normal nerve and muscle activity.

Although an individual's requirement for sodium varies with age, environmental conditions, and level of activity, it is recommended that a healthy sedentary adult consume 500 to 2400 mg per day.[4] This quantity of sodium can generally be met by consuming a typical American diet. However, during prolonged exercise in hot weather, sodium losses in sweat and urine may exceed 10 g per day. For example, assume we are dealing with an athlete who is training 4 hours per day and losing sweat at the relatively modest rate of 1.5 L per hour. The sodium concentration of sweat is approximately 50 mEq/L; consequently, this athlete is losing 300 mEq or 6900 mg of sodium through sweat during his or her workout. If we add to this an average daily urine sodium loss of 120 mEq/L, or 2760 mg, we can see that this athlete loses roughly 9660 mg of sodium, or 24 g of sodium chloride per day. Although concentrated salt tablets are generally unnecessary and may be harmful, a dilute sodium mixture (80 to 120 mg Na per 8 oz), or a slightly more liberal use of sodium with meals, can be helpful to the athlete during and after the workout.

Acclimatization to heat or exercise can compensate for some, although not all, of the sodium loss. For example, an unacclimatized individual may lose 1800 mg (78.26 mEq) of sodium per liter of sweat, while an acclimatized athlete may lose 1100 mg (47.83 mEq) of sodium per liter of sweat.[38] This sodium conservation slightly reduces the need for dietary sodium.

Most foods naturally contain some sodium (see *Table 1.10*). The use of salt in processed foods is the major source of sodium in the US diet. Smoked and preserved meats, canned and ready-to-eat foods, and snack foods reveal additional sources of sodium in various forms including sodium nitrite, sodium phosphate, and sodium ascorbate. Although the current literature pertaining to the effects of sodium on blood pressure is controversial, many Americans consume sodium at a level well beyond physiological need. It is important to be aware of the sodium content of foods and to avoid excessive use of salty products. For most athletes it is important to consider that, in spite of a greater loss of sodium through sweat, the sodium content of the typical American diet is usually sufficient to replace that loss.

For those who require, or are prescribed, a low-sodium diet, the following suggestions may be helpful, particularly when eating in a restaurant:

▶ Order entrées prepared without salt or sodium-containing flavors.
▶ Choose individually prepared items and avoid soups and mixed dishes (eg, casseroles).
▶ Use oil and vinegar for a salad dressing.
▶ Ask for baked or boiled potatoes.
▶ Use salad bars when available, but avoid salt, premixed salads, and dressings.
▶ Avoid fast-food restaurants, or ask that the condiments and grill seasonings be left out during preparation.

REFERENCES

1. Keith RE. Vitamins in sport and exercise. In: Wolinsky I, Hickson JF, eds. *Nutrition in Exercise and Sport*. Boca Raton, Fla: CRC Press; 1989.
2. Williams MH. *Beyond Training: How Athletes Enhance Performance Legally and Illegally*. Champaign, Ill: Human Kinetics; 1989.
3. Krause MV, Mahan LK, eds. *Food, Nutrition, and Diet Therapy*. 7th ed. Philadelphia, Pa: WB Saunders; 1984.
4. National Research Council, Committee on Dietary Allowances. *Recommended Dietary Allowances*. Washington, DC: National Academy of Sciences; 1989.
5. Williams MH. Vitamin and mineral supplements to athletes: do they help? *Clin Sports Med*. 1984;3:623-637.
6. Karpovich P, Millman N. Vitamin B and endurance. *N Engl J Med*. 1942;226:881-882.
7. Archdeacon J, Murlin J. The effect of thiamine depletion and restoration on muscular efficiency and endurance. *J Nutr*. 1944;28:241-254.

TABLE 1.10   Sodium Content of Commonly Consumed Foods

Amount	Food	Sodium (mg)
Cereals		
1 cup	Oatmeal, cooked without salt	2
1 oz	Shredded Wheat	3
1 pkt	Cream of Wheat	241
1 oz	Corn flakes	351
1 cup	Rice, white, cooked without salt	0
1 cup	Spaghetti, cooked without salt, tender	1
Dairy		
1 cup	Yogurt, plain, low-fat	159
1 oz	Cheddar cheese	176
1 cup	Cottage cheese, low-fat	918
1 oz	Swiss cheese	74
1 cup	Whole milk	120
1 cup	Skim milk	126
1 oz	Processed American cheese	406
Meats		
2.5 oz	Sirloin steak, boiled, lean	48
3 oz	Flounder or sole, baked with butter	145
3 oz	Chicken breast, roasted	64
2.5 oz	Fresh ham, roasted, lean	46
2 slices	Salami, cooked	607
1	Frankfurter	504
1	Hamburger (with roll)	463
Vegetables/Fruits		
1 cup	Broccoli, cooked	17
1 cup	Lettuce	5
1 cup	Bean sprouts	6
1 cup	Green beans, cooked from raw	4
1 cup	Green beans, canned	339
1 cup	Squash, baked	2
4 medium	Canned green olives	312
1 medium	Pickles, cucumber, dill	928
1 cup	Chicken soup, canned	1106
1 medium	Orange, raw	1
1 cup	Orange juice	2
1 medium	Tomato, raw	10
1 medium	Apple, raw	1
1/10 medium	Honeydew melon	3
Legumes		
1 cup	Peanuts, oil-roasted, salted	626
1 cup	Peanuts, oil-roasted, unsalted	22
1 cup	Great northern beans, cooked without salt	13
Condiments		
1 tsp	Salt	2132
1 tbsp	Soy Sauce	1029
1 tsp	Mustard	63
1 tbsp	Catsup	156
1 tbsp	Relish, sweet	107
Fats/Oils		
1 tbsp	Margarine, imitation (40% fat)	134
1 tbsp	Margarine, regular, hard	132
1 tbsp	Margarine, regular, soft	151
1 tbsp	Butter, salted	116
1 tbsp	Butter, unsalted	2
1 tbsp	Corn oil	0
1 tbsp	Olive oil	0

Shredded Wheat, Cream of Wheat, Nabisco Brands, Inc, East Hanover, NJ 07936.
Data from Gebhardt SE, Matthews RH. *Nutritive Value of Foods.* Washington, DC: US Dept of Agriculture, Human Nutrition Information Service; 1990. Home and Garden bulletin 72.

8. Lonsdale D, Shamberger RJ. Red cell transketolase as an indicator of nutritional deficiency. *Am J Clin Nutr.* 1980;33:205-221.

9. Hackman, RM. The leading edge: nutrition and athletic performance. In: Katch FI, ed. *1984 Olympic Scientific Congress Proceedings.* Vol 2; *Sport, Health, and Nutrition.* Champaign, Ill: Human Kinetics; 1986.

10. Belko AZ, Obarzanke E, Kalkwarf HJ, et al. Effects of exercise on riboflavin requirements of young women. *Am J Clin Nutr.* 1983;37:509.

11. Bergstrom J, Hultman E, Jorfeldt L, et al. Effect of nicotinic acid on physical working capacity and on metabolism of muscle glycogen in man. *J Appl Physiol.* 1969;26:170-176.

12. Hilsendager D, Karpovich P. Ergogenic effect of glycine and niacin separately and in combination. *Res Quar.* 1964;35(suppl):389-392.

13. Carlson L, Havel R, Ekelund L. Effect of nicotinic acid on the turnover rate and oxidation of the free fatty acids of plasma in man during exercise. *Metabolism.* 1963;12:837-845.

14. McCormick DB. Vitamin B_6. In: Shils ME, Young VR, eds. *Modern Nutrition in Health and Disease.* 6th ed. Philadelphia, Pa; Lea & Febiger; 1988:376-381.

15. Hatcher L, Leklem J, Campbell D. Altered vitamin B_6 metabolism during exercise in man: effect of carbohydrate-modified diets and B_6 supplements. *Med Sci Sports Exer.* 1982;14:112.

16. DeVos A, Leklem J, Campbell D. Carbohydrate loading, vitamin B_6 supplementation and fuel metabolism during exercise in man. *Med Sci Sports Exer.* 1982;14:137.

17. Dalton K. Pyridoxine overdose in premenstrual syndrome. *Lancet.* 1985;18:1168-1169.

18. Tin-May-Than, Ma-Win-May, Khin-Sann-Aung, Mya-Tu M. The effect of vitamin B_{12} on physical performance capacity. *Br J Nutr.* 1978;40:264-273.

19. Herbert V. Vitamin B_{12} plant sources, requirements, and assay. *Am J Clin Nutr.* 1988;48:852-858.

20. Gerster H. The role of vitamin C in athletic performance. *J Am Col Nutr.* 1989;8:636-643.

21. Buzina R, Grgic Z, Jusic M, et al. Nutritional status and physical working capacity. *Hum Nutr Clin Nutr.* 1982;36C:429-438.

22. Buzina R, Sobuticanec K. Vitamin C and physical working capacity in adolescents. *Int J Vitam Nutr Res.* 1985;27(suppl):157-166.

23. Benardot D, Schwarz M, Heller DW. Nutrient intake in young, highly competitive gymnasts. *J Am Diet Assoc.* 1989;89:401-403.

24. Nelson ME, Fisher EC, Catsos PD, Meredith CN, Turksoy RN, Evans, WJ. Diet and bone status in amenorrheic runners. *Am J Clin Nutr.* 1986;43:910-916.

25. Williams MH. *Nutrition for Fitness and Sport.* 3rd ed. Dubuque, Iowa: Wm C Brown Publishers; 1992.

26. Osteoporosis Consensus Conference. *JAMA.* 1984;252:799-802.

27. Vellar OD, Hermansen L. Physical performance and hematological parameters, with special reference to hemoglobin and maximal oxygen uptake. *Acta Med Scand.* 1971;190(suppl 552):1-40.

28. Schoene RB, Escourrou P, Robertson HT, Nelson KL, Parsons JR, Smith NJ. Iron repletion decreases maximal exercise lactate concentrations in female athletes with minimal iron-deficiency anemia. *J Lab Clin Med.* 1983;102:306-312.

29. Buskirk ER. Exercise. In: Brown ML, ed. *Present Knowledge in Nutrition.* 6th ed. Washington, DC: International Life Sciences Institute Nutrition Foundation; 1990.

30. Deuster PA, Kyle SB, Moser PB, Vigersky RA, Sing A, Schoomaker EB. Nutritional survey of highly trained women. *Am J Clin Nutr.* 1986;44:954-962.

31. DeWign JF, DeLongste JL, Mosterd W, Willebrand D. Haemoglobin packed cell volume, serum iron and iron-binding capacity of selected athletes during training. *J Sports Med.* 1971;11:42-51.

32. Berning JR, Steen SN, eds. *Sports Nutrition for the 90s: The Health Professional's Handbook.* Gaithersburg, Md: Aspen Publishers Inc; 1991.

33. Sullivan SN. Exercise-associated symptoms in triathletes. *Phys Sports Med.* 1987;15:105-110.

34. Brune M, Magnusson B, Persson H, Hallberg L. Iron losses in sweat. *Am J Clin Nutr.* 1986;43:438-443.

35. Dressendorfer RH, Sockolov R. Hypozincemia in runners. *Phys Sports Med*. 1980;8:97.

36. Haralambie G. Serum zinc in athletes in training. *Int J Sports Med*. 1981;2:131-138.

37. Lukaski HC, Bolonchuk WW, Klevay LM, Milne DB, Sandstead HH. Maximal oxygen consumption as related to magnesium, copper, and zinc nutriture. *Am J Clin Nutr*. 1983;37:407-415.

38. Morimoto T, Miki K, Nose H, Yamada S, Hirakawa K, Matsubara C. Changes in body fluid and its composition during heavy sweating and effect of fluid and electrolyte replacement. *Jpn J Biometeorol*. 1981;18:31-39.

Fluid and Electrolyte Requirements of Exercise

Steven Fike, Mitchell Kanter, and Elizabeth Markley

▶ WATER BALANCE

Water may be the single most important nutrient for athletic performance. The body may be able to survive weeks or even months without certain vitamins and minerals, but without water, performance may be compromised in as little as 30 minutes. Our bodies are approximately 60% water, and our muscles are approximately 70%. For an athlete exercising vigorously, water's main function is to remove the heat (calories) generated by exercise. The body's metabolic rate may increase 20 to 25 times during intense exercise.[1] The body gets rid of this heat by picking it up in the circulation and transporting it to the skin, where it is lost through evaporation. In addition to dissipating heat, water is the main component of blood. If blood volume gets low, then cardiac output will be compromised and oxygen delivery to the muscles will not be able to meet demand. The result will be less power and endurance.[2] Water, via the bloodstream, also transports electrolytes and other nutrients throughout the body; it gets rid of waste products and it provides shock absorption around tissues and organs.

▶ CONSEQUENCES OF DEHYDRATION

An athlete exercising under hot and humid conditions may lose more than 2 L of water per hour.[3] Research has shown, under experimental conditions in subjects wearing football equipment, a loss of 1.8% of body weight in 30 minutes.[4] Marathon runners have been shown to lose 6% to 10% of body weight during a race.[5] A 2% loss of body weight by dehydration can impair the body's ability to dissipate heat,[6] and a 4% loss can cause exhaustion.[7] Besides impairing the body's thermoregulatory functions, dehydration can harm performance by causing reductions in strength, power, endurance, and aerobic capacity.[8] Unreplaced fluid losses will eventually raise the body's core temperature to the point of heat exhaustion or even life-threatening heat stroke.

▶ FLUID REPLACEMENT GUIDELINES

Fortunately, most coaches and athletes now understand the importance of fluid replacement, and fluid restriction is seldom practiced. An exception is in the sport of wrestling, where fluid restriction or voluntary dehydration still appears prominent.[9] Although the importance of fluid intake may be understood, a recent survey reported that 53% of athletes did not know how much fluid to drink.[10] Thirst is not a reliable indicator of the need for fluid. Individuals exercising in the heat who are given water ad libitum replace only about two thirds of their fluid losses.[11] Exercise blunts the thirst mechanism. Consequently, the most reliable indicator for fluid needs is body weight.

To determine how much fluid an individual should consume during a workout or competition it is best to measure pre- and post-workout weights. Weight should be measured nude or in minimal clothing immediately before and after working out; the weight loss represents fluid loss as sweat. Each pound lost represents 1 p or 16 oz of fluid. Ideally, pre- and post-exercise weights should match, indicating that fluid intake matched fluid loss. In some sports, this may be difficult to achieve, so it is recommended that the maximum allowable weight loss should not exceed 3% of body weight. Use the following formula to estimate the amount of fluid that should be consumed during a workout or competition:

$$\text{Your weight} \times 0.03\ (3\%) = \underline{\hspace{1cm}} \text{lb}$$

This is the maximum amount of weight that should be lost during workout or competition. For each pound over this, 2 extra 8-oz cups of fluid need to be consumed during competition. It is important not to rely on thirst to determine when to drink. A predetermined, measured amount should be consumed in small amounts throughout exercise.

Other factors that may affect fluid consumption include taste and temperature of the beverage. A slightly sweet-tasting beverage may be preferred over that of plain water.[12,13] In addition, sodium and carbohydrate added to beverages may enhance their absorption and prolong the desire to drink.[14] Cooler beverages (at approximately 40°F) are preferred over warmer drinks and are absorbed more quickly.[12,15] A good practice would be to offer a choice of both water and carbohydrate-electrolyte (sport drinks) beverages during practice and competition due to the variation in individual preferences (see *Table 1.11*).

▶ SPECIAL CONSIDERATIONS

Special consideration should be given to environmental conditions that increase the risk for dehydration and to individuals who are at greater risk for heat illness. As temperature increases, so does the risk for heat illness. Water loss through sweat increases approximately 13% for each 1-degree rise on the Centigrade scale.[3] Relative humidity is an even more significant risk factor in heat-related illness. As humidity increases, the body's ability to dissipate heat (by evaporation of sweat) decreases.[1] When sweat beads up and rolls off the body, it does not release heat. Another condition that may affect fluid balance is air travel. Since the passenger compartment of an airplane is very dry, evaporation will cause significant moisture to be lost from the body during air travel.[16] The longer the flight the greater the potential for becoming dehydrated. Consequently, one should make a special effort to drink extra fluids during and immediately following air travel.

Alcoholic and caffeinated beverages should be avoided because of their diuretic properties. People who are at particular risk for dehydration and heat illness include the following:

TABLE 1.11   Fluid-Replacement Beverages

Beverages	Flavors	CHO Type	% CHO	Na/8oz (mg)	K/8oz (mg)	Other Vitamins/ Minerals	Osmolality
Gatorade (Quaker Oats Co)	Many	Sucrose/ glucose	6	110	25	Cl, P	320–360
Gatorade Light	Many	Glucose	2.5	80	25	Trace	200
Quickick (Cramer Products, Inc)	Many	Fructose/ sucrose	4.7	116	23	Ca, Cl, P	305
Sqwincher (Univ Prod, Inc)	Many	Glucose/ fructose	6.8	60	36	Vit C, Cl, P, Ca, Mg	470
Exceed (Ross Labs)	Lemon/ lime, orange	Glucose polymer/ fructose	7.2	50	45	Ca, Mg, P, Cl	250
PowerBurst (PowerBurst Corp)	Many	Fructose	6.0	35	55	Vit B, C, A, E; Cl; Mg; Ca; pantothenic acid; folic acid; biotin	433
Body Fuel 450 (Vitex Foods, Inc)	Orange	Maltodextrin/ fructose	4.2	80	20	P; Cl; Fe; vit A, B, C	210
10-K (Bev Prod, Inc)	Many	Sucrose, glucose, fructose	6.3	52	26	Vit C, Cl, P	350
Mountain Dew Sport (PepsiCo, Inc)	Regular	High fructose Corn syrup/ sucrose	10	60	40	Vit C, Cl, Ca	674
Soft drinks	Many	High fructose Corn syrup/ sucrose	10.2-11.3	9.2-28	Trace	P	600–715
Diet soft drinks	All	None	0	0-25	Low	P	<50
Fruit juice	Many	High fructose/ sucrose	11–15	0–15	61-150	P; vit C, A, B; Ca; Fe	690–890
Water	–	–	0	Low	Low	Low	10–20

Adapted from *Gatorade Thirst Quencher*, copyright 1990, Quaker Oats Company.

1. Obese and overweight individuals, due to the insulation of fat. Because of their uniforms and higher body fat, football linemen appear to be at greater risk.[17]
2. Children, because they generate more heat, sweat less, take longer to acclimatize, and gain more heat from the environment.[18,19]
3. Nonacclimatized individuals.
4. Individuals who have had a previous incident of heat illness.
5. Out-of-shape individuals, due to their less-efficient thermoregulatory mechanisms.

One of the best assurances of competing at full potential is to avoid dehydration. Follow these guidelines:

▶ Drink plenty of water or fluid-replacement beverages before, during, and after exercise.
▶ Don't wait until you are thirsty to drink. Thirst is a symptom of dehydration.
▶ Drink cool beverages.
▶ Drink 16 oz for every pound lost in exercise or competition.
▶ Begin replacing fluid losses immediately after exercise for quickest recovery. If weight on the following day is not within 1% of the pre-exercise weight of the previous day, it may not be advisable for the athlete to work out.
▶ Closely supervise children participating in sports or other activities in hot and humid conditions. Make sure they have scheduled fluid breaks.

▶ DEHYDRATION

Dehydration is the result of a loss of intracellular, interstitial, and intravascular water. It can be acute, occurring from one bout of exercise, or chronic, reflecting losses from moderate exercise and an inadequate intake of water over a period of time. Acute dehydration is defined as a loss of at least 1% body weight.[20] Chronic dehydration may be seen as a gradual loss of body weight over time, resulting in a 1% or greater reduction in total body weight.[21]

The desire to drink fluids does not adequately prevent dehydration. Thirst may not be triggered until a deficit of approximately 700 mL of water, equivalent to an approximately 1% loss of body weight.[20,22] Despite ad libitum fluid replacement, dehydration (ranging from 1% to 4% of body weight) is commonly reported in individuals participating in cycling, running, and canoeing events.[23-26] This phenomenon is referred to as voluntary dehydration[12] and is not inconsequential with respect to performance. A reduction in plasma volume equivalent to a 1% to 2% loss of body weight has been shown to impair exercise performance.[8,21] Although maximum oxygen uptake may not be affected by dehydration, both speed and endurance are known to decrease.[27,28] More important, dehydration prevents adequate thermoregulation due to a decrease in plasma volume and an increase in serum osmolality.[24,29] Consequently, dehydration contributes to a rise in core body temperature and an increased risk for hyperthermia.[28,30]

Sweat Production and Temperature Regulation

The primary cause of dehydration during exercise is an increase in sweat production along with inadequate fluid replacement. The purpose of sweating is to regulate body temperature via evaporation. Muscular work causes heat to be produced as a result of an increased rate of energy metabolism. This heat production causes an increase in body temperature that is directly proportional to exercise intensity. At very low exercise intensities, heat is transferred to the environment via convection and radiation without the use of sweating. Very little water is lost to the environment and there is minimal risk for dehydration. At higher exercise intensities, convection and radiation are inadequate for body cooling. Sweat is produced, and heat and water are lost through the skin via evaporation.

Water and Electrolyte Losses From Sweat

Sweat is composed of water and electrolytes in a concentration that is hypotonic to body fluids. It contains approximately 15 to 120 mEq sodium per liter, 5 to 110 mEq chloride per liter, and 3 to 10 mEq potassium per liter.[31] In comparison, extracellular fluid (plasma and interstitial fluid) contains an average of 135 to 145 mEq sodium per liter, 95 to 105 mEq chloride per liter, and 3.05 to 5.0 mEq potassium per liter. Generally, sweating results in a proportionately greater loss of water than electrolytes.

In exercise-induced sweating, both plasma and interstitial fluid volumes decrease and there is a concurrent increase in extracellular electrolyte concentration.[23,28] As the level of body water loss increases, intracellular water moves into the extracellular space, although this may not occur until the cessation of exercise. There is conflicting evidence regarding the maintenance of plasma volume. Most studies report significant reductions in plasma volumes with exercise and dehydration.[24,31-33] However, plasma volume appears to be preserved in some dehydrated individuals who are heat-acclimatized.[34] Overall, there appears to be tremendous variability in the intravascular response depending on a number of factors, including type and intensity of exercise, state of hydration, and heat acclimatization.[28]

It is estimated that moderate to heavy exercise can produce 1 to 1.5 L of sweat per hour, which is equal to approximately 1% to 2% loss of body weight.[25,35] A marathon lasting 4 hours could easily produce 5 to 6 L of sweat, creating severe dehydration if water is not replaced. Sodium and chloride losses in an exercise session lasting 1 hour or less are generally small and easily replaced by a diet providing about 5 g salt.[29] However, sodium losses can be significant in exercise lasting more than 2 hours. Three liters of sweat contain between 2.4 to 12 g salt. Even greater losses may be expected during marathons, ultramarathons, triathlons, and events lasting longer than 8 hours, particularly if these events are conducted in the heat.[36,37] Hiller reports that a sweat loss of 1.5 L per hour for 12 hours will result in a loss of 36 g NaCl.[36] These losses can result in hyponatremia and dehydration if both sodium and water are not replaced.[38]

Research on electrolyte balance during exercise in the heat suggests that loss of potassium via sweat is negligible and that heavy sweating, under most exercise conditions, is unlikely to create a potassium deficiency.[22,39,40] In a study of eight men consuming a diet restricted to 25 mmol potassium per day, 4 days of strenuous exercise did not result in a decrease in muscle or serum potassium.[40] However, there is always the risk that heavy sweating combined with an inadequate intake of dietary potassium could result in potassium depletion. Armstrong and colleagues conclude that potassium depletion may be more of a risk than sodium depletion during extended exercise and heat exposure, because ingested food is often supplemented with sodium.[39]

To avoid any potential problem, athletes should be counseled to consume regularly foods that are known to be good sources of potassium. Luckily, many of these foods (fruits, vegetables, low-fat dairy products) are consistent with the general recommendation for a high-carbohydrate, low-fat energy intake.

Dehydration and Thermoregulation

A loss of 1% to 4% body weight has been shown to reduce plasma volume by 8% to 16%.[21,23,27,33] This reduced plasma volume is associated with a decrease in cardiac output, an increase in heart rate, an elevation in blood pressure, and a reduction in peripheral vascularization.[30,32,41] Inadequate peripheral blood flow prevents heat transfer to the skin for cooling and is associated with decreased sweating and an elevated core body temperature.[28]

Impaired thermoregulation has been associated with both the state of dehydration and an increase in plasma hemoconcentration. Sweat inhibition in severe dehydration has been shown to be selective, resulting in reduced sweating on the body, but not on the forehead, where evaporation is needed for cooling of the brain.[42] Although some investigators have reported no change in sweat rates with dehydration,[32] impaired sweating is commonly associated with loss of body water.[8,43,] This impairment is thought to be related to an increase in plasma sodium concentration that increases the threshold for sweating to a higher core temperature.[30,43]

The relationship between dehydration and maintenance of core body temperature remains controversial. Normal internal body temperatures have been reported with increasing losses of percent body weight.[25] However, in most studies, significant increases in core temperature occur with severe dehydration.[32,44]

Dehydration With Exercise in the Heat

The greatest risk for dehydration occurs with exercise in the heat. Heat removal via convection and radiation requires a large increase in skin temperature when the ambient air temperature is high. Skin temperature rises when there is an increase in peripheral blood flow. This is difficult to accomplish during exercise, since blood is diverted to muscles for oxygen delivery. Consequently, heat storage increases and there is an increase in sweat production and in the fluid requirements for cooling.

Heat acclimatization results in an expansion of plasma volume at rest and maintenance of plasma volume during exercise.[27,34] It also is characterized by an increased capacity to produce sweat. These changes are partially due to an increase in extracellular sodium in response to aldosterone and a reduction in sodium excretion by the kidney.[40] Both high plasma volumes and elevated sweat rates increase fluid requirements. Thus, although there is improved cooling and a smaller rise in internal body temperature, the risk for dehydration becomes even greater with heat acclimatization.

In non-heat-acclimatized individuals exercising in the heat, sodium requirements increase along with fluid requirements, because increased sweat production results in increased NaCl losses. Although heat acclimatization tends to reduce the total loss and concentration of sodium in sweat,[22,40,45] exercise in the heat appears to increase the risk for salt-depletion dehydration. As mentioned earlier, hyponatremia has been reported in individuals experiencing large sweat losses associated with high losses of NaCl and inadequate intake of dietary NaCl.[36,37]

It has been suggested that a high-sodium diet and the retention of sodium with heat acclimatization may interfere with potassium conservation and lead to potassium depletion. However, there is evidence that potassium retention is not affected by the ingestion of either high or low intakes of sodium during heat acclimatization.[22] Heat acclimatization causes retention of both urinary sodium and potassium, and any increase in potassium requirements is most likely due to large increases in sweat production.

Dehydration and Gastrointestinal Disturbances

Runners often complain of gastrointestinal (GI) symptoms while exercising. A study of 1000 marathon runners found that 40% of those surveyed had GI complaints.[46] Recent evidence suggests that dehydration greater than 4% of body weight is related to an increased frequency of GI symptoms.[47] This is likely to be caused by ischemia of the GI tract due to a severe reduction in blood flow to allow for increased skin perfusion.[29]

Another source of gastrointestinal symptoms with severe dehydration may be the presence of gastric residuals from incomplete gastric emptying. It appears that once a person has become severely dehydrated while running in warm temperatures, gastric emptying is inhibited.[48,49] This same inhibition of gastric emptying has not been shown to occur if the person remains hydrated by drinking fluids during running or cycling in the heat.[48,50]

Heat Cramps

The major cause of heat cramps is whole-body salt deficiency that is characterized by hyponatremia and hypochloremia.[38] Heat cramps are frequently a complication of heat exhaustion, but may appear alone without other symptoms of dehydration. They usually occur in individuals exercising for several hours in a hot climate who have large sweat losses and have consumed a large volume of unsalted water.[29] It is important not to confuse heat cramps with other forms of muscle cramps, such as those caused by GI upset. Heat cramps occur in voluntary skeletal muscles, including those of the abdomen and the extremities. They consist of a contraction for 1 to 3 minutes at a time of a few muscle bundles that can be accurately located. The cramp actually moves down the muscle from one bundle to another and is associated with excruciating pain.

Treatment for heat cramps consists of administering a 1% oral NaCl solution (two 10-grain salt tablets crushed in 1 L of water). If symptoms include nausea and vomiting, an intravenous solution of 0.5 to 1.0 L normal saline may be necessary.[38] Since heat acclimatization results in sodium conservation, the best way to prevent heat cramps is to exercise moderately at first in the heat with adequate salt intake before engaging in long, strenuous exercise.

▶ HEAT STROKE

Of all the complications that result from excessive heat stress, heat stroke is the most serious and, potentially, the most life-threatening. When heat stroke occurs, sweating generally ceases, and the body temperature may rise to dangerously high levels. If left untreated, circulatory collapse, central nervous system damage, and death are likely sequelae. When individuals are suffering from heat stroke they often faint, and their skin becomes hot and dry. Ice packs or cold water immersion are usually recommended as immediate treatment steps until medical personnel can be summoned. Intelligent rehydration habits and careful attention to rapid body-weight changes, as well as avoidance of exercise under extremely hot, humid conditions, are recommended for decreasing the risk of developing heat stroke and other related illnesses.

▶ HYPONATREMIA

Hyponatremia, or low serum sodium (less than 130 mEq Na per liter), is not commonly associated with physical exercise. Nonetheless, a number of recent reports have indicated the occurrence of hyponatremia in athletes who consumed salt-free fluids during prolonged exercise. With the number of long-distance and ultraendurance events on the rise, it is likely that the incidence of hyponatremia will increase as well. Acute hyponatremia generally occurs as a result of excessive sodium loss, excessive intake of salt-free water, or both. Mental confusion, disorientation, and restlessness are often early signs of hyponatremic encephalopathy. Consumption of a beverage containing sodium (4 to 8 oz per 15 minutes; 100 to 120 mg Na per 8 oz) is usually sufficient to slow the progression of hyponatremic symptoms.[51,52]

REFERENCES

1. McArdle WD, Katch FI, Katch VL. *Exercise Physiology-Energy, Nutrition, and Human Performance.* 2nd ed. Philadelphia, Pa: Lea & Febiger; 1986.
2. Rowell LB, Marx HJ, Bruce RA, Conn RD, Kusumi F. Reductions in cardiac output, central blood volume and stroke volume with thermal stress in normal men during exercise. *J Clin Invest.* 1966;45:1801-1816.
3. Hayes MA, Williamson RJ, Heidenreich WF, et al. Endocrine mechanisms involved in water and sodium metabolism during operation and convalescence. *Surgery.* 1957;41:343-386.
4. Matthews DK, Fox EL, Tanzi D. Physiological responses during exercise and recovery in a football uniform. *J Appl Physiol.* 1969;26:611.
5. Pugh LCGE, et al. Rectal temperatures, weight losses and sweat rates in marathon running. *J Appl Physiol.* 1966;21:1251.
6. Sawka MN, Francesconi RP, Young AJ, Pandolph KB. Influence of hydration level and body fluids on exercise performance in the heat. *JAMA.* 1984;252:1165-69.
7. Adolph EF. *Physiology of Man in the Desert.* New York, NY: Interscience Publications; 1949:231-232.
8. Armstrong LE, Costill DL, Fink WJ. Influence of diuretic-induced dehydration on competitive running performance. *Med Sci Sports Exer.* 1985;17:456-461.
9. Steen SN, Brownell KD. Patterns of weight loss and regain in wrestlers: has the tradition changed? *Med Sci Sports Exerc.* 1990;22:762-768.
10. Grandjean AC. Fluid and electrolytes. In: Mellion MB, ed. *Office Management of Athletic Injuries.* Philadelphia, Pa: Hanley & Belfus; 1987:59.
11. Pitts GC, Johnson RE, Consolazio FC. Work in the heat as affected by intake of water, salt, and glucose. *Am J Physiol.* 1944;142:253.
12. Hubbard RW, Sandick BL, Matthew WT, et al. Voluntary dehydration and allesthesia for water. *J Appl Physiol.* 1984;57:868.
13. Costill DL, Cote R, Miller T, et al. Water and electrolyte replacement during repeated days of work in the heat. *Aviat Space Environ Med.* 1975;46:795.
14. Nose H, Mack GW, Shi X, Nadel ER. Role of osmolality and plasma volume during rehydration in humans. *J Appl Physiol.* 1988;65:325.
15. Murray R. The effects of consuming carbohydrate-electrolyte beverages on fluid absorption during and following exercise. *Sports Med.* 1987;4:322-351.
16. Sports Medicine Council. *Jet Lag and Athletic Performance.* Colorado Springs, Colo: US Olympic Committee; 1986.
17. Wailgum TD, Paolone A. Heat tolerance of college football lineman and backs. *Phys Sports Med.* 1984;12:81.
18. American Academy of Pediatrics. Climatic stress and the exercising child. *Pediatrics.* 1982;69:808-809.
19. Bar-Or O. Climate and the exercising child—a review. *Int J Sports Med.* 1980;1:53-65.
20. Brooks GA, Fahey TD. *Exercise Physiology: Human Bioenergetics and Its Applications.* New York, NY: John Wiley & Sons; 1984.
21. Kristal-Boneh E, Glusman JG, Chaemovitz C, Cassuto Y. Improved thermoregulation caused by forced water intake in human desert dwellers. *Eur J Appl Physiol.* 1988;57:220-224.
22. Armstrong LE, Costill DL, Fink WJ, et al. Effects of dietary sodium on body and muscle potassium content during heat acclimation. *Eur J Appl Physiol.* 1985;54:391-397.
23. Wells CL, Stern JR, Kohrt WM, Campbell KD. Fluid shifts with successive running and bicycling performance. *Med Sci Sports Exerc.* 1987;19:137-141.
24. Carter JE, Gisolfi CV. Fluid replacement during and after exercise in the heat. *Med Sci Sports Exerc.* 1989;21:532-539.

25. Noakes TD, Adams BA, Myburgh KH, Greeff C, Lotz T, Natham M. The danger of an inadequate water intake during prolonged exercise: a novel concept revisited. *Eur J Appl Physiol*. 1988;57:210-219.

26. Myhre LG, Hartung GH, Nunneley SA, Tucker DM. Plasma volume changes in middle-aged male and female subjects during marathon running. *J Appl Physiol*. 1985;59:559-563.

27. Armstrong LE, Pandolf KB. Physical training, cardiorespiratory physical fitness, and exercise-heat tolerance. In: Pandolf KB, Sawka MN, Gonzalez RR, eds. *Human Performance Physiology and Environmental Medicine at Terrestrial Extremes*. Indianapolis, Ind: Benchmark Press, Inc; 1988.

28. Sawka MN. Body fluid responses and hypohydration during exercise-heat stress. In: Pandolf KB, Sawka MN, Gonzalez RR, eds. *Human Performance Physiology and Environmental Medicine at Terrestrial Extremes*. Indianapolis, Ind: Benchmark Press, Inc; 1988.

29. Hubbard RW, Armstrong LE. The heat illnesses: biochemical, ultrastructural, and fluid-electrolyte considerations. In: Pandolf KB, Sawka MN, Gonzalez RR, eds. *Human Performance Physiology and Environmental Medicine at Terrestrial Extremes*. Indianapolis, Ind: Benchmark Press, Inc; 1988.

30. Nielsen B. Temperature regulation: effects of sweat loss during prolonged exercise. *Acta Physiol Scand*. 1986; 128(suppl 556):105-109.

31. Brandenberger G, Candas V, Follenius M, Libert JP, Kahn JM. Vascular fluid shifts and endocrine responses to exercise in the heat: effect of rehydration. *Eur J Appl Physiol*. 1986;55:123-129.

32. Bothorel B, Follenius M, Gissinger R, Candas V. Physiological effects of dehydration and rehydration with water and acidic or neutral carbohydrate electrolyte solutions. *Eur J Appl Physiol*. 1990;60:209-216.

33. Nielsen B, Sjogaard G, Ugelvig J, Knedusen B, Dohlmann B. Fluid balance in exercise dehydration and rehydration with different glucose-electrolyte drinks. *Eur J Appl Physiol*. 1986;55:318-325.

34. Sawka MN, Toner RP, Francesconi RP, Pandolf KB. Hypohydration and exercise: effects of heat acclimation, gender, and environment. *J Appl Physiol*. 1983;55:1147-1153.

35. Pivarnik JM. Water and electrolytes during exercise. In: Hickson JF, Wolinsky I. *Nutrition in Exercise and Sport*. Boston, Mass: CRC Press; 1989.

36. Hiller WDB. Dehydration and hyponatremia during triathlons. *Med Sci Sports Exerc*. 1989;21:S219-S221.

37. Noakes TD, Norman RJ, Buck RH, Godlonton J, Stevenson K, Pittaway D. The incidence of hyponatremia during prolonged ultraendurance exercise. *Med Sci Sports Exerc*. 1990;22:165-170.

38. Hubbard RW, Armstrong LE. Hyperthermia: new thoughts on an old problem. *Phys Sports Med*. June 1989;17.

39. Armstrong LE, Hubbard RW, Szlyk PC, Matthew WT, Sils IV. Voluntary dehydration and electrolyte losses during prolonged exercise in the heat. *Aviat Space Environ Med*. 1985;56:765-770.

40. Costill DL. Muscle metabolism and electrolyte balance during heat acclimation. *Acta Physiol Scand*. 1986;128(suppl 556):111-118.

41. Baum K, Essfeld D, Stegemann J. Reduction in extracellular muscle volume increases heart rate and blood pressure response to isometric exercise. *Eur J Appl Physiol*. 1990;60:217-221.

42. Caputa M, Cabanac M. Precedence of head homeothermia over trunk homeothermia in dehydrated men. *Eur J Appl Physiol*. 1988;57:611-615.

43. Sawka MN, Young AJ, Francesconi RP, Muza SR, Pandolf KB. Thermoregulatory and blood responses during exercise at graded hypohydration levels. *J Appl Physiol*. 1985;59:1394-1401.

44. Candas V, Libert JP, Brandenberger G, Sagot JC, Amoros C, Kahn JM. Hydration during exercise: effects on thermal and cardiovascular adjustments. *Eur J Appl Physiol*. 1986;55:113-122.

45. Kirby CR, Convertino VA. Plasma aldosterone and sweat sodium concentrations after exercise and heat acclimation. *J Appl Physiol*. 1986;61:967-970.

46. Keeffe EB, Lowe DK, Goss JR, Wayne R. Gastrointestinal symptoms of marathon runners. *West J Med*. 1984;141:481-484.

47. Rehrer NJ, Janssen GME, Brouns F, Sarts HM. Fluid intake and gastrointestinal problems in runners competing in a 25-km race and a marathon. *Int J Sports Med*. 1989;10:S22-S25.

48. Neufer PD, Young AJ, Sawka MN. Gastric emptying during exercise: effects of heat and hypohydration. *Eur J Appl Physiol*. 1989;58:433-439.

49. Owen MD, Dregel KC, Wall PT, Gisolfi CV. Effects of ingesting carbohydrate beverages during exercise in the heat. *Med Sci Sports Exerc*. 1986;18:568-575.

50. Ryan AJ, Bleiler TL, Carter JE, Gisolfi CV. Gastric emptying during prolonged cycling exercise in the heat. *Med Sci Sports Exerc*. 1989;21:51-58.

51. Noakes TD, Goodwin N, Rayner B, Branken T, Taylor R. Water intoxication: a possible complication during endurance exercise. *Med Sci Sports Exer*. 1985;17:370-375.

52. Barr S, Costill D. Water: can the endurance athlete get too much of a good thing. *J Am Diet Assoc*. 1989;89:1629-1635.

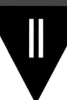
Assessment of Nutritional Status

Melinda Manore, Editor

Assessment of nutritional status has become a standard aspect of practice for the nutrition professional. Increasingly, clients are requesting information on risk of nutritional deficiency, body composition, and general physical fitness. Athletes are more interested than most in these indexes, and are likely to consider any evaluation that does not supply information on body composition as inadequate. Because of the availability of many techniques and formulas, the nutrition practitioner may find it difficult to select the most appropriate one for the individual being evaluated. This section provides information on a variety of methods for the assessment of nutritional status, and offers guidance on their potential limitations and inherent advantages.

Medical and Nutrition Assessment

Melinda Manore and Monique Ryan

Prior to beginning a fitness program, it is desirable for adults to have a complete medical and nutrition assessment. This assessment is a tool for screening and identifying medical problems and their nutritional relationships. Identification of problems is the first step in planning an appropriate and safe exercise program and nutrition regimen. A complete medical assessment should include measurements that lead to a better understanding of physical fitness and nutritional status. The assessment may include some or all of the following components:

▶ Cardiorespiratory fitness
▶ Muscular strength
▶ Endurance
▶ Flexibility
▶ Body composition
▶ Biochemical tests (eg, blood glucose, blood lipids)
▶ Health history
▶ Medication history
▶ Diet history

▶ PHYSICAL EXAM

The physical examination should be conducted by a properly licensed physician, nurse practitioner, or physician assistant. Vital signs (ie, temperature, heart rate, blood pressure, respiration), head-to-toe inspection, resting 12-lead electrocardiogram (ECG), stress test, heart sounds, anthropometric measurements, laboratory (biochemical) data, and physical fitness evaluation are all components of this examination. (A more in-depth description of physical fitness assessment, anthropometric assessment, and interpretation of biochemical data is provided later in this section.)

The frequency with which a person should have a physical examination depends on the individual's medical history, age, and physical condition. The generally healthy person aged 30 years or younger probably does not require a physical examination more often than once every 2 to 3 years. As age increases, so does the recommended frequency of the physical examination. Persons aged 30 to 35 years should be examined every 2 years; persons aged 36 to 40 years should be examined every 18 months (the exam should include a resting ECG); persons aged 40 years and older should be examined (including an ECG and stress test) every 18 months; and persons aged 50 years and older should have an annual exam that includes a resting and stress ECG if symptoms indicate their necessity.

▶ MEDICAL AND NUTRITION HISTORY

The assessment of an individual's nutrition and health status is not complete until a medical and nutrition history has been taken by a registered dietitian or other appropriately certified or licensed health professional. This history should be sufficiently comprehensive so as to give the health professional a good understanding of the individual's *risk* of developing an illness.

Medical History

The purpose of the medical history is to help identify, in advance, people who are at high risk for stress testing and exercise participation. As part of their medical assessments, clients should complete medical history questionnaires (see the sample questionnaire in appendix 4). This questionnaire should address the following areas[1]:

- ▶ Personal history of coronary artery disease
- ▶ Family history of coronary artery disease
- ▶ The presence of risk factors associated with coronary artery disease (hypertension, diabetes, obesity, blood lipids, stress, and smoking history)
- ▶ Exercise history
- ▶ Allergies
- ▶ Chronic illnesses or conditions
- ▶ Past surgeries or injuries or both
- ▶ Current medications
- ▶ Current treatment for illness
- ▶ Fat and cholesterol content of the diet
- ▶ Evaluation of cardiac, pulmonary, and gastrointestinal symptoms

Using information from the health history questionnaire, dietitians can classify clients according to health status prior to their beginning an exercise program, by using guidelines and categories established by the American College of Sports Medicine.[1] These categories are outlined in *Table 2.1*. The

TABLE 2.1   Classification of Individuals by Health Status Prior to Exercise Testing or Exercise Prescription

Category	Description
Apparently healthy	Those who are apparently healthy and have no major coronary risk factors
Individuals at higher risk	Those who have symptoms suggestive of possible metabolic disease or coronary disease and/or at least two of the following major coronary risk factors: 1. History of high blood pressure (≥160/90 or on antihypertensive medication) 2. Elevated serum cholesterol ≥6.20 mmol/L (≥240 mg/dL) 3. Cigarette smoking 4. Abnormal resting ECG–including evidence of old myocardial infarction, left ventricular hypertrophy, ischemia, conduction defects, dysrhythmias 5. Family history of coronary or other atherosclerotic disease prior to age 55 6. Diabetes mellitus
Patients with disease	Those with known cardiac, pulmonary, or metabolic disease (diabetes, thyroid disorders, renal disease, liver disease)

Adapted with permission from American College of Sports Medicine. *Guidelines for Exercise Testing and Prescription.* Philadelphia, Pa: Lea & Febiger; 1991.

TABLE 2.2   Categorization of the Primary Risk Factors for Cardiovascular and Blood Values

Risk Factor	Optimal Value	Moderately High Risk	High Risk
Blood pressure	<120/80 mm Hg	140/90 to 160/95 mm Hg	>160/95 mmHg
Cigarettes/d	0	10-20	>20
Cholesterol, mg/dL			
Age 20-29	<160	160-220	>220
Age 30-39	<180	180-240	>240
Age 40+	<190	190-260	>260
NIH* values	<200	200-239	≥240
Chol/HDL ratio	<3.5	4.5-5.0	>5.0

Data from Nieman DC. *Fitness and Sports Medicine, An Introduction.* Palo Alto, Calif: Bull Publishing Co; 1990.
  *National Cholesterol Education Program.

questionnaire is especially useful in assessing risk factors for cardiovascular disease. *Table 2.2* categorizes blood pressure, cigarette smoking, and serum cholesterol into risk levels for developing cardiovascular disease.

Diet History

The medical history should include, as an integral piece, an in-depth assessment of the client's nutritional status. This assessment usually includes an interview to obtain diet and activity information, and is a means of predicting energy intake and requirement.

For the athlete, the diet history data can be gathered through the medical (patient) chart or interview or both. (Sample diet history questionnaires are included in appendix 5.) It is especially important that information be obtained on the type, duration, and intensity of activity the athlete is engaged in. This information will assist the health professional in assessing the dietary and nutrient problems commonly associated with the activity. The following diet-history interview format, outlined in The American Dietetic Association's *Manual of Clinical Dietetics,*[2] has been adapted for use with athletes:

1. *Weight:* Current weight, usual weight, weight goal for sport and/or weight suggested by coach or trainer, recent weight loss or gain, percent body fat, goal body fat, and frequency of dieting for weight loss.
2. *Appetite/intake:* Appetite changes and factors affecting appetite/intake–such as preferences, training routine, activity level, anorexia, stress, allergies, medications, chewing/swallowing problems (bulimia, oral health), gastrointestinal problems (gastritis, laxative abuse, constipation).
3. *Eating patterns:* Typical patterns (weekdays/weekends); primary eating place (dorm, home, cafeteria, training table); primary food shopper at home; dietary restrictions (understanding of and compliance with these restrictions); frequency of eating out; effect of training, precompetition, competition, and travel on typical eating patterns; ethnicity of diet; and food preferences.

4. *Estimation of typical energy and nutrient intake:* Standards include the 1989 Recommended Dietary Allowances[3] (see appendix 6), recommended macronutrient intakes for athletes (see section I), *Dietary Guidelines for Americans,*[4] and the American Heart Association guidelines.[5] Food intake information may be obtained from a 24-hour recall, food frequency questionnaire, and/or food diary.

5. *Psychosocial data:* Economic status, occupation, educational level, living/cooking arrangements, and mental status.

6. *Medication and/or supplemental use:* Current medications and supplements used, including amounts and reason for use. Drug-nutrient or nutrient-nutrient interactions may necessitate special dietary considerations[6,7] (see appendix 7). Effect of medication on physical performance and eating habits (some medications are taken with food; others, without food).

7. *Other:* Age; sex; level (minutes per day, miles per week) and types of physical activity engaged in during competition, training, and nontraining periods; fitness level ($\dot{V}O_2$max; strength tests; and flexibility).

REFERENCES

1. American College of Sports Medicine. *Guidelines for Exercise Testing and Prescription.* 4th ed. Philadelphia, Pa: Lea & Febiger; 1991.

2. Chicago Dietetic Association, South Suburban Dietetic Association. *Manual of Clinical Dietetics.* 3rd ed. Chicago, Ill: The American Dietetic Association; 1988.

3. Food and Nutrition Board. *Recommended Dietary Allowances.* 10th ed. Washington, DC: National Academy Press; 1989.

4. *Nutrition and Your Health: Dietary Guidelines for Americans.* 3rd ed. Washington, DC: US Dept of Agriculture, US Dept of Health and Human Services; 1990. Home and Garden bulletin 232.

5. American Heart Association. *Dietary Guidelines for Healthy American Adults.* Dallas,Tex: American Heart Association; 1986. AHA publication 21-0030.

6. Allen AM. *Food-Medication Interactions.* 7th ed. Pottstown, Pa: Food Medication Interactions; 1991.

7. Krause MV, Mahan LK. *Food, Nutrition and Diet Therapy.* 7th ed. Philadelphia, Pa: WB Saunders Co; 1984.

Nutrient Intake Assessment

Melinda Manore and Monique Ryan

Assessment of dietary intake is one of the most frequently used procedures in dietetics and human nutrition research. In both of these settings, the goal is to achieve the most accurate description of an individual's (or group's) typical food and nutrient intake. Therefore, the diet data collection method must be as accurate, precise, and reliable as possible for the population being assessed. In addition, a variety of other factors (eg, interviewer's time, cost, purpose of the assessment) must be addressed. *Table 2.3* lists a variety of diet-assessment methods with the advantages and disadvantages associated with each.

Collection of the diet data is only one part of dietary intake assessment. Once the information has been collected, it must be analyzed for nutrient content and then compared with a nutrient standard or goal. Today, most diets are analyzed for nutrient content by commercially available computerized nutrient-analysis programs.[1] To avoid introducing additional error into the diet-assessment technique, care should be taken in the selection and use of these computer programs. (See additional information on the selection of diet-analysis computer programs later in this section.)

Although a variety of dietary standards are available, those most commonly used are the latest (1989) RDAs[2] (see appendix 6), the 1990 *Dietary Guidelines for Americans,*[3] the 1986 American Heart Association guidelines,[4] and the food exchange system[5] (see appendix 8). Research on the nutrient needs of athletes has also produced dietary recommendations (see section I). These dietary standards and goals can be tailored to meet the needs of a particular client.

▶ METHODS FOR COLLECTION OF NUTRIENT INTAKES

Three methods are used for collecting information on clients' nutrient intakes.

24-Hour Recall

The 24-hour recall is the easiest and fastest method available for assessing food and nutrient intake. This method requires that a client recall, in detail, all the foods and beverages consumed during the previous 24 hours. Knowing the preparation methods, the brand names of foods and beverages, and any vitamin-mineral supplements is critical to an effective evaluation.

Two major limitations of the 24-hour recall are (1) its reliance on memory (people forget what and how much they ate) and (2) the tendency of some clients to minimize poor food choices and overstate good food choices.[6,7] To increase accuracy, a skilled interviewer can ask key questions to help the client remember all the foods and amounts of foods consumed. Measuring devices and food models can also be used in the interview process. Due to the limitations mentioned, the success of the 24-hour recall will depend, in large

TABLE 2.3   Diet-Assessment Methods

Strengths	Limitations
24-Hour Recall Respondent burden is low. Well accepted by most respondents. No record keeping by respondent is required. Time for administration is short. Probability sampling within populations and individuals is possible. Bias introduced by record keeping is avoided. Costs are low, especially for computerized versions. Useful in clinical situations. More objective than dietary history. Does not alter usual diets. Serial 24-hour recalls can provide estimates of usual intakes in individuals.	Single 24-hour recall does not represent individual's usual intake. Interviewers must be trained. Some, such as the very young or old, cannot remember their intakes. Forgetting may introduce bias and may lead to incomplete records, especially for those who have poor memories. Desire to please interviewer may result in distorted intakes. Recalls are likely to be incomplete for certain items and nutrients. Forgetting is especially high for liquids, snacks, alcohol, fats, and sweets, leading to errors in calories, fat, and alcohol. Group means of single 24-hour recalls are reliable, but individual rankings vary from one day to the next and cannot identify individuals whose intakes are consistently high or low. Serial recalls are needed in this situation. Often used incorrectly in surveys to identify individuals with inadequate intakes or to identify associations with other risk factors.
Food Frequency Questionnaires Provides description of how often foods are eaten. Easy to standardize. Does not require highly trained interviewers, and some types may be self-administered. Rapid Inexpensive Useful for describing food intake patterns for diet and meal planning. Useful when purpose is to study associations of a specific food or small number of foods and disease, such as artificially sweetened beverages and bladder cancer, coffee and birth defects or pancreatic cancer, or alcohol and birth defects. Correlations with other methods or food is good when group is focus of analysis. Limited information about nutrient intakes may be obtained. Useful when purpose is to establish relative rankings with respect to intakes of certain food items or groups. Does not alter usual diets. Helpful for rapid estimates of single nutrients or food groups.	Lists compiled for the general population are not useful for obtaining information on groups with different eating patterns (eg, vegetarians or those on special ethnic or therapeutic diets). Difficult to obtain information on total consumption because some foods are not included in lists. Respondent burden rises as number of items queried increases. Many assumptions are necessary if food frequency estimates are to be used to estimate nutrient intakes, and special computer programs must be used. Reliability is lower for individual foods than for groups of foods. Foods differ in extent to which they are over- or underreported. Amount and frequency with which a food is consumed influence errors in estimation, staples and large quantities being better estimated than accessories or items eaten less frequently. Intakes are underestimated because not all foods eaten are listed; forgetting occurs. Translation from intakes of food groups to nutrients requires that many assumptions be made. Validity must be established for each questionnaire. Longer lists may agree well with diet histories for single nutrients.
Semiquantitative Questionnaires Rapid to administer. Sometimes possible to self-administer. Do not alter usual diets. Precoding and direct data entry to computer available to speed analysis on some versions. Correlations between these questionnaires and other methods are satisfactory for food items and targeted nutrients when groups are the focus of analysis. Permit investigators in large epidemiologic investigations to obtain dietary information that would not be possible with longer methods. Costs of analysis are relatively low.	Utility in dietary assessment of individuals not yet ascertained. Existing questionnaires differ as to their purpose and should only be used for their intended purposes. Most instruments currently available are only for adults. Must be periodically updated. Specific nutrient intakes, rather than all nutrient intakes or food constituents, are measured. General population, not specific subgroups with different diets, is suitable target group. As food consumption patterns change, questionnaires must be updated. Not yet validated for those who eat modified or unusual diets. Ability to monitor short-term changes in food intake (weeks or months) is unknown. Correlations for individual nutrient intakes obtained with semiquantitative food frequency questionnaires are poor when compared to diet histories and food records in household measures. Correlations between existing semiquantitative food frequency questionnaires and diet histories may be poor for ethnic groups eating unusual diets and for those on special diets.

(continued)

TABLE 2.3   Diet-Assessment Methods (continued)

Strengths	Limitations
Burke-type Dietary History	
Provides a more complete and detailed description of both qualitative and quantitative aspects of food intake than do food records, 24-hour recalls, or food frequency questionnaires. Correlations with other measures of nutritional status are good. Accounts for seasonal and other systematic variations in diet. Useful in longitudinal studies. Does not alter usual diets. Provides some description of previous diet before beginning prospective studies.	Highly skilled research nutritionists are required to administer it. Highly dependent on subject's memory. Time-consuming (1 to 2 hours). Difficult to standardize. Differences among interviewers can be considerable. Costs of analysis are high because records must be checked, coded, and entered appropriately. Time frame actually used by subject for reporting intake history is uncertain. Subjects usually overestimate intakes owing to overestimating frequency and portion size and forgetting missed meals and sick days, so that dietary histories tend to be higher than food records collected over same period. Validity must be established in each study.
Food Diary	
Record of what is eaten is recorded at time of consumption. Subject can be instructed in advance so that recording errors are minimized. Errors of recall are less than with retrospective methods.	Food intake may be altered during reporting periods. Respondent burden is great. Literacy required. Respondent may not record intakes on assigned days, compromising representativeness. Portion sizes are difficult to estimate. Measuring helps. Models, pictures, or abstract shapes for sizing overcome some but not all inaccuracies. Underreporting is common. Number of days must be sufficient to provide usual intakes. Records must be checked and coded in a standardized manner. Measured food intakes are more valid than records above. Costs of coding and analysis are high.
Weighed Food Diary	
Increased accuracy over food diaries with estimates of portions or household measures.	Increased respondent burden. May alter consumption, especially away from home and may increase number of dropouts.
Telephone Interviewers	
Face-to-face interviews are eliminated. Respondent burden lowered. Effects of forgetting minimized. Validity good. Respondent acceptance good.	Validation studies incomplete.
Photographic Records	
Validity good.	Technical problems with estimating portion size and some foods from photographs. Necessary details may be lacking. Food waste may be ignored, leading to overestimates.
Electronic Records (specially programmed portable computer)	
Decrease respondent burden. Preliminary validations good.	Require considerable instruction. Special food groups must be constructed for population to be studied. Portion size estimates may be imprecise.
Duplicate Portion Collection and Analysis	
Highly accurate in metabolic research studies. Duplicate portion can be analyzed chemically. Helpful for validating other methods for constituents on which food composition data are incomplete.	May alter intakes. High respondent burden. Expensive and time-consuming to analyze. Differences between duplicate portions and weighed records large (7% for energy, larger for other nutrients).

From ME Shils and VR Young: *Modern Nutrition in Health and Disease,* 7th edition. Philadelphia, Lea & Febiger, 1988. Reprinted with permission.

part, on the client's memory, motivation to respond accurately, and ability to convey precise information. The persistence and skill of the interviewer is also a critical factor in obtaining accurate information from a 24-hour recall.[6,8]

A single 24-hour recall is most useful for estimating the nutrient intake of a group or population, but may not be an appropriate tool for assessing the usual food and nutrient intake of an individual.[6,9,10] If the 24-hour recall is to be used for estimating individual food intakes, the US Committee on Food Consumption Patterns recommends that a minimum of four 24-hour recalls be collected over a 1-year period.[9] (See appendix 9 for a sample 24-hour recall form.)

Another approach to obtaining a representative estimate of an individual's average food intake is to combine the 24-hour recall with a food frequency questionnaire or checklist. Combining these two methods of diet assessment can provide a more complete picture of an individual's typical diet pattern and nutrient intake.[11]

Food Frequency Questionnaire

A food frequency questionnaire (FFQ) is designed to provide descriptive information about an individual's usual dietary pattern. It consists of a list of foods and inquires about the number of times specific foods are consumed per day, per week, or per month. The information collected can then be used to assess the food patterns and preferences that may not be evident from a food recall or diet record. For best results, the FFQ should be brief, requiring less than 20 to 25 minutes for administration and completion.[11] As with the 24-hour recall, the FFQ relies on memory; therefore, it is inappropriate for use with young children or with individuals who have poor memories.

The format of the FFQ can be designed to provide either qualitative or semiquantitative information on a client's typical food intake.[8,9,12] Questionnaires that provide qualitative data (ie, they only list typical foods consumed) are most useful for obtaining general descriptive information about an individual's dietary patterns or for comparing consumption of certain foods before and after nutrition intervention.[9,11] Semiquantitative FFQs not only list typical foods consumed, but also attempt to quantify the usual intake of these foods. This type of questionnaire allows the assessment of specific nutrient intakes in addition to dietary patterns. Selective FFQs can also be created to inquire about specific nutrient concerns, such as fat,[13] carbohydrate,[14] and cholesterol.[15]

Because the aim of the FFQ is to assess the frequency with which certain food items or food groups are consumed during a specified period, it is important that the questionnaire be designed and tested specifically for the population and nutrient being measured. A variety of FFQs have been designed and validated for various populations.[12,14,16] For example, Moses and Manore[14] have developed and tested a FFQ to monitor carbohydrate intake in athletes. (An example of an FFQ is provided in appendix 10.)

Food Records

A food record is a list of all foods consumed, including a description of food preparation methods and brand names used, over a specified time period (typically 3 to 7 days). To predict nutrient content accurately, it is best if the foods consumed are weighed or measured. However, it is most common for consumed foods to be recorded by common portion sizes expressed in common household measure units. More in-depth information on eating habits can also be included on a food record, such as time, place, feelings, and behaviors associated with eating.[11,17] When the records are completed, the nutrient contribution from each food is determined, and average nutrient intake for the time period being monitored can be calculated.

Food records are generally considered the most precise and accurate method for monitoring food intake because they do not rely on the client's memory or the interviewer's ability to jog a person's memory.[6,8] In addition, food records can be used for measuring either individual or group food intake.[6,9] However, the accuracy of a food record is still reliant on the individual's cooperation and skill in recording the foods consumed.

Determining the number of days food intake should be recorded to give an accurate and reliable assessment of typical dietary intake has been addressed by a number of researchers.[18-24] Schlundt determined that, for most purposes, diet records collected for 3 to 14 days will provide accurate estimates of nutrient intake.[22] However, within this range both reliability and accuracy increase with each additional day up to day 7.[21,22] For most nutrients, there was little advantage to measuring intakes beyond 2 or 3 weeks.[22,23] The disadvantage to longer periods of recording food consumption is that the increased respondent burden decreases accuracy.[6] For shorter records (3 to 4 days), at least one weekend day should be included.[10,21]

Specific guidelines for keeping records should be included in the instruction sheet given to the client, and these instructions should also be reviewed verbally. (A sample food record/diary form is provided in appendix 11.) Guidelines for clients who are recording foods in a food record follow:

1. Record items immediately after they are consumed. Use common measures, such as cups and tablespoons, to describe the amount consumed, and, whenever possible, measure or weigh the food items being consumed.
2. Record all beverages and all items added to them, such as sugar and cream added to coffee. Include the beverages (eg, water) taken with medications.
3. Include condiments, such as butter, margarine, mustard, mayonnaise, and salad dressing.
4. Completely describe the foods consumed, eg, "whole wheat bread," "white turkey meat without skin," and "meatless spaghetti sauce."
5. Indicate how the food was prepared, eg, *fried* chicken, *broiled* beef steak, and *steamed* vegetables.
6. Record all foods and beverages consumed as snacks.
7. Keep the food record diary sheet(s) accessible at all times so that items can be recorded immediately.
8. Write down any nutritional supplements consumed, such as sports drinks consumed during training or a race.
9. When using convenience foods, save the food label and return it with the completed food diary.
10. Whenever possible, note the brand names of food items (eg, canned foods, convenience foods, deli items).
11. If food is consumed at a restaurant or fast-food establishment, record the name of the restaurant and the product purchased.

▶ ANALYSIS AND INTERPRETATION OF FOOD INTAKE DATA

Once food intake information has been collected, it should be translated into nutrition terms based on an accepted standard.[17] This will make the information understandable to the client and help set the groundwork for formulating dietary goals.

There are several methods used for dietary interpretation. A simple and quick method is to check to see if any major food groups (meat, poultry, fish, dry beans, eggs, and nuts; milk, yogurt, and cheese; bread, cereal, rice, and pasta; fruit; vegetable) are not consumed or are consumed infrequently. It is assumed that, if adequate calories and a variety of foods are being consumed from each group, the nutrients provided by these food groups will be adequately represented in the diet. Since no single food can provide all the nutrients needed, the diet must also be checked for variety within each food group. As a general rule it could be said that a monotonous diet will increase the risk of poor nutritional status. In addition, foods within each group vary in their fat and sodium content, so the frequency of consumption of foods high in fat and/or sodium within each group should also be checked. Finally, if an individual consistently consumes foods high in simple sugars and/or fats (eg, rich desserts, high-fat spreads, highly processed foods), fat and caloric intake can be high, even though he or she is eating a variety of other foods.

The food Exchange Lists (see appendix 8) categorize foods that are similar in calories, carbohydrates, protein, and fat content for specified portion sizes. These lists can also be used to estimate the nutritional adequacy of the diet.

Some practitioners tally nutrient intake using food composition tables, and then they compare the nutrient totals to the 1989 RDAs (see appendix 6). The RDAs are a well-accepted guide for planning and evaluating diets of population groups and individuals, including athletes. In addition, the 1990 Dietary Guidelines for Americans,[3] the 1986 American Heart Association guidelines,[4] and/or specific diet recommendations for athletes (see section I) can be used.

Currently, computerized diet analysis is a popular and quick means of analyzing energy and nutrient intakes from diet records. This method, when properly applied, is considered to be the most efficient, accurate, and timely means available for analyzing the nutrient content of consumed foods. Recorded foods are entered into a computerized nutrient-analysis program. A computer printout is then generated, allowing both the registered dietitian (or qualified nutritionist) and client to review the calculated information and establish dietary goals. Most programs will calculate total calories, as well as grams and percentages of carbohydrates, protein, and fat. In addition, most programs will also compare calculated vitamin and mineral intakes to the appropriate RDA based on age and sex. Some programs may also give information regarding the type of fat and sugar consumed, the polyunsaturated/saturated fat ratio, or the cholesterol-saturated fat index[25] of the diet. Some offer specific recommendations for improving nutrient intake.

REFERENCES

1. Byrd-Bredbenner C. Computer nutrient analysis software packages: considerations for selection. *Nutr Today.* Sept/Oct 1988:13-21.
2. Food and Nutrition Board. *Recommended Dietary Allowances.* 10th ed. Washington, DC: National Academy Press; 1989.
3. *Nutrition and Your Health: Dietary Guidelines for Americans.* 3rd ed. Washington, DC: US Dept of Agriculture, US Dept of Health and Human Services; 1990. Home and Garden bulletin 232.
4. American Heart Association. *Dietary Guidelines for Healthy American Adults.* Dallas, Tex: American Heart Association; 1986. AHA publication 21-0030.
5. Hamilton EMN, Whitney EN, Sizer FS. *Nutrition: Concepts and Controversies.* 5th ed. New York, NY: West Publishing Co, 1991.
6. Dwyer JT. Assessment of dietary intake. In: Shils ME, Young VR, eds. *Modern Nutrition in Health and Disease.* 7th ed. Philadelphia, Pa: Lea & Febiger; 1988.

7. Karvetti R, Knuts L. Validity of the 24-hour dietary recall. *J Am Diet Assoc.* 1985;85:1437-1444.
8. Krall EA, Dwyer JT. Validity of a food frequency questionnaire and a food diary in a short-term recall situation. *J Am Diet Assoc.* 1987;87:1374-1376.
9. Gibson RS. *Principles of Nutritional Assessment.* New York, NY: Oxford University Press; 1990.
10. Todd KS, Hudes M, Calloway DH. Food intake measurement: problems and approaches. *Am J Clin Nutr.* 1983;37:139-146.
11. Kris-Etherton P, ed. *Cardiovascular Disease: Nutrition for Prevention and Treatment.* Chicago, Ill: The American Dietetic Association; 1990.
12. Willett WC, Reynolds RD, Cottrell-Hoehner S, Sampson L, Browne ML. Validation of a semi-quantitative food frequency questionnaire: comparison with a 1-year diet record. *J Am Diet Assoc.* 1987;87:43-47.
13. Block G, Clifford C, Naughton MD, Henderson M, McAdams M. A brief dietary screen for high fat intake. *J Nutr Ed.* 1989;21:199-207.
14. Moses K, Manore MM. Development and testing of a carbohydrate monitoring tool for athletes. *J Am Diet Assoc.* 1991;91:962-965.
15. Lee J, Kolonel LN, Hankin JH. Cholesterol intake as measured by unquantified and quantified food frequency interviews: implications for epidemiological research. *Int J Epidemiol.* 1985;14:249-253.
16. Block G, Hartman AM, Dresser CM, Carroll MD, Gannon J, Gardner L. A data-based approach to diet questionnaire design and testing. *Am J Epidemiol.* 1986;124:453-469.
17. Peterson M, Peterson K. *Eat to Compete: A Guide to Sports Nutrition.* Chicago, Ill: Year Book Medical Publishers Inc; 1988.
18. Acheson KJ, Campbell IT, Edholm OG, Miller DS, Stock MJ. The measurement of food and energy intake in man–an evaluation of some techniques. *Am J Clin Nutr.* 1980;33:1147-1154.
19. Basiotis PP, Welsh SO, Cronin FJ, Kelsay JL, Mertz W. Number of days of food intake records required to estimate individual and group nutrient intakes with defined confidence. *J Nutr.* 1987;117:1638-1641.
20. Heaney RP, Davies KM, Recker RR, Packard PT. Long-term consistency of nutrient intakes in humans. *J Nutr.* 1990;120:869-875.
21. Jackson B, Dujovne CA, DeCoursey S, Beyer P, Brown EF, Hassanein K. Methods to assess relative reliability of diet records: minimum records for monitoring lipid and calorie intake. *J Am Diet Assoc.* 1986;86:1531-1535.
22. Schlundt DG. Accuracy and reliability of nutrient intake estimates. *J Nutr.* 1988;118:1432-1435.
23. Sempos CT, Johnson NE, Smith EL, Gilligan C. Effects of intraindividual and interindividual variation in repeated dietary records. *Am J Epidemiol.* 1985;121:120-130.
24. White EC, McNamara DJ, Ahrens EH. Validation of a dietary record system for the estimation of daily cholesterol intake in individual outpatients. *Am J Clin Nutr.* 1981;34:199-203.
25. Conner SL, Gustafson JR, Artaud-Wild SM, Classick-Kohn CJ, Conner WE. The cholesterol-saturated fat index for coronary prevention: background, use, and a comprehensive table of foods. *J Am Diet Assoc.* 1989;89:807-816.

Physical Fitness Assessment

Melinda Manore and Monique Ryan

▶ HEART RATE

Determination of both resting heart rate (RHR) and maximal heart rate (MHR) are necessary for planning and implementing a cardiovascular fitness program. MHR is the fastest heart rate measured when a client is brought to total exhaustion during a graded exercise test. This method of determining MHR is preferred because individuals of the same sex and age have heart rates that vary greatly.[1,2] When measured MHR is unavailable, an estimation[3] can be made by subtracting age in years from 220:

$$MHR = 220 - age \text{ (years)}$$

Note: Because this formula provides only an estimate of MHR, caution should be used when using it to develop a fitness program. For example, a 45-year-old individual may have a true heart rate of 145 to 205 beats per minute, rather than the estimated 175 beats per minute. However, two thirds of the population at this age would have MHRs of 165 to 185 beats per minute.[4] Although heart rate will increase in direct proportion to the intensity of exercise, MHR changes little with training. To monitor heart rate before, during, and after exercise, count the number of heart beats (starting with zero) in 10 seconds and multiply by six. Estimated maximal attainable heart rates for various age groups are given in *Table 2.4.*

▶ BLOOD PRESSURE

In addition to determining MHR, the dietitian should pay careful attention to the client's blood pressure measurement. The upper limits of normal blood

TABLE 2.4 Maximal Attainable Heart Rates (MHR) for Various Age Groups

Age	Predicted MHR	Target Heart Rate		
		60%	70%	80%
20-29	200-191	120-114	140-134	160-153
30-39	190-181	114-109	133-127	152-145
40-49	180-171	108-103	126-120	144-137
50-59	170-161	102-97	119-113	136-129

Data from Kris-Etherton P, ed. *Cardiovascular Disease: Nutrition for Prevention and Treatment.* Chicago, Ill: The American Dietetic Association; 1990.

pressure are 140 mm Hg systolic and 90 mm Hg diastolic. Pressures above this are classified as mildly hypertensive. Severe hypertension is indicated if diastolic blood pressure exceeds 115 mm Hg.

Table 2.5 provides a profile of blood pressure risk factors for coronary artery disease. A variety of factors affect blood pressure. These include:

- ▶ Age
- ▶ Sex
- ▶ Time of day
- ▶ Physical discomfort
- ▶ Apprehension
- ▶ Bladder fullness
- ▶ Body position
- ▶ Surroundings
- ▶ Method of measurement

Blood pressure is usually obtained with the client sitting or standing. More detailed information on procedures for obtaining proper blood pressure measurement can be obtained elsewhere.[5,6]

During exertion, diastolic blood pressure should remain relatively constant, while systolic blood pressure rises linearly as work load increases.[7] An exercise test should be terminated if the systolic blood pressure exceeds 250 mm Hg or the diastolic pressure exceeds 120 mm Hg. During a test, blood pressure should be obtained every 1 to 2 minutes or at each test stage. If hypotensive or hypertensive readings are present, blood pressure should be checked at more frequent intervals.[8] During recovery, blood pressure should be monitored every 2 to 3 minutes until resting levels are reached.

▶ STRESS TESTING

A maximal exercise test (stress test) is an important way to determine cardiovascular fitness. More important, it is used in the detection of cardiovascular disease and to assess a client's exercise capacity prior to starting an exercise program. Stress testing can also be used in the treatment and rehabilitation of clients who have cardiovascular disease. A variety of tests have been developed to diagnose cardiovascular disease and formulate exercise prescriptions for exercise training programs.[9,10]

For individuals of all ages, a maximal graded exercise test can provide valuable information that can be used in developing a safe and effective exercise prescription.[7] Healthy individuals younger than 45 years of age can usually begin a moderate exercise program without a graded exercise test. Those older than 45 years should have a complete medical/physical examination, including a maximal graded exercise test, prior to starting an exercise program. A physician should be present at all maximal graded exercise tests for individuals older than 35 years of age. In addition, all high-risk individuals, regardless of

TABLE 2.5 Profile of Blood Pressure Risk Factors of Coronary Heart Disease

	Very Low	Low	Moderate	High	Very High
Blood pressure, mm Hg					
Systolic	<110	120	130-140	150-160	>170
Diastolic	<70	76	82-88	94-100	>106

Adapted with permission from Pollock ML, Wilmore JH. *Exercise in Health and Disease: Evaluation and Prescription for Prevention and Rehabilitation.* 2nd ed. Philadelphia, Pa: WB Saunders Co; 1990.

age, should be given a physician-supervised maximal graded exercise test prior to beginning an exercise program.[8] *Table 2.6* summarizes the American College of Sports Medicine (ACSM) guidelines for exercise testing. ACSM has also developed guidelines for contraindications to exercise and exercise testing, as the risks for these people may outweigh the benefits. *Table 2.7* summarizes these contraindications.[8]

During a maximal stress test, the client reaches a plateau in oxygen consumption before the test is terminated.[10,11] To ensure that maximal exertion has been achieved, serial measurements of oxygen can be obtained. If maximal exertion cannot be achieved due to various health limitations, maximum effort can be approximated by having the client exercise to symptom-limited exercise tolerance.[12] The exercise test ends when the client indicates that he or she can

TABLE 2.6 Guidelines for Exercise Testing and Participation

Classification	Apparently Healthy Younger Men (≤40 y) Women (≤50 y)	Older Adults	Higher Risk* No Symptoms	Symptoms	With Disease†
Medical exam and diagnostic exercise test recommended prior to:					
Moderate exercise‡	No‖	No	No	Yes¶	Yes
Vigorous exercise§	No	Yes	Yes	Yes	Yes
Physician supervision recommended during exercise test:					
Submaximal testing	No	No	No	Yes	Yes
Maximal testing	No	Yes	Yes	Yes	Yes

*Persons with two or more risk factors or symptoms (see Table 2.1).

†Persons with known cardiac, pulmonary, or metabolic disease.

‡Moderate exercise (exercise intensity, 40% to 60% $\dot{V}o_2$ max)—Exercise intensity well within current capacity and can be comfortably sustained for a prolonged period, eg, 60 min.

§Vigorous exercise (exercise intensity >60% $\dot{V}o_2$ max)—Exercise intense enough to represent a substantial challenge and would ordinarily result in fatigue within 20 min.

‖The "no" responses in this table mean that an item is not necessary. The "no" response does not mean that the item should not be done.

¶A "yes" response means that an item is recommended.

Adapted with permission from American College of Sports Medicine: *Guidelines for Exercise Testing and Prescription.* Philadelphia, Lea & Febiger, 1991.

TABLE 2.7 Contraindications for Entry Into Inpatient and Outpatient Exercise Programs

1. Unstable angina
2. Resting diastolic blood pressure >100 mg Hg or resting systolic blood pressure >200 mm Hg
3. Orthostatic blood pressure drop of ≥20 mm Hg
4. Moderate to severe aortic stenosis
5. Acute systemic illness or fever
6. Uncontrolled atrial or ventricular dysrhythmias
7. Uncontrolled sinus tachycardia (>120 beats/min)
8. Uncontrolled congestive heart failure
9. Third-degree AV heart block
10. Active pericarditis or myocarditis
11. Recent embolism
12. Thrombophlebitis
13. Resting ST displacement (>3 mm)
14. Uncontrolled diabetes mellitus
15. Orthopedic problems that would prohibit exercise

From American College of Sports Medicine: *Guidelines for Exercise Testing and Prescription.* Philadelphia, Lea & Febiger, 1991. Reprinted with permission.

no longer continue. The stress test generally consists of a 12-lead ECG, with blood pressure and heart rate readings taken at rest and while exercising. The test is usually graded at several levels of physical work, each of 3 to 5 minutes duration.

When a stress test is completed, the following information should be included in the laboratory report:

1. Preexercise heart rate and blood pressure in both the exercise posture and recovery posture
2. Maximum exercise level achieved and the energy cost of the maximum work load
3. Heart rate and blood pressure at each stage of the test
4. Heart rate and blood pressure during recovery
5. ECG abnormalities noted on the preexercise recording, at any test stage, and during recovery
6. Any symptoms that occurred during the testing period, and the test stage at which they appeared
7. Reason for termination of the test (eg, target achieved, symptoms, volitional exhaustion, ECG findings)
8. Test interpretations, including risks and the likelihood of disease, and any relevant findings and their significance

This information can then be used in client education and for advising the client on an exercise regimen.[13]

During exercise of submaximal intensity, maximal oxygen uptake is predicted from heart rate and ventilation rate, both of which increase in proportion to increases in oxygen uptake.[4,11] Although the use of submaximal tests may not be appropriate for research purposes, their use in assessment of cardiovascular capacity is justified when financial, personal safety, or time considerations become prohibitive.[11]

▶ STRENGTH AND FLEXIBILITY TESTING

Both strength and flexibility are an important part of any exercise program. Maintenance of flexibility is especially important for the role it plays in the prevention of injury.[14] The assessment of flexibility has been reviewed in detail by Corbin.[15] In general, assessment of flexibility is uncomplicated, and can be done with minimal equipment (tape and measuring stick) and cost. The most common flexibility test used for mass screening is the "sit-and-reach" test.[14]

Muscular strength can be defined as the maximum amount of force that can be exerted by a muscle, while *muscular endurance* is the ability of a muscle to exert a force repeatedly over a period of time.[4] Because of the interrelationship between muscular strength and endurance, an increase in one of these components usually results in some degree of improvement in the other. The assessment of muscular strength has been recently reviewed by Skinner and colleagues[14] and Howley and Franks.[4]

▶ MAXIMAL OXYGEN CONSUMPTION ($\dot{V}O_2$max)

Direct measurement of maximal oxygen consumption during maximal exercise is regarded as the best laboratory measure of heart and lung capacity.[7] In healthy individuals, oxygen consumption increases as work load increases, until a plateau is reached. This threshold is referred to as $\dot{V}O_2$max. Thus, $\dot{V}O_2$max is the greatest rate of oxygen consumption attained during exercise and is usually expressed in liters per minute (L/min) or millimeters per kilogram of body weight per minute (mL•kg^{-1}•min^{-1}).[16] It is also the measure of maximal aerobic metabolism of the body. Prior to this plateau, aerobic work that can be maintained for a long period is referred to as a steady-state threshold.

Maximal aerobic capacity is often assessed in athletes to predict performance, with direct measurement of $\dot{V}O_2$max preferred over an estimation. The higher the $\dot{V}O_2$max value obtained, the greater the client's potential for performing high-intensity aerobic work.[2] However, many factors (not just $\dot{V}O_2$max) may contribute to an individual's exercise performance.

Percent of $\dot{V}O_2$max utilized during exercise is the amount of oxygen consumed relative to $\dot{V}O_2$max, and is useful for determining how stressful the exercise is with respect to one's maximum capacity. Percent $\dot{V}O_2$max is calculated by dividing the oxygen consumption during exercise by the $\dot{V}O_2$max and multiplying by 100:

$$\%\dot{V}O_2\text{max} = \left(\frac{\dot{V}O_2 \text{ during exercise}}{\dot{V}O_2\text{max}} \right) \times 100$$

The athlete with a higher $\dot{V}O_2$max would find an exercise requiring a specific $\dot{V}O_2$ easier than an athlete with a lower $\dot{V}O_2$max. Lactic acid accumulation begins after a certain percent of $\dot{V}O_2$max is reached. In nonathletes, lactic acid accumulation will occur at a lower level (approximately 65% $\dot{V}O_2$max), while in trained distance runners it will occur at a higher level (approximately 80% $\dot{V}O_2$max). The higher the $\dot{V}O_2$max without lactic acid accumulation, the more successful the endurance exercise will be. While $\dot{V}O_2$max appears to be genetically influenced, training improves the ability to utilize a higher percent of $\dot{V}O_2$max without lactic acid accumulation.[1,17]

▶ POWER

Power, by definition, is work produced per unit time, and can be expressed[3] as force (f) times distance (d) divided by time (t):

$$P = \frac{f \times d}{t}$$

Power, therefore, is a combination of both speed and strength, and refers to the rate at which one performs work.[7]

Some simple anaerobic tests for power consist of running up a flight of stairs or timing a 50-yard dash with a 15-yard running start.[3] Tests (such as the Wingate Anaerobic Test) have been developed to measure peak power, mean power, and rate of fatigue by using a predetermined force to produce a supramaximal effort.[7]

▶ ANAEROBIC THRESHOLD

The anaerobic threshold occurs when the ventilatory response during graded exercise is no longer linear.[18] The physiological mechanism behind anaerobic threshold is not fully understood. It usually occurs close to the work rate at which blood lactic acid concentrations start to accumulate.[16]

Regular exercisers may perceive anaerobic threshold as the exercise intensity at which breathing and talking become somewhat difficult. In most individuals, the onset of blood lactic acid accumulation is a marker for determining the upper end of the intensity range for "aerobic" exercise programs.[18] Fitness programs emphasizing aerobic exercise will want exercise intensity to be below the anaerobic threshold. This will prevent the rapid accumulation of lactic acid, which usually causes discomfort and necessitates an earlier termination of the exercise.

▶ LACTATE THRESHOLD

The lactate threshold occurs when the relatively constant blood lactate level observed during graded exercise suddenly increases. Endurance training programs can increase the lactate threshold, thereby delaying fatigue.[4]

▶ METABOLIC EQUIVALENTS

Metabolic equivalents (METs) are often used to measure the work load at various stages of a graded exercise test. One MET is equal to the resting oxygen consumption of the "average human" and equals $3.5 \text{ mL} \bullet \text{kg}^{-1} \bullet \text{min}^{-1}$ or approximately 1 kcal/kg per hour of oxygen consumed.[7] The formula that can be used to determine the MET level for a particular exercise follows[8]:

$$\text{METs} = \frac{\text{oxygen required for exercise}}{\text{oxygen required at rest } (3.5 \text{ mL} \bullet \text{kg}^{-1} \bullet \text{min}^{-1})}$$

Healthy, sedentary people can usually exercise up to 10 to 12 METs, while well-conditioned athletes often exercise above 15 METs.

▶ RATE OF PERCEIVED EXERTION

A valuable parameter for determining exercise intensity is subjective exertion or effort level.[12] The Rating of Perceived Exertion Scale developed by Borg[19] was based on a scale of 6 to 20. This roughly corresponds to a maximal heart rate of 60 to 200. A revised scale of 0 to 10 points was developed to contain ratio properties (a logical zero point) and account for variables such as lactic acid and excessive ventilation, which rise in a nonlinear fashion[7] (see *Table 2.8*).

Either scale can be used during a graded exercise test to provide useful information for determining exhaustion or prescribing exercise.[12,20] Clinical studies have found that the Rate of Perceived Exertion Scale provides a reproducible measure of effort within a wide range. The scale has been found to correlate with heart rate, ventilation, lactate production, and percent $\dot{V}O_2$max.[12] Clients perceive intensity at the lactate threshold to be "somewhat hard or strong" or a 13 to 14 on the original scale (4 on the newer scale). Exercising at the "somewhat hard" level correlates with the lactate threshold or the level of exercise intensity that is recommended.[21]

▶ ELECTROCARDIOGRAM (ECG)

Heart rate during exercise is best determined by an ECG, which records the electrical activity of the heart. During this procedure, a visible record of the heart's electrical activity is provided by a stylus, which traces this activity on a

TABLE 2.8 Rated Perceived Exertion (RPE) Scales*

RPE		New Rating Scale	
6		0	Nothing at all
7	Very, very light	0.5	Very, very weak
8		1	Very weak
9	Very light	2	Weak
10		3	Moderate
11	Fairly light	4	Somewhat strong
12		5	Strong
13	Somewhat hard	6	
14		7	Very strong
15	Hard	8	
16		9	
17	Very hard	10	Very, very strong
18			Maximal
19	Very, very hard		

Adapted with permission from Borg GA. Psychological bases of physical exertion. *Med Sci Sports Exerc.* 1982;14:377-387, © The American College of Sports Medicine. Also adapted from Nieman DC. *Fitness and Sports Medicine: An Introduction.* Palo Alto, Calif: Bull Publishing Co; 1990.

*Original scale (6-19) on left; revised (0-10) on right.

moving strip of heat-sensitive paper. When the heart is stimulated, a wave of depolarization passes through it and moves toward a positive skin electrode, which results in a positive upward deflection recorded on the ECG.[7]

A diagnostic test should be performed with a multiple ECG system that, ideally, uses 12 skin electrodes.[7] In young, healthy populations, a single-lead system may be adequate if the primary purpose of the test is to measure fitness. A standard resting ECG should be taken before the test is begun, with a recording of the ECG taken at periodic intervals. Clients should be monitored 10 minutes into recovery, since changes may occur during the cool-down phase,[8] and more frequent readings should be secured if heart abnormalities appear.

One of the major reasons for providing a treadmill ECG stress test in high-risk populations is to load the heart muscle beyond normal demands to see if any obstruction in blood flow to the coronary arteries can be detected.[10] An ECG provides information on heart rate, rhythm, and conduction pathways, along with signs of ischemia or infarction.[4]

▶ EXERCISE PRESCRIPTION

A recommended program of exercise should be designed to meet an individual's objectives for fitness, as modified for reasonableness by a properly certified and licensed health professional. Due to individual variation in many factors (eg, health, goals, education), the exercise prescription should be tempered to meet the individual's needs in a safe and effective manner. Prior to giving the client an exercise prescription, the health professional should obtain information on the client's medical history, current health, and fitness. Under ideal circumstances, it is best for the exercise prescriber to know the client, discuss the client's goals at length, be aware of the client's interests, understand the client's scheduling limitations, and be familiar with the client's motivation for fitness. It is also important to know the results of the client's physical fitness test.[7] Specific exercise elements (such as intensity, duration, and frequency of activity) should be prescribed with a knowledge of how these affect energy expenditure and fitness. Both long-term and short-term goals should be considered with specific plans and activities.

Aerobic activity should be a major part of the exercise prescription because of its association with cardiovascular fitness. Most commonly, the aerobic activity will include walking, jogging, cycling, swimming, stepping, rowing, aerobic dancing, or some combination of these. Specific strength and flexibility exercises should be included to improve performance and prevent injury.

A minimum of 3 and a maximum of 6 days per week is recommended for exercise, depending on the fitness level of the client and the intensity of the exercise.[7] The exercise session should begin with a 5- to 10-minute warm-up that includes stretching exercises, 20 to 60 minutes of cardiovascular conditioning, and a 5- to 10-minute cool-down period to slow the heart rate.[22] It should be understood by clients, especially those at a low fitness level, that any amount of cardiovascular conditioning is beneficial, and that the recommended times are for maximal aerobic benefit. The client should be encouraged to do any amount of cardiovascular conditioning possible, even if the client is capable of doing only 5 minutes initially. The recommended time investment of 30 to 80 minutes per session should, therefore, be thought of as a goal rather than an immediate necessity for the improvement of cardiovascular fitness.

Strength training to develop and maintain fat-free weight can be done at moderate intensity a minimum of 2 days per week. One set of 8 to 12 repetitions of 8 to 10 exercises that condition the major muscle groups is the recommended minimum.[22]

Clients who know their maximal heart rate (MHR) from a treadmill test or an age-based average should exercise from 60% to 85% of MHR. Exercising at 60% of MHR for longer duration will achieve the same training effect as a higher percentage for shorter duration. Low-intensity exercise, such as walking, can begin at just a few minutes for the overweight or unfit person and be gradually increased to 40 to 60 minutes.

An effective physical activity program should include methods for keeping clients motivated and preventing relapse to old and potentially unhealthy habits. Ways for making exercise more enjoyable should be encouraged, with an emphasis on periodic follow-ups for fitness assessment, positive reinforcement, and permanent life-style change.[7]

A prescribed weekly exercise calorie level can be helpful for achieving weight-loss goals, and it helps to clarify the need for exercise at a recommended frequency, intensity, and duration. The caloric output recommended for maintaining optimal cardiovascular health is, on average, about 2000 kcal per week. This level can be easily achieved by most fit people with regular exercise that achieves the target heart rate, along with a generally more active life-style.[23]

REFERENCES

1. Pollock ML, Wilmore JH. *Exercise in Health and Disease: Evaluation and Prescription for Prevention and Rehabilitation.* 2nd ed. Philadelphia, Pa: WB Saunders Co; 1990.
2. Åstrand PO, Rodahl K. *Textbook of Work Physiology.* 3rd ed. New York, NY: McGraw-Hill; 1986.
3. McArdle WD, Katch FI, Katch VL. *Exercise Physiology: Energy, Nutrition, and Human Performance.* 3rd ed. Philadelphia, Pa: Lea & Febiger; 1991.
4. Howley ET, Franks BD. *Health/Fitness Instructor's Handbook.* Champaign, Ill: Human Kinetics Publishers Inc; 1986.
5. Gifford RW. Hypertension: current view of diagnostic evaluation. In: *The Hypertension Handbook.* West Point, Pa: Merck & Co; 1974.
6. Maxwell MH. Hypertension: a functional approach to screening. In: *The Hypertension Handbook.* West Point, Pa: Merck & Co; 1974.
7. Nieman DC. *Fitness and Sports Medicine.* Palo Alto, Calif: Bull Publishing Co; 1990.
8. American College of Sports Medicine. *Guidelines for Exercise Testing and Prescription.* 4th ed. Philadelphia, Pa: Lea & Febiger; 1991.

9. Blair SN, Painter P, Pate RR, Smith LK, Taylor CB. *Resource Manual for Guidelines for Exercise Testing and Prescription.* American College of Sports Medicine. Philadelphia, Pa: Lea & Febiger; 1988.

10. Ellestad MH. *Stress Testing Principles and Practice.* 3rd ed. Philadelphia, Pa: FA Davis Co; 1986.

11. Lamb DR. *Physiology of Exercise: Responses and Adaptations.* New York, NY: Macmillan Publishing Co; 1978.

12. Hanson P. Clinical exercise testing. In: Blair SN, Painter P, Pate RR, Smith LK, Taylor CB. *Resource Manual for Guidelines for Exercise Testing and Prescription.* American College of Sports Medicine. Philadelphia, Pa: Lea & Febiger; 1988.

13. Paolone AM. Prescribing exercise programs. In: Bove AA, Lowenthal DT, eds. *Exercise Medicine: Physiological Principles and Clinical Applications.* New York, NY: Academic Press; 1983.

14. Skinner JS, Baldini FD, Gardner AW. Assessment of fitness. In: Bouchard C, Shephard RJ, Stephens T, Sutton JR, McPherson BD, eds. *Exercise, Fitness, and Health: A Consensus of Current Knowledge.* Champaign, Ill: Human Kinetics Books; 1990.

15. Corbin C. Flexibility. *Clin Sports Med.* 1984;3:101-117.

16. Pate RR, Lonnett M. Terminology in exercise physiology. In: Blair SN, Painter P, Pate RR, Smith LK, Taylor CB. *Resource Manual for Guidelines for Exercise Testing and Prescription.* American College of Sports Medicine. Philadelphia, Pa: Lea & Febiger; 1988.

17. Smith ML, Mitchell JH. Cardiorespiratory adaptations to training. In: Blair SN, Painter P, Pate RR, Smith LK, Taylor CB. *Resource Manual for Guidelines for Exercise Testing and Prescription.* American College of Sports Medicine. Philadelphia, Pa: Lea & Febiger; 1988.

18. Durstine JL, Pate RR. Cardiorespiratory responses to acute exercise. In: Blair SN, Painter P, Pate RR, Smith LK, Taylor CB. *Resource Manual for Guidelines for Exercise Testing and Prescription.* American College of Sports Medicine. Philadelphia, Pa: Lea & Febiger; 1988.

19. Borg GAV. Psychophysical bases of perceived exertion. *Med Sci Sports Exerc.* 1982;14:377-381.

20. Carton RL, Rhodes EC. A critical review of the literature on ratings scales for perceived exertion. *Sports Med.* 1985;2:198-222.

21. Demello JJ, Cureton KJ, Boineau RE, Singh MM. Ratings of perceived exertion at the lactate threshold in trained and untrained men and women. *Med Sci Sports Exerc.* 1987;19:354-362.

22. American College of Sports Medicine. Position stand: the recommended quantity and quality of exercise for developing and maintaining cardiorespiratory and muscular fitness in healthy adults. *Med Sci Sports Exerc.* 1990;22:265-274.

23. Kris-Etherton P, ed. *Cardiovascular Disease: Nutrition for Prevention and Treatment.* Chicago, Ill: The American Dietetic Association; 1990.

Body Measurements

Melinda Manore, Dan Benardot, and Page Love

An important component to the assessment of nutritional status is the determination of body size. This is done through a variety of techniques in which anthropometric measures are secured. Anthropometric measurements are defined as indexes of body stature, weight, and fatness, which are then compared with gender-specific, age-specific, and sport-specific standards. These measurements can be obtained at either one point in time or over a designated period, such as a training season.

▶ MEASUREMENT TECHNIQUES

This section describes and defines various anthropometric measurement techniques (eg, stature, weight, circumferences, skinfolds, body widths, elbow breadth) used in the assessment of body size. Some of these measurements can also be used in the assessment of body composition. For a more complete review of specific anthropometric measurement techniques, see the *Anthropometric Standardization Reference Manual* by Lohman and colleagues.[1]

Stature/Height

The most appropriate way to measure stature or height is with a measuring stick or measuring tape attached to a true vertical flat surface with a fixed horizontal headboard. Typically, this is a wall or a freestanding measuring device such as a "stadiometer," or movable anthropometer (see *Figure 2.1*). The headboard should be moved downward so that it comes in contact with the most superior part of the head, with the hair slightly compressed. The client should be barefoot and should stand on a flat surface that is at a right angle to the vertical board. The client's weight should be distributed evenly on both feet, heels together, and arms hanging freely on the side. The scapula, buttocks, and heels touch the vertical wall or surface, and the client should hold his or her head straight. The measurement is made within the nearest 0.125 in or 0.5 cm (2.54 cm = 1 inch).[2]

Weight

The most appropriate way to measure weight accurately is to use a beam scale with nondetachable weights, eg, a platform scale that is calibrated with a known weight every 3 or 4 months (see *Figure 2.2*). If possible, the client should be weighed before breakfast and after the bladder has been emptied, and the client should wear underwear or light clothing with no shoes. Before weighing the client, the health professional must first calibrate the scale to zero. The client

FIGURE 2.1   Anthropometer; used for length, height, breadth, and width measurements.

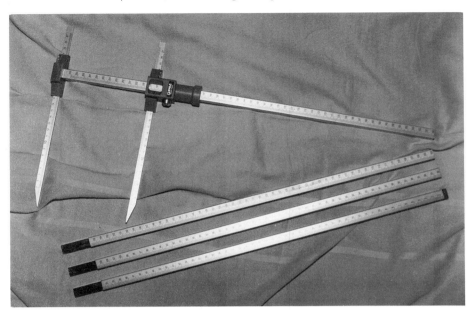

FIGURE 2.2   Platform scale

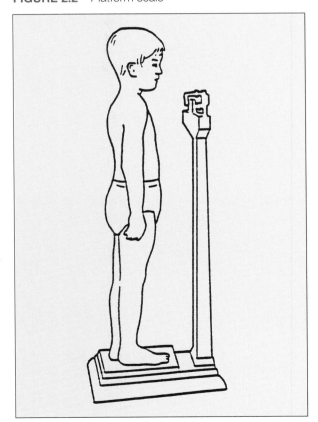

From *Anthropometric Standardization Reference Manual* (p 7) by T.G.
Lohman, A.F. Roche, and R. Martorell (eds), 1988, Champaign, IL: Human
Kinetics. Copyright 1988 by Timothy G. Lohman, Alex F. Roche, and
Reynaldo Martorell. Reprinted by permission.

should then stand with body weight distributed evenly between both feet on the center of the platform. The measurer stands between the measuring beam and the client so that the movable beam can be shifted with ease. Weight is measured to the nearest 0.5 lb or 0.2 kg (2.2 lb = 1 kg).[2] If weight needs to be converted to kilograms, divide weight in pounds by 2.2.

Body Circumferences

The measurement of body girth or circumference can be made around the following sites: head, neck, mid-upper arm, forearm, wrist, chest, abdomen, hips, buttocks, upper thigh, and calf. These measurements are made with a flexible, but inelastic, cloth or plastic tape. The zero end of the tape is held in the left hand of the measurer and the other end of the tape held in the measurer's right hand. For each circumference, the plane of the tape around the body is perpendicular to the long axis of the body. With the client standing erect for all of the circumference measurements, the tape should also be parallel to the floor. The tension applied to the tape as each circumference is being measured is snug around the body part but not tight enough to compress subcutaneous body fat (see *Figure 2.3*). The measurement is made to the nearest 0.125 in or 0.1 cm.[3] The sequence of measurements should be repeated three times, starting from upper-body measurements through lower-body measurements so that the chance of

FIGURE 2.3 Circumference measurements

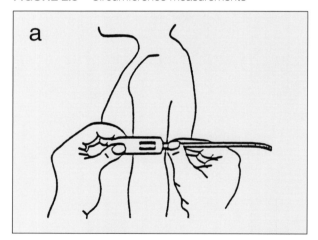

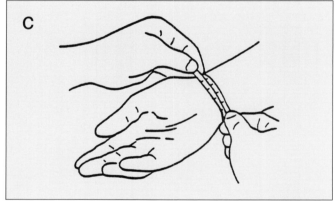

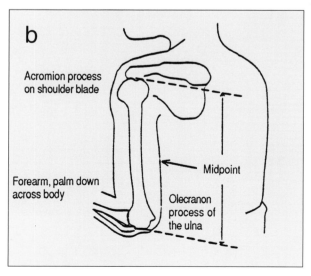

(a) Use of insertion tape to measure mid-upper-arm circumference. (b) Location of the midpoint of the upper arm. Figure 2.3a and b reprinted from *Nutrition Assessment: A Comprehensive Guide for Planning Interventions* by M.D. Simko, C. Cowell, and J.A. Gilbride with permission of Aspen Publishers, Inc. © 1984. (c) Positioning for the measurement of wrist circumference. Figure 2.3c from *Anthropometric Standardization Reference Manual* (p 53) by T.G. Lohman, A.F. Roche, and R. Martorell (eds), 1988 Champaign, IL: Human Kinetics. Copyright 1988 by Timothy G. Lohman, Alex F. Roche, and Reynaldo Martorell. Reprinted by permission.

intrameasurer bias is lessened. This method should be used with discretion in the obese population because of the increased compressibility factor of fat tissue with this body type.[4] See *Table 2.9* for specific criteria on measurement of body-circumference sites.

TABLE 2.9 Body Composition Measurements

Height	The distance from the bottom of the subject's heel to the top of the head. Recorded in inches and/or centimeters
Weight	Weight in pounds and/or kilograms
Skeletal Measurements, cm	
Elbow breadth	With the right arm bent at a 90-degree angle and perpendicular to the body, the greatest breadth across the elbow joint is measured along the axis of the upper arm*
Biacromial width	The distance between the most lateral projections of the acromial process
Bi-iliac width	The maximal diameter between the iliac crests
Bitrochanteric width	The maximal diameter between the greater trochanters
Bideltoid width	Maximal diameter between one side of the rib cage and the other
Wrist circumference	Wrist is measured where it bends distal to styloid process on the right arm
Knee circumference	With the knee flexed, the measuring tape measures across the middle of the patella and around the diameter of the leg from this point
Circumferences, cm	
Mid upper arm	With the right arm hanging loosely, the circumference of the midpoint of the posterior of the upper arm between the acromial process of the scapula and the olecranon process of the elbow
Forearm	Maximal circumference of the lower arm below the elbow joint with the elbow extended and hand supinated
Abdomen	At the level of the iliac crests, and anteriorly, the circumference at the umbilicus
Buttocks	Anteriorly at the symphysis pubis, and posteriorly, the circumference at the maximal protrusion of the gluteal muscles
Thigh	The circumference just below the gluteal fold or the maximal thigh girth
Calf	The maximal girth of the midgastrocnemius muscle
Skinfolds, mm†	
Chest	A diagonal fold taken midway between the anterior axillary line and the nipple line
Abdomen	A vertical fold taken a small distance laterally from the umbilicus
Thigh	A vertical fold on the anterior side of the thigh, midway between the hip and knee joints
Triceps	A vertical fold on the posterior midline of the upper arm, midway between the acromial and the olecranon processes
Suprailium	A diagonal fold above the crest of the ilium
Subscapular	A fold taken on the diagonal line on the vertebral border of the inferior angle of the scapula

From *Anthropomeric Standardization Reference Manual* by T.G. Lohman, A.F. Roche, R. Martorell (eds), 1988; Champaign, Ill: Human Kinetics. Copyright 1988 by Timothy G. Lohman, Alex F. Roche, and Reynaldo Martorell.

*This measurement is taken on the right side of the body.

†All measurements are taken on the right side of the body.

Katch and McArdle[5] have developed regression equations that use measurements of body circumferences on the upper, middle, and lower body (ie, midarm, chest, waist, iliac, thigh, and calf) and measurements of height and weight to estimate body fat (see *Table 2.10*). In addition, Tran and Weltman[6] have published equations for predicting body density in women from measurement of abdomen, hips, iliac, and thigh circumferences (see *Table 2.11*). Although the prediction of body fat from circumference measurements in the obese population is more difficult, Weltman and colleagues[7] have developed regression equations for predicting body composition from circumference measurements in obese adult men (see *Table 2.12*).

TABLE 2.10   Prediction of Body Density From Anthropometric Measurements in Men and Women

Equation for men	
Body density = 1.10986 – (0.00083 $\times$ tricep skinfold) – (0.00087 $\times$ subscapular skinfold) – (0.00098 $\times$ abdomen circumference) + (0.00210 $\times$ forearm circumference)	
Equation for women	
Body density = 1.09246 – (0.00049 $\times$ scapula skinfold) – (0.00075 $\times$ iliac skinfold) + (0.00710 $\times$ elbow diameter) – (0.00121 $\times$ thigh circumference)	
Circumferences	
Abdomen (cm)	Mean of abdomen 1 and abdomen 2
Abdomen 1	Laterally midway between the lowest lateral portion of the rib cage and iliac crest, and anteriorly midway between the oyphoid process of the sternum and the umbilicus
Abdomen 2	Laterally, at the level of the iliac crests, and anteriorly, at the umbilicus
Forearm	Maximal circumference of the lower arm below the elbow joint with elbow extended and hand supinated
Thigh	Circumference just below the gluteal fold or the maximal thigh girth
Skinfolds	
Triceps (mm)	A vertical fold on the posterior midline of the upper arm, midway between the acromial and the olecranon processes
Iliac (cm)	A diagonal fold above the crest of the ilium
Body fat	(4.570/body density – 4.142) x 100

From Katch FI, McArdle WD. Prediction of body density from simple anthropometric measurements in college-age men and women. *Hum Biol.* 1973;45:445-454.

TABLE 2.11   Generalized Regression Equation for Predicting Body Density in Adult Women Using Circumferences*

Body density = 1.168297 – (0.002824 $\times$ abdomen) + (0.0000122098 $\times$ abdomen^2) – (0.000733128 $\times$ hips) + (0.000510477 $\times$ height) – (0.000216161 $\times$ age).

$r = 0.889$; adjusted $r^2 = 0.787$; SEE = 4.2% body fat

Abdomen (cm)	Mean of abdomen 1 and abdomen 2
Abdomen 1 (cm)	Laterally, midway between lowest portion of the rib cage and iliac crest, and anteriorly, midway between the xiphoid process of the sternum and the umbilicus
Abdomen 2 (cm)	Laterally at the level of the iliac crest and anteriorly at the umbilicus
Hips (buttocks) (cm)	Anteriorly at the level of the symphysis pubis and posteriorly at the maximal protrusion of the gluteal muscles
Age	Age in y
Height	Height in cm

From Tran ZV, Weltman A. Generalized equation for predicting body density of women from girth measurements. *Med Sci Sports Exerc.* 1989;21:101-104.

*r indicates correlation coefficient; SEE, standard error of estimation.

TABLE 2.12   Prediction of Body Composition in Adult Obese Males Using Body Circumference Measurements*

Body density = (– 0.00040 × abdomen) – 1.063
  r = 0.50   SEE = 0.0067 g/cc
Percentage body fat = (0.31457 × abdomen) – (0.10969 × weight) + 10.8336
  r = 0.54   SEE = 2.88% fat
Fat weight (kg) = (0.22753 × weight) + (0.3134 × abdomen) – 22.608
  r = 0.90   SEE = 2.86 kg
Lean body weight (kg) = (0.77249 × weight) – (0.31353 × abdomen) + 22.620
  r = 0.94   SEE = 2.86 kg

Abdomen (cm)	Mean of abdomen 1 and abdomen 2
Abdomen 1 (cm)	Laterally, midway between the lowest lateral portion of the rib cage and iliac crest, and anteriorly, midway between the xyphoid process of the sternum and the umbilicus
Abdomen 2 (cm)	Laterally, at the level of the iliac crests, and anteriorly, at the umbilicus
Weight	Weight in kilograms (2.2 kg = 1 lb)

From Weltman A, Seip RL, Tran ZV. Practical assessment of body composition in adult obese males. *Hum Biol.* 1987;59:523-535.
   *r indicates correlation coefficient; SEE, standard error of estimation.

Recent interest has focused on the waist/hip ratio (WHR) as a risk factor predicting heart disease. Significant correlations have been found between WHR and diabetes mellitus, heart disease, hypertension, hyperlipidemia, and stroke.[8-10] WHR can be determined by measuring the circumference of the abdomen (waist) and the circumference of the hips, and calculating the ratio from these two measures. Bray[11] outlines the procedure:

> The abdominal or waist circumference is measured with a flexible tape placed in a horizontal plane at the level of the natural waist line or narrowest part of the torso as seen from the anterior view. The hip circumference is measured in the horizontal plane at the level of maximal circumference, including the maximum extension of the buttocks posteriorly.

A WHR >0.80 in women or >0.95 in men places them at greater risk for heart disease. Increased abdominal obesity is called android obesity.[11,12] A WHR lower than these values, but also associated with excessive body weight, is referred to as gynoid obesity (see *Figure 2.4*). See the new recommended height/weight charts by the USDA[13] in appendix 12.

FIGURE 2.4   Distribution of waist-to-hip circumference ratios.

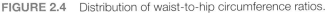
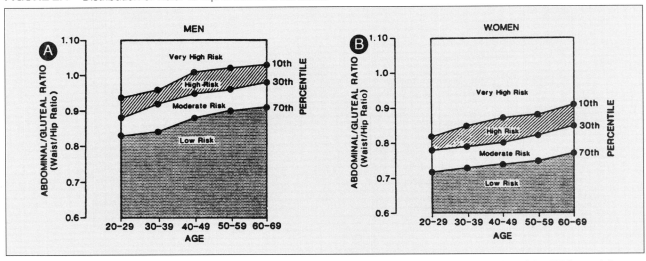

These data are adapted from the Canadian Fitness survey. The estimates of risk are those of the author. A men; B women. (copyright 1988 George A Bray, MD; reproduced with permission). From Bray GA, Gray DS. Obesity Part 1, pathogenesis. *West J Med. 1988; 149:429-441.*

A new application of abdominal girth measurements in determining changes in body fat is reported in research conducted with the military.[14] Group data from military measurements were used to derive target abdominal girths for desired body-fat percentages at specific heights (20% for males, 30% for females). These same target girths have been calculated for professional football players, longshoremen, shot-put and weight-lifting athletes, and obese men and women. Changes in abdominal girth have been shown to be proportional to changes in total body-fat loss.

Skinfolds

Skinfold thicknesses can be measured using devices such as the spring-loaded Harpenden or Lange skinfold calipers (see *Figure 2.5*). These measure the thickness of a double layer of skin and fat that is pulled away from the muscle at selected sites. Common sites for measurement of skinfold thicknesses are the chest, midaxilla, abdomen, ilium, triceps, subscapular, and midthigh (see *Figure 2.6*). These measurements are then used in body-fat prediction equations. Each site is palpated before measurement so that the measurer becomes familiar with the area. The thumb and index finger pull the double fold of skin and subcutaneous fat tissue forward to the site by 1 cm. This separation is necessary so that the fingers do not affect the measurement. As the skinfold is elevated, the thumb and the index finger are approximately 8 cm apart on a line perpendicular to the long axis of the skinfold, and the fold is held firmly between these two fingers. Only skin and adipose tissue are elevated. The caliper is held in the right hand as the skinfold is elevated in the left hand. Pressure is exerted to separate the caliper arms as the instrument is slipped over the skinfold, and the arms are located at equal distance on each side of the skinfold. The pressure of the caliper arms is released gradually, and the measurement should be made within 4 seconds to the nearest 0.5 mm.[15] The sequence of measurements is repeated three times, starting from upper-body

FIGURE 2.5 Lange skinfold caliper used for assessing thickness of subcutaneous fat.

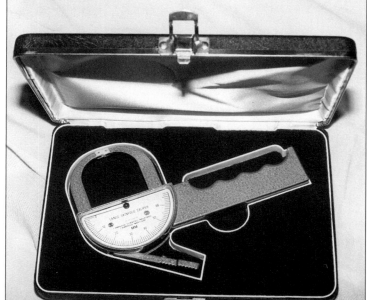

Caliper maintains constant jaw pressure of 10 g/m² regardless of jaw opening. Measuring range of 0-60 mm.

FIGURE 2.6   Commonly used anthropometric measurement sites.

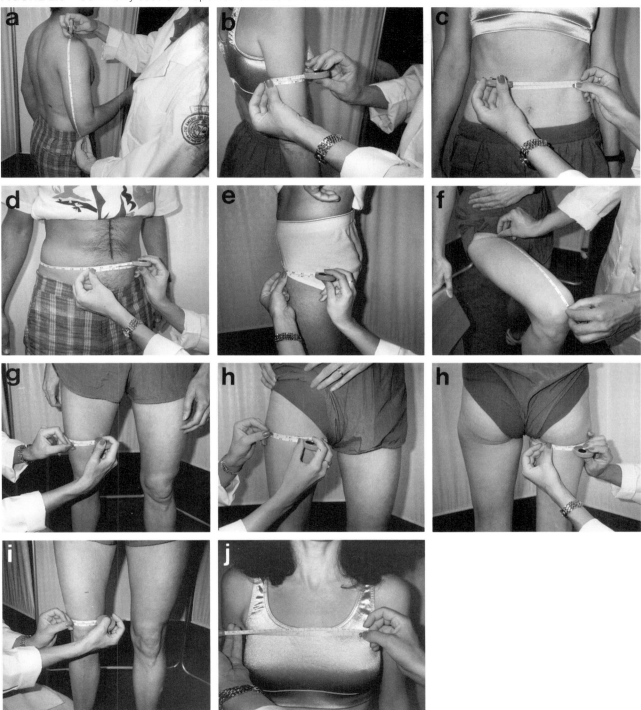

Circumference measurements taken with a flexible steel anthropometric tape. All circumference measurements of arms or legs taken on subject's right side. (a) *Upper-arm midpoint* used for taking triceps skinfold and mid-upper-arm circumference; made midway between the acromion and olecranon processes, with the arm held at a right angle from the elbow. (b) *Midarm circumference* taken at the marked midpoint between the acromion and olecranon processes. (c) *Waist circumference* taken at the smallest circumference of the torso. (d) *Abdomen circumference* taken at the maximal circumference of the abdomen. (e) *Hip (buttocks) circumference* taken over the maximal circumference of the buttocks. (f) *Midthigh midpoint* used for midthigh circumference and midthigh skinfold. (g) *Midthigh circumference* taken midway between the inguinal crease and the proximal border of the patella. (h) *Proximal thigh circumference* (front and rear view) taken horizontally, just distal to the gluteal fold. (i) *Distal thigh circumference* taken just proximal to the femoral epicondyles. (j) *Chest circumference* taken horizontally at the 4th costosternal joints (at the level of the 6th ribs), after normal expiration. (*Continued.*)

FIGURE 2.6 Commonly used anthropometric measurement sites (continued).

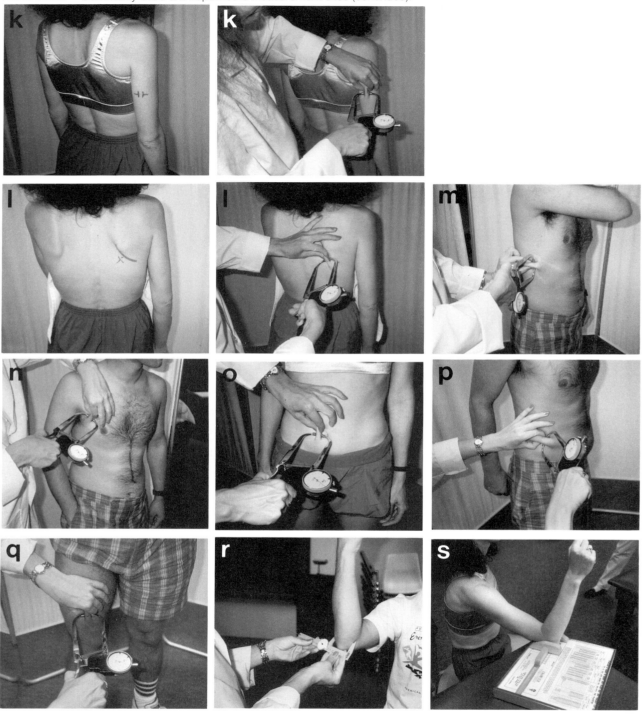

Skinfold measurements, taken with a skinfold caliper that exerts a standard amount of compression per unit size of jaw surface area. All skinfolds taken on the subject's right side. (k) *Triceps skinfold* taken on the midline posterior surface of the arm over the triceps muscle, at midpoint between the acromial and olecranon processes. (l) *Subscapular skinfold* taken just inferior to the lower angle of the scapular, following the natural plane of the scapula. (m) *Midaxillary skinfold* taken at the level of the sternum, on the midaxillary line. (n) *Chest (pectoral) skinfold* taken, for males, midway between the nipple and the arm fold and, for females, adjacent to the arm fold. (o) *Abdomen skinfold* taken immediately lateral of the umbilicus. (p) *Suprailiac skinfold* taken on the midaxillary line just superior to the iliac crest. (q) *Midthigh skinfold* taken midway between the inguinal crease and the proximal border of the patella.

Elbow breadth measurement for estimation of body frame size. (r) *Sliding caliper* measures distance between the epicondyles of the humerus. (s) *Frameter* simplifies measurement of distance between the epicondyles of the humerus.

measurements through lower-body measurements, so that the chance of intrameasurer bias is lessened (see Figure 2.6). Skinfolds may not be appropriately used to predict body fat levels for the elderly because suitable regression equations are not available for this population. In addition, skinfold calipers may be difficult to use with morbidly obese clients because the double fold of subcutaneous fat may exceed the jaw width of standard calipers.

Body Diameters and Widths

Despite morphological changes in bone, the external size of the skeleton remains fairly constant throughout adulthood.[16] Some of the earliest anthropometric studies incorporated body diameters (biacromial width, chest width, knee width, and elbow width) to predict skeletal weight and lean body weight.[17] A broad-blade anthropometer was used for measuring chest width, and all other diameters were made with a narrow blade anthropometer (see *Figure 2.7*). These calipers consist of a base measuring rod, one fixed blade, and a movable blade that slides up and down the caliper. The body-width sites are defined by bony landmarks and are palpable. The caliper is held so that the fingers of the measurer are holding the measuring blades, compressing the subcutaneous tissue around the body projections. The measurements are made within 0.1 cm.[18] The sequence of measurements is repeated three times, starting with upper-body measurements through lower-body measurements, so that the chance of intrameasurer bias can be lessened.

FIGURE 2.7   Calipers for measuring body diameters.

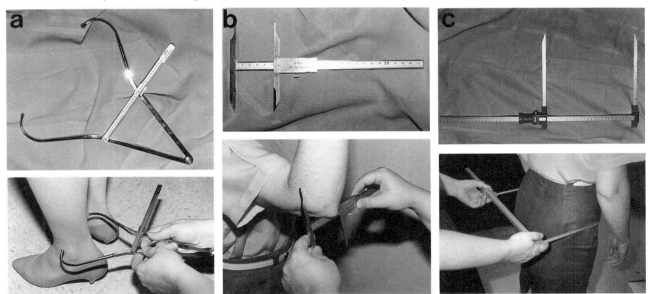

(a) Spreading caliper used for measuring chest breadth, chest depth, ankle breadth, and wrist breadth. Example–measurement of ankle breadth. (b) Small sliding caliper used for measuring elbow breadth. Example–measurement of elbow breadth. (c) Large sliding caliper used for measuring large skeletal breadths and knee height. Example–measurement of bitrochanteric breadth.

Elbow Breadth

The measurement of elbow breadth is simplified with the use of a flat, sliding-blade caliper attached to a baseboard. The client raises his or her right arm with the elbow fixed in a 90-degree angle (see *Figure 2.8*). The arm is then placed in the caliper, and the caliper blade slides until the lateral and medial epicondyle cannot be compressed any more. The measurement is made to the nearest 0.1 cm.[18] See appendix 13 for companies that provide anthropometric measuring equipment.

► ASSESSMENT OF BODY SIZE

Body-size determination requires estimations of both body frame size and body weight. Behnke's[17,19] work in the 1950s and 1960s established the first estimations of body size using skeletal measurements and developed a somatogram of the "reference" man. The measurement of body size–as opposed to body weight alone–incorporates the influence of body stature, age, body width, bone thickness, muscularity, and body proportions on body weight.[20]

Body Frame Size

Body frame size is primarily determined through measurement of skeletal dimensions or bony breadths and circumferences. Body frame size is not, however, a measure of relative leanness or fatness of the body. Two main methods of determining body frame measurements are well accepted in the literature. These are height/wrist circumference[21] and elbow breadth.[22] See appendix 14 for standards on measuring body frame size based on height/wrist circumference and elbow breadth.

Height/Wrist Circumference Ratio

The height/wrist circumference ratio is commonly used for determining frame size. Measurements can be easily made with a plastic measuring tape. The wrist is measured where it bends distal to the styloid process on the right arm.[3] The

FIGURE 2.8 Elbow breadth measurement using a Frameter.

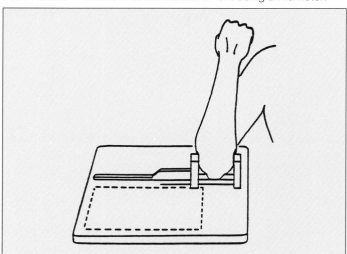

From *Anthropometric Standardization Reference Manual* (p 37) by T.G. Lohman, A.F. Roche, and R. Martorell (eds), 1988, Champaign, IL: Human Kinetics. Copyright 1988 by Timothy G. Lohman, Alex F. Roche, and Reynaldo Martorell. Reprinted by permission.

ratio of height to wrist circumference has been categorized into three frame-size categories: small, medium, and large (appendix 14).

Elbow Breadth

This method has become the standard "marker" for determining frame size.[21] Frisancho and Flegel[22] used elbow breadth to develop weight tables based on National Health and Nutrition Examination Survey (NHANES) I (1971-1974) and NHANES II (1976-1980) data[23] (see appendix 14).

Elbow breadth can be measured by a Frameter, a device designed by Frisancho, or by a sliding anthropometric caliper (see Figure 2.8). This measurement is taken with the right arm bent at a 90-degree angle and perpendicular to the body. The greatest breadth across the elbow joint is measured with the caliper along the axis of the upper arm.[21,24] Elbow breadth has become the most accepted method of determining frame size because it represents stable body dimensions and is easy to measure. It is less affected by body fat than any other dimension, having a low correlation coefficient ($r = 0.42$) with percentage body fat.[24] Values measured for elbow breadth form a normal distribution, and resulting frame-size categories have been statistically derived from this distribution.

Determination of Healthy Body Weight

Weight is influenced by sex, age, height, body width, bone thickness, lean/fat ratio, and length of trunk relative to height.[25] The most commonly used standards for ideal body weight (adjusted for sex, height, and body frame size) are the 1959 and 1983 Metropolitan Life Insurance Company weight tables[26,27] (see appendix 15). These were established in 1959 and updated in 1983. The weights in these tables were those of healthy policyholders and are, therefore, weights associated with low mortality rates. The tables should not be used to represent the US population as a whole because of the selective criteria used in their development. It is also important to consider that the weights listed do not discriminate between fat weight and lean weight, nor do the original charts offer guidelines for discriminating between small, medium, and large body-frame-size categories.

Another way of determining healthy or good body weight is to use weights that are associated with the most favorable mortality experience. The Diet and Health Report (1989) produced by the National Research Council provides a critique of this approach. The council developed "good" body weight tables for Americans (see appendix 12), which were subsequently published in the *Dietary Guidelines for Americans*.[28]

Body Mass Index (Quetelet's Index) (kg/m²)

Weight differences at a given height are assumed to be attributable to frame-size differences assessed from different anthropometric measurements.[29] Body mass index (BMI), however, is more representative of body-fat weight than other frame-size techniques. BMI has a correlation coefficient of $r = 0.57$ to body-fat percentage when calculated by regression equations based on skinfold thickness measurements.[30] When male pelvic and hip diameters are included with BMI, the correlation to body-fat percentage increases ($r = 0.63$).[31] Therefore, increasing fatness may be a factor of accelerating skeletal growth. Radiographs (x-ray films) can show to what extent certain body diameters are related to body fatness. *Table 2.13* compares BMI with different levels of obesity.[32]

TABLE 2.13 Comparison of Body Mass Index (BMI) Calculations Using Standard and Conversion Formulas for Different Levels of Obesity

Level of Obesity	(Metric) Standard Formula			(US units) Conversion Formula			Differences,[c] %
	kg	in	BMI[a]	lb	in	BMI[b]	
Very obese	100	1.651	36.686	220	65	36.710	+0.065
Obese	75	1.651	27.515	165	65	27.532	+0.062
Nonobese	60	1.651	22.012	132	65	22.026	+0.064
Nonobese	50	1.651	18.343	110	65	18.355	+0.065

From Stensland SH, Margolis S. Simplifying the calculation of body mass index for quick reference. Copyright The American Dietetic Association. Reprinted by permission from *J Am Diet Assoc.* 1990;90:856.

[a] Standard formula: kg/m^2

[b] Conversion formula: $(lb/in^2) \times 705$

[c] $([BMI^b - BMI^a]/BMI^a) \times 100$

A number of studies have shown higher mortality rates for persons at either end of the weight spectrum. However, because of uncontrolled risk factors, the increased risk of mortality for those at the lower-weight end of the spectrum is debatable. A recent study shed light on this issue by comparing the highest and lowest BMIs with mortality rates.[33] It was found that those at the lowest BMI (<20 kg/m^2) were not at risk for higher mortality. This study demonstrates the usefulness of using BMI as a means of viewing body weight. See *Table 2.14* for minimum BMI values in obesity. BMI is calculated as follows:

$$BMI = \frac{\text{pounds weight} \times 0.4536}{(\text{inches height} \times 0.0254)^2}$$

or

$$BMI = \frac{\text{kilogram weight}}{\text{meters height}^2}$$

A nomogram can be used to locate BMI and obesity ranges without performing manual calculations (see *Figure 2.9*). The generally accepted "good" BMI is 19 to 25 kg/m^2 for men and women aged 19 to 34 years, and 21 to 27 kg/m^2 for those older than 35 years of age. Overweight is represented by a BMI of 25 kg/m^2 (for those aged 19 to 34 years) and 27 to 30 kg/m^2 (for those 35 years of age and older) and is associated with low risk. A BMI >30 kg/m^2 is almost always associated with increased body fat, except in bodybuilders and other highly muscular athletes.[11] For example, a bodybuilder who is 200 lb (90.9 kg), 68 in tall (171.5 cm), and 6% body fat would have a BMI of 30.9 kg/m^2.

TABLE 2.14 General Population Guidelines and Gender-Specific Desirable Ranges for Body Mass Index (kg/m^2)

General Guidelines
Underweight: ≤20
Normal: 20.1–25.0
Overweight: 25.1–30.0
Obese: >30

Desirable Ranges
Males: 21.9-22.4
Females: 21.3-22.1

Adapted from: Millar WJ, Stephens T. The prevalence of overweight and obesity in Britain, Canada, and the United States. *Am J Public Health.* 1987;77:38-41. National Research Council. *Diet and Health: Implications for Reducing Chronic Disease Risk.* Washington DC: National Academy Press; 1989

FIGURE 2.9   Nomogram for predicting body mass index (BMI).

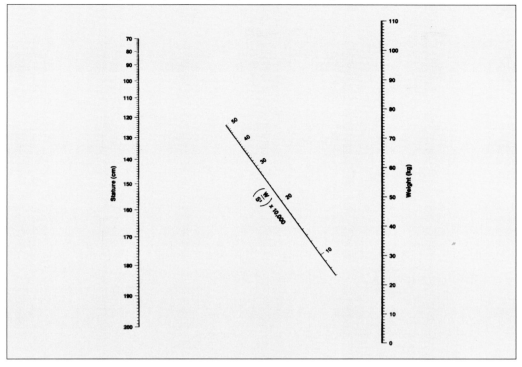

Directions
1. Locate the person's stature on the left column. Numbers in this column *increase* going down the scale.
2. Locate the person's weight on the right column. Numbers in this column *decrease* going down the scale.
3. Lay a ruler or straightedge so that it touches these two points–stature and weight.
4. Note where the straightedge crosses the slanted line between these two columns. This is the person's W/S² value.
5. Enter the W/S² value in the person's record.

Used with permission of Ross Laboratories, Columbus, OH 43216, from *Nutritional Assessment of the Elderly Through Anthropometry.* © 1984 Ross Laboratories. (Adapted from *Am J Clin Nutr.* 1981;34:2831.)

Figure 2.10 gives the proposed classifications by Bray[11] of obesity and the increased risk of disease based on the BMI.

▶ ASSESSMENT OF BODY COMPOSITION

The assumption used by most body-composition assessment methods is that the body is made of two compartments: *fat* and *fat-free* weight. The fat-free portion of the body is assumed to be relatively constant and have a density of 1.1 g/cc at 37°C, a water content of 72% to 74%, and a potassium content of 60 to 70 mmol/kg in men and 50 to 60 mmol/kg in women.[34] Fat weight, or stored triglyceride, is also assumed to be constant with a density of 0.900 g/cc at 37°C and void of both water and potassium. All body-composition methods use either this two-compartment model or further divide the fat and fat-free weight into four compartments: water, protein, ash or bone mineral, and fat.

The traditional and more established methods for body composition are total body water, total body potassium, densitometry (underwater weighing), urinary creatinine excretion, and anthropometry (bone measurements, skinfold, arm circumference; see appendix 16). Newer body-composition methods frequently use a multicompartment model (eg, measuring bone, fat, water, and protein content of the body). Some of these newer methods include urinary 3-methylhistidine excretion (3-MH), bioelectrical impedance (BIA), near infrared interactance (NIR), total body electrical conductivity (TOBEC), dual-photon

FIGURE 2.10 Proposed Classification of Obesity and
Increased Risk of Disease Based on BMI

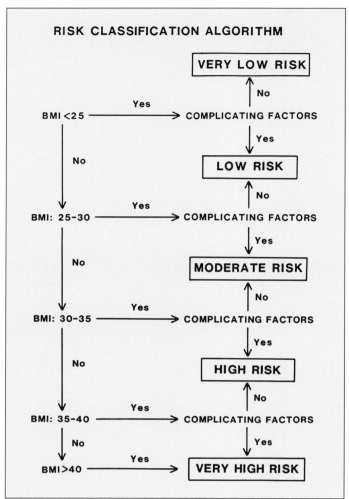

After measuring the BMI, the individual risk is increased or decreased based on the
presence of complicating factors. These would be age under 40, a high WHR (>0.95 for
men; > 0.80 for women), and male. From Bray GA. Pathophysiology of obesity. *Am J
Clin Nutr.* 1992;55:488S-494S. Copyright 1988 George A. Bray, MD; reproduced with
permission.

absorptiometry (DPA), and dual energy x-ray absorptiometry (DEXA). As
newer methods are developed they are usually validated against one or more of
the three more established methods (total body water, total body potassium,
underwater weighing), in spite of the fact that these methods have known
inaccuracies. For instance, underwater weighing equations for predicting body
density are based on the analysis of three young, white, male cadavers. It is clear
that these tissue densities may not be representative of all populations. The
DEXA methodology holds promise in providing a means of direct assessment of
tissue densities in a low-radiation environment, so this system may eventually
be considered the standard with which other newer methods are compared.

This section briefly outlines the traditional methods of body composition,
giving the degree of precision and the limitations of use associated with each. In
addition, the newer methods will be reviewed, with an emphasis placed on
those methods that are most practical for field measurements. Again, degree of
precision associated with each will be given along with limitations of use. For a
more complete review of body-composition measurement methods and the

assumptions associated with each, see the reviews by Brodie,[35] Lukaski,[34] or Lohman.[36] In addition, a book by Lohman[37] reviews new developments in body composition.

Densitometry: Underwater Weighing

In underwater (or hydrostatic) weighing, body volume and density are estimated by the difference between the client's weight on land and in water. Body-density estimations are based on the assumption that lean tissue and fat tissue measurements, derived from a small number of human cadaver dissections, are constant.[38] However, Martin and colleagues demonstrated, through work on human cadavers, that densities of both lean and fat tissues vary.[39] In addition, lower bone-mineral content and total body water in younger and older populations can lead to overestimations of body fat because the density of the lean component is underestimated.[40] Due to the errors associated with variations of water and bone-mineral content, the error associated with this method is 2.5%.[41] The error is greatest in populations with lower bone density (children, women, elderly) or heavier bone density (athletes). Clinical and field use of this method is limited because equipment mobility is difficult and for some populations total or partial submersion in water is impractical. In addition, this technique does not differentiate fat deposition sites.

Anthropometry: Skinfold Thickness Measurements

Measurement of skinfolds is one of the most commonly used anthropometry techniques. This method is based on two assumptions: the thickness of the subcutaneous adipose tissue reflects a constant proportion of the total body fat, and the sites selected for measurement represent the average thickness of the subcutaneous adipose tissue.[34] The potential error associated with the use of skinfolds, assuming the correct equation is used, the technician is well trained, and appropriate skinfold sites chosen, is 3% to 4%.[41] This means that if an individual is actually 20% body fat, predicting body fat with skinfolds and a regression equation could produce a figure as low as 16% or as high as 24% fat.

Many regression equations have been developed to predict body density and body-fat percentage from skinfold measurements.[42] For example, Jackson and Pollock[43] and Jackson and colleagues[44] published equations for predicting body density in men and women (see *Table 2.15*). These equations, using three

TABLE 2.15 Generalized equations for Predicting Body Density Based on Age and Sum of Three Skinfolds

Male	BD =	$1.1093800 - 0.0008267 (X_1) + 0.0000016 (X_1)^2 - 0.0002574 (X_3)$
	r =	0.905
	SEE =	0.0077
Female	BD =	$1.0994921 - 0.0009929 (X_2) + 0.0000023 (X_2)^2 - 0.0001392 (X_3)$
	r =	0.842
	SEE =	0.0086

Percentage body fat = [(4.95/BD) - 4.50] × 100

Where	BD =	Body density
	X_1 =	Sum of chest, abdomen, and thigh skinfolds, mm
	X_2 =	Sum of triceps, thigh, and suprailium skinfolds, mm
	X_3 =	Age (y)

Data from Jackson AS, Pollock ML. Generalized equations for predicting body density of men. *Br J Nutr.* 1978;40:497-504. Jackson AS, Pollock ML, Ward A. Generalized equations for predicting body density of women. *Med Sci Sports Exerc.* 1980;12:175-182.

to five skinfold measurements, have been more recently revised by Jackson and Pollock[45] and are best suited for use with adults aged 20 to 50 years (see appendix 17). However, these equations overestimate fatness in elderly individuals. More accurate formulas have not yet been developed for the elderly.[41] Other formulas developed for the YMCA[46] that estimate body fat using measurements at four and six sites have norms based on more athletic populations. In addition, Sinning and colleagues[40,47] have developed equations for young adult athletes. The most appropriate equation to use is one based on populations similar in age, sex, and activity level to the group being studied. (See *Tables 2.16* and *2.17* for anthropometric estimation of body fat for women and men.)

Total Body Water (TBW)

Since fat is mainly anhydrous (containing no water), and water is a relatively constant component in fat-free mass (72% to 74%), determining the amount of water contained in a client's body provides an estimate of fat-free mass. The technique for obtaining this information is to give a dose of water that contains a tracer element. The ideal tracer should not be metabolizable (ie, it should remain in the same form) or toxic, and it should evenly distribute itself throughout the entire body water in 3 to 4 hours. Traditionally, this tracer has been tritium or deuterium; occasionally, it has been oxygen 18 (^{18}O), an isotope of oxygen. Once the tracer is given and 3 to 4 hours have passed, a sample of body water is taken (saliva, urine, or blood) and analyzed for the concentration of this tracer. A high concentration is an indication of low body water (and thus a low level of lean mass), while a low concentration is an indication of a high body water (and a high level of lean mass).[34,48] Some general assumptions of this technique are that the tracer has the same distribution volume as water, is exchanged by the body in a manner similar to water, and is nontoxic in the

TABLE 2.16 Anthropometric Estimation of Body Fat for Women

For women, the sum of five *or* three skinfolds

Sum of Five	Sum of Three
1. Thigh	1. Triceps
2. Ilium	2. Abdomen
3. Abdomen	3. Ilium
4. Tricep	
5. Scapula	

Equations for women:

Sum of five: Percentage fat = $0.29731 (X_1) - 0.00053 (X_1)^2 + 0.03037 (X_2) - 0.63054$
Where X_1 = Sum of 5 skinfolds (mm)
X_2 = Age (y)
$r = 0.848$ SE = 3.76% fat

Sum of three: Percentage fat = $0.41563 (X_1) - 0.00112 (X_1)^2 + 0.03661 (X_2) + 4.03653$
Where X_1 = Sum of 3 skinfolds (mm)
X_2 = Age (y)
$r = 0.825$ SE = 3.98% fat

Data from Jackson AS, Pollock ML. Practical assessment of body composition. *Phys Sports Med.* 1985;13(5):76-90. Golding L, Myers C, Sinning W. *The Y's Way to Physical Fitness.* 3rd ed. Champaign, Ill: Human Kinetics Publishers Inc; 1989.

TABLE 2.17 Anthropometric Estimation of Body Fat for Men

For men, the sum of six *or* four skinfolds

Sum of Six	Sum of Four
1. Chest	1. Chest
2. Thigh	2. Ilium
3. Ilium	3. Abdomen
4. Abdomen	4. Axilla
5. Tricep	
6. Scapula	

Equations for men:

Sum of six: Percentage fat = $0.21661 (X_1) - 0.00029 (X_1)^2 + 0.13341 (X_2) - 5.72888$
Where (X_1) = Sum of 6 skinfolds (mm)
(X_2) = Age (y)
$r = 0.904$ SE = 3.42% fat

Sum of four: Percentage fat = $0.27784 (X_1) - 0.00053 (X_1)^2 + 0.12437 (X_2) - 3.28791$
Where (X_1) = Sum of 4 skinfolds (mm)
(X_2) = Age (y)
$r = 0.892$ SE = 3.63% fat

Data from Golding L, Myers C, Sinning W. *The Y's Way to Physical Fitness.* Rosemont, Ill: National Board of the YMCA; 1982.

amounts used.[34] The precision associated with measuring body fat by the TBW method is relatively high, producing an error of about 3% to 4%.[34]

Total Body Potassium

Potassium 40 is a naturally occurring isotope of potassium, and it exists in the body at a known concentration of 0.012% of total body potassium. Since most (>90%) potassium is in the fat-free mass, measuring potassium 40 is a means of predicting fat-free mass. This technique requires a specially constructed room or chamber designed to reduce background radiation, and scintillation counters to measure the high-energy gamma radiation emitted by potassium 40. Although the potassium 40 method is an accurate way to predict body fat (precision is approximately equal to 3% in humans) and is useful for validating other body-composition techniques, the cost and space associated with the equipment can be prohibitive for use in standard practice.[34]

Urinary Creatinine Excretion

Creatine is produced by the liver and kidney and taken up by many body tissues. Most (98%) creatine, however, is located in skeletal muscle in the form of creatine phosphate. Creatinine is released from the muscle via the nonenzymatic hydrolysis of free creatine liberated during the dephosphory-lation of creatine phosphate.[34] Therefore, urinary creatinine excretion is related to fatfree mass and muscle mass.

The major limitation of this method is the large intraindividual variability of daily urinary creatinine excretion, which can range from 11% to 20% for individuals on a free-living diet.[34] In addition, other factors (such as diet, exercise, and the accuracy of urine collections) can affect this method. The precision of this technique is low compared with other traditional methods of body-composition assessment described earlier, and it is best used in a research setting where confounding factors can be controlled.

Bioelectrical Impedance Analysis (BIA)

Bioelectrical impedance analysis, one of the newer methods of body-composition assessment, is based on the principle that impedance to an electrical flow of an applied current is related to the volume of the conductor (the human body) and the square of the conductor's length (height). BIA results are based on the greater electrolyte content of fat-free mass and its greater conductivity of electricity compared with that of adipose tissue and bone.[49,50] The client lies on a table or flat surface with extremities not touching the body trunk. Electrodes are placed on the phalangeal-metacarpal joint of the dorsal right hand (wrist) and below the metatarsal arch on the superior side of the right foot (ankle). A low-dose 50-KHz current is passed through the client for approximately 15 seconds. The electrical conductance of the body is detected as the lean component of the body, muscle tissue, carries this current. Selected equations are then used to estimate fatfree and fat mass.

BIA has considerable potential as a field method for measuring body composition because it is noninvasive, convenient, quick and easy, and applicable to individuals of almost all ages.[51,52] Many systems are available for purchase in the market and are currently being used in a number of clinical settings worldwide. Prediction equations derived from impedance analysis have standard errors of estimate of 3% to 5%.[34,50,53,54] The reliability of the prediction equations is improved when population-specific (ie, age-specific and fatness-specific) equations are used.[55-60] Houtkooper and colleagues[61,62] have validated the BIA technique for children and adolescents, and they have developed equations for predicting fat-free body mass.

One factor that will significantly affect results, and that is of particular concern with athletes, is the hydration state of the individual. Lower resistances are expected with relative overhydration and higher resistances with relative underhydration.[55] Several hours should be allowed before BIA measurements are made on clients who have had significant physical activity or fluid intake.[50] Most studies show that BIA is accurate in estimating total body water, but accuracy may be lost as body-composition results are extrapolated. BIA tends to overestimate body fat in the lean and underestimate body fat in the obese. Thus, very lean and obese clients are susceptible to inaccurate measurements.[63] However, Kushner and colleagues have validated the BIA technique using TBW for measurement of changes in body composition in obese females losing 5% to 20% of total body weight.[64]

Near Infrared Interactance (NIR)

Infrared interactance was developed from agriculture research conducted at the USDA. This method is based on the principles of light absorption and reflection. When light strikes a material, the energy is reflected, absorbed, or transmitted, depending on the scattering and absorption properties of the sample.[34] The currently available NIR equipment is the Futrex-5000 (Futrex Inc, Gaithersburg, Md). The equipment is portable, quick, noninvasive, and estimates body composition by application at a single site. A fiberoptic probe is positioned at midbiceps (upper arm) and an electromagnetic radiation wave (light beam) is emitted. Reflected energy or light absorption is monitored as the light beam penetrates subcutaneous fat and muscle and is reflected off the bone and conducted to the optical detector in the probe. This electromagnetic signal penetrates a 1-cm depth into upper-arm tissue, and interactance is calculated based on the energy transmission received by the optical probe. This method is still in the developmental stages, and limited research is available validating this method with various populations. Current estimated error ranges are from 2% to 15%.[34,50,63,65] Subject sample size for the original research and development was small, but a strong correlation has been observed between NIR and underwater weighting ($r = 0.79$).[66]

Two recent studies examined the validity of NIR as compared with underwater weighing (McLean and Skinner,[67] and Houmard and colleagues[65]). McLean and Skinner[67] found skinfold measures better predictors of body fat than the Futrex-5000, using underwater weighing as the criterion for body fat measurement. In addition, the Futrex-5000 overestimated body fat in lean subjects with <8% body fat and underestimated body fat in subjects with >30% body fat. Houmard and colleagues[65] used the Futrex-5000 to determine body fat in collegiate football players and found that NIR underestimated body fat by approximately 5% as compared with underwater weighing and three- and seven-site skinfold measures. Thus, more studies are needed to validate this tool for use with both the general population and athletes.

Total Body Electrical Conductivity (TOBEC)

This technique is based on the principle that the electrical conductivity of lean tissue is greater than that of fat tissue because of the higher electrolyte content of lean tissue.[68] To estimate body composition using the TOBEC principle, the client lies on a flat surface and is transported inside a small chamber that emits electrical impulses and measures responses to these impulses.[68] The TOBEC instrument is a large container with a solenoidal coil driven by a 5-MHz oscillating radio frequency current. The difference between impedance when the client is inside the coil versus when the coil is empty is an index of the TOBEC of the body. Several readings are taken, each approximately 15 seconds long, and the entire assessment takes only a few minutes. The TOBEC value is proportional to the fat-free mass of the client, and the total body fat is estimated to be the difference between fatfree mass and total body weight.

It has been found that TOBEC estimates of fat-free weight have high correlations with muscle mass estimated from urinary 3-MH and creatinine excretion ($r = 0.86$). TOBEC has also been found to be statistically identical to underwater weighting ($r = 0.97$) and whole-body potassium 40 counting ($r = 0.98$) in estimating body composition.[34] The prediction error for TOBEC as compared with underwater weighing is approximately 4%. Thus, TOBEC is an accurate noninvasive technique for estimating body composition.[69,70] However, because TOBEC is expensive and the equipment is not portable, the application of this technique in field settings is limited.

Other Body-Composition Assessment Methods

Besides the body-composition assessment methods already discussed in this section, a variety of other techniques are available. Some of these include: ultrasound, 3-methylhistidine excretion, neutron activation analysis, computed tomography (CT), magnetic resonance imaging (MRI), dual-photon absorptiometry (DPA), and dual-energy x-ray absorptiometry (DEXA). Because these techniques are not easily adapted to the clinical or consultation setting, and because they are expensive or are still being perfected or both, they are not covered in detail here. For more information on these methods, see reviews by Brodie,[35] Lukaski,[34] Lohman,[71] and Heymsfield and colleagues.[72]

Body-Composition Assessment of Athletes

Several body-composition assessment studies have pointed out differences in normal populations when compared with athletes. Using Behnke's studies of the military, Willowby[73] found that the athletes he assessed had larger girth measurements, especially in the upper-body extremities, representing muscular hypertrophy. A similar study using anthropometric data collected on 39 male bodybuilders and weight lifters, following Behnke's protocol,[74] reported no differences in frame size, percentage body fat, lean body weight, and diameter measurements between the two athletic groups. Increased levels of lean body weight and muscular build enlargement were also observed in that study. The average lean body weights were 20 lb above those of the normal reference man, indicating that this population has 30% greater average body weight for height than the population in the standard height/weight tables. Sinning and colleagues[40,47] have validated skinfold measurement equations for athletic men and women. See appendix 18 for a list of studies in which anthropometric measurements have been measured in a variety of athletes.

Limitations of Methods for Determining Body Composition

The existing methods for predicting composition all have relative strengths and weaknesses. These may be different for each user, because a method's strengths

TABLE 2.18 Limitations of Methods for Determining Human Body Composition*

| | | | Precision | |
| | | | Fat-free | |
Method	Cost	Technical Difficulty	Mass	% Fat
Water				
Deuterium	2	3	3	3
Oxygen-18	5	5	4	4
Tritium	3	3	3	3
Potassium	4	4	4	3
Creatinine	2	3	2	1
Densitometry				
Immersion	3	4	5	5
Plethysmography	4	3	5	5
Skinfold thickness	1	2	2	2
Arm circumference	1	3	2	2
Neutron activation	5	5	5	5
Photon absorptiometry	4	4	4	4
3-Methylhistidine	2	3	3	?†
Electrical				
Conductivity	5	1	4	4
Impedance	2	1	4	4
Computed tomography	5	5	?	?
Ultrasound	3	3	3	3
Infrared interactance	4	3	3	3
Magnetic resonance	5	5	?	?

From Lukaski HC. Methods for the assessment of human body composition: traditional and new. © *Am J Clin Nutr.* 1987;46:537-56. American Society for Clinical Nutrition.

*Ranking system: ascending scale, 1 = least and 5 = greatest.

†Unknown at this time.

and weaknesses relate to a variety of factors, including ease of use, intended use, cost, equipment availability, portability, size, ease of calibration, trained operators, and precision. Other factors relate to whether the technique will be used to obtain an absolute value in a population once, or to monitor change in body composition over time. Consider these factors prior to deciding on the best technique for you. See *Table 2.18* for a list of the limitations and precision levels of the current methods used in determining human body composition, as compiled by Lukaski.[34]

REFERENCES

1. Lohman TG, Roche AF, Martorell R, eds. *Anthropometric Standardization Reference Manual.* Champaign, Ill: Human Kinetics Books; 1988.
2. Gordon CC, Chumlea WC, Roche AF. Stature, recumbent length, and weight. In: Lohman TG, Roche AF, Martorell R, eds. *Anthropometric Standardization Reference Manual.* Champaign, Ill: Human Kinetics Books; 1988.
3. Callaway CW, Chumlea WC, Bouchard C, et al. Circumferences. In: Lohman TG, Roche AF, Martorell R, eds. *Anthropometric Standardization Reference Manual.* Champaign, Ill: Human Kinetics Books; 1988.
4. Becque MD, Katch VL, Moffatt RJ. Time course of skin-plus-fat compression in males and females. *Hum Biol.* 1986;58:33-42.
5. Katch FI, McArdle WD. Prediction of body density from simple anthropometric measurements in college-age men and women. *Hum Biol.* 1973;45:445-454.
6. Tran ZV, Weltman A. Generalized equation for predicting body density of women from girth measurements. *Med Sci Sports Exerc.* 1989;21:101-104.
7. Weltman A, Seip RL, Tran ZV. Practical assessment of body composition in adult obese males. *Hum Biol.* 1987;59:523-535.

8. Bouchard C, Bray GA, Hubbard VS. Basic and clinical aspects of regional fat distribution. *Am J Clin Nutr.* 1990;52:946-50.

9. Seidell JC, Cigolini M, Charzewska J, Contaldo F, Ellsinger B-M, Bjorntorp P. Measurement of regional distribution of adipose tissue. Presented at the First European Congress on Obesity; June 5-6, 1988; Stockholm, Sweden.

10. Sjöström L. Morbidity of severely obese subjects. *Am J Clin Nutr.* 1992;55:508S-515S.

11. Bray GA. Pathophysiology of obesity. *Am J Clin Nutr.* 1992;55:488S-494S.

12. Kris-Etherton P, ed. *Cardiovascular Disease: Nutrition for Prevention and Treatment.* Chicago, Ill: The American Dietetic Association; 1990.

13. US Dept of Health and Human Services, National Center for Health Statistics. *Anthropometric Reference Data and Prevalence of Overweight: United States, 1976-1980, Data from the National Health Survey.* Washington, DC: US Govt Printing Office; 1987;series 11 (238).

14. Katch FI, Katch VL, Behnke AR. New approach for estimating excess body fat from changes in abdominal girth. *Am J Hum Biol.* 1990;2:125-131.

15. Harrison GG, Buskirk ER, Lindsay Carter JE, et al. Skinfold thicknesses and measurement technique. In: Lohman TG, Roche AF, Martorell R, eds. *Anthropometric Standardization Reference Manual.* Champaign, Ill: Human Kinetics Books; 1988.

16. Åstrand P, Rodahl K. *Textbook of Work Physiology.* 3rd ed. New York, NY: McGraw Hill; 1986.

17. Behnke AR. The estimation of lean body weight from "skeletal" measurements. *Hum Biol.* 1959;32:295-315.

18. Wilmore JH, Frisancho RA, Gordon CC, et al. Body breadth equipment and measurement techniques. In: Lohman TG, Roche AF, Martorell R, eds. *Anthropometric Standardization Reference Manual.* Champaign, Ill: Human Kinetics Books; 1988.

19. Behnke AR. Anthropometric estimate of body size, shape, and fat content. *Postgrad Med.* 1963;34:190-198.

20. Himes JH, Frisancho RA. Estimating frame size. In: Lohman TG, Roche AF, Martorell R, eds. *Anthropometric Standardization Reference Manual.* Champaign, Ill: Human Kinetics Books; 1988.

21. Frisancho AR. *Standards of Weight, Fat, and Muscle by Frame Size for the Assessment of Nutritional Status of Adults and the Elderly Developed for Use With the Frameter.* Ann Arbor, Mich: Health Products; 1985.

22. Frisancho AR, Flegel PN. Elbow breadth as a measure of frame size for US males and females. *Am J Clin Nutr.* 1983;37:311-314.

23. Frisancho AR. New standards of weight and body composition by frame size and height for assessment of nutritional status of adults and the elderly. *Am J Clin Nutr.* 1984;40:808-819.

24. Frisancho AR. Nutritional anthropometry. *J Am Diet Assoc.* 1988;88:553-555.

25. Forbes G. *Human Body Composition.* New York, NY: Springer-Verlag; 1987.

26. Metropolitan Life Insurance Company. New weight standards for men and women. *Stat Bull Metrop Insur Co.* 1959;40:1-4.

27. Metropolitan Life Insurance Company. 1983 Metropolitan height and weight tables. *Stat Bull Metrop Insur Co.* 1983;64:2-9.

28. *Nutrition and Your Health: Dietary Guidelines for Americans.* 3rd ed. Washington, DC: US Dept of Agriculture, US Dept of Health and Human Services; 1990. Home and Garden bulletin 232.

29. Hertzberg HTE. The conference on standardization of anthropometric techniques and terminology. *Am J Phys Anthropol.* 1967;28:1-16.

30. Durnin JVGA, Wormersley J. Body fat assessed from total body density and its estimation from skinfold thickness: measurements on 481 men and women aged 16 to 72 years. *Br J Nutr.* 1974;32:77-97.

31. Rookus MA, Burema J, Deurenberg P, Van Der Wiel-Wetzels WAM. The impact of adjustment of a weight-height index (W/H^2) for frame size on the prediction of body fatness. *Br J Nutr.* 1985;54:335-342.

32. Stensland SH, Margolis S. Simplifying the calculation of body mass index for quick reference. *J Am Diet Assoc.* 1990;90:856.

33. Lindsted K, Tonstad S, Kuzma JW. Body mass index and patterns of mortality among Seventh-Day Adventist men. *Int J Obes.* 1991;15:397-406.
34. Lukaski HC. Methods for the assessment of human body composition: traditional and new. *Am J Clin Nutr.* 1987;46:537-56.
35. Brodie DA. Techniques of measurement of body composition. *Sports Med.* 1988;5:11-40,74-98.
36. Lohman TG. Skinfolds and body density and their relation to body fatness: a review. *Hum Biol.* 1981:53;181-225.
37. Lohman TG. *New Developments in Body Composition.* Champaign, Ill: Human Kinetics Publishers Inc; 1992.
38. Wilmore JH, Behnke AR. An anthropometric estimation of body density and lean body weight in young women. *Am J Clin Nutr.* 1970;23:267-274.
39. Martin A, Clarys J, Drinkwater D. Gross tissue weights in the human body by cadaver dissection. *Hum Biol.* 1984;56:459-473.
40. Sinning WE, Wilson JR. Validity of "generalized" equations for body composition analysis in women athletes. *Res Quar Exerc Sport.* 1984;55:153-160.
41. Lohman TG. Body composition assessment in sports medicine. *Sports Med Digest.* 1990;12:1-2.
42. Katch FI, Katch VL. Measurement and prediction errors in body composition assessment and the search for the perfect prediction equation. *Res Quar Exerc Sport.* 1980;51:249-260.
43. Jackson AS, Pollock ML. Generalized equations for predicting body density of men. *Br J Nutr.* 1978;40:497-504.
44. Jackson AS, Pollock ML, Ward A. Generalized equations for predicting body density of women. *Med Sci Sports Exerc.* 1980;12:175-182.
45. Jackson AS, Pollock ML. Practical assessment of body composition. *Phys Sports Med.* 1985;13:76-90.
46. Golding L, Myers C, Sinning W. *The Y's Way to Physical Fitness.* Rosemont, Ill: National Board of the YMCA; 1982.
47. Sinning WE, Dolny DG, Little KD, et al. Validity of "generalized" equations for body composition analysis in male athletes. *Med Sci Sports Exerc.* 1985;17:124-130.
48. Lukaski HC, Johnson PE. A simple, inexpensive method of determining total body water using a tracer dose of D2O and infrared absorption of biological fluids. *Am J Clin Nutr.* 1985;41:363-370.
49. Segal KR, Gutin B, Presta E, Wang J, Van Itallie TB. Estimation of human body composition by electrical impedance methods: a comparative study. *J Appl Physiol.* 1985;58:1565-1571.
50. Keller B, Katch FI. Validity of bioelectrical resistive impedance resistance for estimation of body fat in lean males. *Med Sci Sports Exerc.* 1985;17:272. Abstract.
51. Deurenberg P, Weststrate JA, Hautvast JGAJ. Changes in fat-free mass during weight loss measured by bioelectrical impedance and by densitometry. *Am J Clin Nutr.* 1989;49:33-36.
52. Deurenberg P, van der Kooij K, Evers P, Hulshof T. Assessment of body composition by bioelectrical impedance in a population aged >60 y. *Am J Clin Nutr.* 1990;51:3-6.
53. Malina RM. Bioelectric methods for estimating body composition: an overview and discussion. *Hum Biol.* 1987;59:329-335.
54. Chumlea WC, Baumgartner RN, Roche AF. Specific resistivity used to estimate fat-free mass from segmental body measures of bioelectric impedance. *Am J Clin Nutr.* 1988;48:7-15.
55. Jackson AS, Pollock ML, Graves JE, Mahar MT. Reliability and validity of bioelectrical impedance in determining body composition. *J Appl Physiol.* 1988;64:529-534.
56. Segal KR, Van Loan M, Fitzgerald PI, Hodgdon JA, Van Itallie TB. Lean body mass estimation by bioelectrical impedance analysis: a four-site cross-validation study. *Am J Clin Nutr.* 1988;47:7-14.
57. Baumgartner RN, Chumlea WC, Roche AF. Bioelectric impedance phase angle and body composition. *Am J Clin Nutr.* 1988;48:16-23.
58. Guo S, Roche AF, Houtkooper L. Fat-free mass in children and young adults predicted from bioelectric impedance and anthropometric variables. *Am J Clin Nutr.* 1989;50:435-443.

59. Lukaski HC, Johnson PE, Bolonchuk WW, Lykken GI. Assessment of fat-free mass using bioelectrical impedance measurements of the human body. *Am J Clin Nutr.* 1985;41:810-817.

60. Lukaski HC, Bolonchuk WW, Hall CB, Siders WA. Validation of tetrapolar bioelectrical impedance method to assess human body composition. *J Appl Physiol.* 1986;60:1327-1332.

61. Houtkooper LB, Lohman TG, Going SB, Hall MC. Validity of bioelectric impedance for body composition assessment in children. *J Appl Physiol.* 1989;66:814-821.

62. Houtkooper LB, Going SB, Lohman TG, Roche AF, Van Loan M. Bioelectrical impedance estimation of fat-free body mass in children and youth: a cross-validation study. *J Appl Physiol.* 1992;72:366-373.

63. Nieman DC. *The Sports Medicine Fitness Course.* Palo Alto, Calif: Bull Publishing Co; 1986.

64. Kushner RF, Kunigk A, Alspaugh M, Andronis PT, Leitch CA, Schoeller DA. Validation of bioelectrical-impedance analysis as a measurement of change in body composition in obesity. *Am J Clin Nutr.* 1990;52:219-223.

65. Houmard JA, Israel RG, McCammon MR, O'Brien KF, Omer J, Zamora BS. Validity of a near-infrared device for estimating body composition in a college football team. *J Appl Sport Sci Res.* 1991;5:53-59.

66. Israel RG, Houmard JA, O'Brien KF, McCammon MR, Zamora BS, Eaton AW. Validity of a near-infrared spectrophotometry device for estimating human body composition. *Res Quar Exerc Sport.* 1989;60:379-383.

67. McLean KP, Skinner JS. Validity of Futrex-5000 for body composition determination. *Med Sci Sports Exerc.* 1992;24:253-258.

68. Presta E, Wang J, Harrison GG, Bjorntorp P, Harker WH, Van Itallie TB. Measurement of total body electrical conductivity: a new method for estimation of body composition. *Am J Clin Nutr.* 1983;37:735-739.

69. Van Loan MD, Belko AZ, Mayclin PL, Barbieri TF. Use of total-body electrical conductivity for monitoring body composition changes during weight reduction. *Am J Clin Nutr.* 1987;46:5-8.

70. Cochran WJ, Wong WW, Fiorotto ML, Sheng HP, Klein PD, Klish WJ. Total body water estimated by measuring total-body electrical conductivity. *Am J Clin Nutr.* 1988;48:946-950.

71. Lohman TG. Research progress in validation of laboratory methods of assessing body composition. *Med Sci Sports Exerc.* 1984;16:596-603.

72. Heymsfield SB, Smith R, Aulet M, et al. Appendicular skeletal muscle mass: measurement by dual-photon absorptiometry. *Am J Clin Nutr.* 1990;52:214-218.

73. Willowby D. An anthropometric method for arriving at the optimal proportions of the body in any adult individual. *Res Quar.* 1932;3:48-77.

74. Katch VL, Katch FI, Moffatt R, Gittlelson M. Muscular development and lean body weight in bodybuilders and weight lifters. *Med Sci Sports Exerc.* 1980;12:340-344.

Computer Programs for Nutrition, Diet, Fitness, and Body-Composition Assessment

Marie Dunford and Melinda Manore

One of the most efficient and effective uses of computerization in the dietetics profession is computerized dietary analysis. Originally limited to mainframe computers, diet-assessment programs are now well suited and generally available to microcomputer users. At a minimum, computerized nutrition and diet-assessment programs analyze dietary intakes and compare intakes with standards. Additionally, programs can identify trends, create diets, and provide clients with nutrition information.

The determination of the "best" computer program is never an easy task. Potential users can gather written information about available programs and, in some cases, view program demonstrations. It is important to ask specific questions about the program's capabilities. Ultimately, the evaluation of computer software for diet assessment should focus on two major areas, database quality and program features.

▶ EVALUATION OF COMPUTERIZED NUTRIENT DATABASES

The initial step in software evaluation is the evaluation of the nutrient database. The nutrient database contains the numerical values that are the foundation of all calculations performed by the computer program, and is the basis for estimating nutrient intake. Therefore, an accurate nutrient database is essential.

The inherent limitations of all nutrient databases, computerized or not, are well recognized.[1-5] It serves professionals and clients alike to keep the following in mind:

> ▶ Many foods listed in a nutrient database have not been evaluated for nutrient content.
> ▶ The nutrient values associated with many foods may be estimates or predictions derived from other foods that have been biochemically analyzed for nutrient content.
> ▶ Many foods listed in a nutrient database have missing values because they were never analyzed for certain nutrients, and there are no similar foods that have been analyzed from which to project nutrient content.
> ▶ The methods used for chemically evaluating the nutrient content of foods are of variable sophistication and accuracy for different nutrients.
> ▶ Nutrient databases do not consider the variability of nutrient content for foods grown in different areas.
> ▶ The bioavailability of any nutrient may be influenced by the food in which it resides and the other foods that are consumed at the same meal, neither of which are considered in a nutrient database.

Results of research comparing computerized databases have been mixed. Taylor and colleagues[4] analyzed 24-hour dietary records using three computerized nutrient databases. Results of this study demonstrated that 9 of the 19 nutrient value means differed, although no database consistently reported high or low values. Another study of four computerized databases revealed no statistically significant differences between three of the databases when analyzing 60 24-hour recalls.[1] There were significant differences ($P<.01$) between one database and the other three, but the reasons for the differences could not be detected. A recent review by Nieman and colleagues[3] compared six popular microcomputer dietary-analysis systems with the USDA Nutrient Data Base for Standard Reference (USDA NDB). A 3-day food record with 73 food items was entered into each program, and nutrient averages were compared with USDA NDB. All six programs were within 7% of the USDA NDB for energy, protein, total fat, and total carbohydrate; however, the other nutrients varied more than 15% from the USDA NDB. Variability between programs was even greater. These studies emphasize the fact that, in general, the nutrient values associated with foods are, at best, estimates of the actual nutrient content.

When reviewing a computer program, the health professional should consider a number of database issues:

▶ Source(s) and currency of data
▶ Missing values
▶ Number of nutrients associated with each food
▶ Number of foods in the database
▶ Portion size units available for each food
▶ Dietary standards against which nutrient intake is related

Sources and Currency of Data

The most commonly cited source of nutrient values is the USDA Handbook 8 series (USDA Nutrient Data Base for Standard Reference), *Nutrient Composition of Foods*. Many databases rely on Home and Garden Bulletin 72, *Nutrient Values of Foods*, which is a subset of USDA Handbook 8. These databases are generally accepted as valid. Both have the limitation, however, that no brand-name food values (with the exception of ready-to-eat cereals) are included. This limitation has encouraged software developers to add nutrient values of brand-name food items that have been derived from other sources.[5,6]

Data may also be derived from manufacturer's information, journal articles, food composition tables from other countries, and unpublished sources. Separate, specialized databases (eg, frozen convenience foods, school lunch) are available from some companies. Because the database serves as the basis for every analysis, each data source should be valid and identified.[2,3,5,6]

The number of data sources has increased dramatically over the years. One computer program, with nearly 6000 foods in the database, lists more than 450 data sources. As additional research is undertaken and advanced analytical techniques become available, nutrient values will change. When purchasing a computer program, one must consider these important questions:

▶ How frequently are updates offered?
▶ What is the additional cost of an update?
▶ Will installing the update disrupt or alter user-entered changes in the current database?

Missing Values

The extent of missing values in the database cannot be overlooked. Calculations for those nutrients with missing data must be interpreted with caution, because missing values may be calculated as zeros.[5] Examining the data output may offer some clues as to how missing data are treated (eg, if saturated, monounsaturated, and polyunsaturated fatty acids do not equal total fatty acids, or if the foods consumed appear to be adequate, but some nutrient totals are low).[6]

Programs advertised as containing "no missing values" should beg the question: are values imputed? It is interesting to note that figures released in 1987 by the US Department of Agriculture indicated that the percentage of nutrient values that have been determined by direct chemical analysis varies. Nutrients for which approximately half of the values are either unknown or are imputed in the USDA Nutrient Database for Standard Reference include[6]:

▶ All the individual amino acids (but not total protein)
▶ Folacin
▶ Pantothenic acid
▶ Vitamin A (expressed as retinol equivalents)
▶ Vitamin B_6
▶ Vitamin B_{12}

Number of Nutrients in the Database

Potential users must determine the number of nutrients essential to best serve their populations.[7] Some programs offer a small number (12 to 15 nutrients), while other programs contain more than 50 nutrients per food. Programs analyzing large numbers of nutrients can be cumbersome and may serve to confuse clients. On the other hand, the additional nutrients may be helpful for certain clients, and some programs may be customized so that a limited number of nutrients are routinely analyzed.

Types of Foods in the Database

Program information usually includes a statement of the number of foods contained in the database. Although the total number of foods in the database is important, the breadth and depth of the foods included should also be considered. Evaluation should be based on the number of foods in the database that most completely reflect the diets of the client population. In some work environments, a database with a strong list of ethnic and regional foods may be a necessity. In other work environments, it is essential to have a database that includes many fast foods, convenience foods, or both. Dietitians working with athletes may want to include in the database frequently used sports food products and sport supplements (protein powders, amino acid supplements).

In some databases, the actual number of different foods may be inflated because a single food is listed several times with different portion sizes. Thus, a stick of butter, a pat of butter, and a tablespoon of butter may be counted as three different foods. In reality, these entries represent one food item with three different portion sizes. Similarly, there may be separate entries for foods that differ little in nutrient value (eg, cakes made from cake mixes and commercially prepared cakes).[6] In addition, some users may want to have the capacity to analyze recipes. If this is the case, the database should be viewed from this perspective.

In many cases, foods can be added by the user as a means of enhancing the database. However, this can be an extremely time-consuming task if a substantial number of foods must be added to make the database usable. If foods are added by the user, extreme care must be taken to ensure that data are entered accurately.

Portion Size

The accuracy of any nutrient calculation is dependent on the accuracy of the portion-size estimates. The serving sizes used in the database must be represented by common household or other widely used measures. Some entries appear as "one piece" or "one serving." While this may be an appropriate description for some foods, such measures may leave the user guessing, which increases the chance of error.[6]

Standards Used

All programs will include some basis for comparison. Commonly used standards include the Recommended Dietary Allowances, the US Dietary Guidelines, the Exchange Lists, and the American Heart Association recommendations. Energy requirements are often determined using height, weight, gender, age, and activity levels. Check to be certain that the appropriate standards for the client populations served are included, and if standards can be altered by the user. Although there is no "athletic RDA," some clients may wish to set their own standards based on an understanding of what is required by a specific athletic population (eg, 1.5 g protein per kilogram of body weight per day, or 70% of calories derived from carbohydrate).[7]

Evaluation of Program Features

In addition to data analysis, it is important to evaluate a variety of program features. These include data entry, verification and correction procedures, help features, cost, and printout format and design. Demonstration diskettes may be helpful in the evaluation process.[8]

Method of Data Entry

Always a tedious task, data entry deserves close attention. Evaluate the data entry features with efficiency in mind. Coding, whether it be on- or off-screen, is a routine and time-consuming task and is not a good use of a dietitian's time. Also, if coding is necessary, it must be accurate to ensure valid results.[9]

Most newer programs are menu-driven, allowing the user to highlight and select a food, which then appears on the screen. Foods are selected from the database by entering a complete or partial name of the food, or by accessing food categories and viewing a list of foods. Portion sizes are displayed when a food is selected.

Data entry may also be achieved by entering food codes. Numeric codes are most common, but other coding schemes may exist. Coding materials (eg, pages containing food lists with associated code numbers) should be checked to determine if the food items are arranged in a logical format. If recipe analysis is of prime importance, consider whether common basic ingredients can be entered and assigned a single code. Off-screen coding may be an advantage if computer access is limited, but the chance of error is increased.[6,10]

Data Verification and Correction Procedures

Careful data entry can minimize errors, but the need to verify and correct data will always be present. Some programs have built-in error-detection functions that flag potential data-entry errors (eg, values that appear to be out of normal range, such as 100 lb of ground beef). When errors are not so obvious, the user must detect incorrect entries and edit them. Editing procedures may be cumbersome, and are an important consideration. Determine if there are any limits on the editing that can be done on a list of foods selected for analysis.[6]

Help Features

No matter how experienced, all users rely on help features to some degree. On-screen help menus are handy features that briefly explain or clarify the information appearing on the screen and increase the user's efficiency. Inexperienced users often rely on manuals and other printed material if questions arise. Do not assume that written documentation will be accurately and clearly presented. Manuals should be reviewed for their clarity. The degree of technical support offered by software companies varies. Some software companies offer toll-free phone numbers to reach knowledgeable staff and on-site programmers who can answer questions. Others offer only written materials.

Cost

The cost of the software program cannot be overlooked, but price should not be the only consideration. Software prices run the gamut, and high-priced packages do not necessarily ensure a comprehensive, high-quality product. It is important to choose the program that has the most desirable features, and the fewest limitations, and that is priced within an acceptable range. Planning a budget for program updates in addition to the initial expenditure is also a consideration.[6]

Printout Format and Design

The end product of most computerized nutrient analyses will be a printout. Printout formats and designs will vary, but all formats should be clear, concise, interpretable, accurate, and appropriate for the intended audience. Most software programs offer samples of printouts, so this is one feature that can easily be reviewed.

Clarity of information is an important issue. Too much information on a page or the presence of many symbols will only serve to confuse the client trying to read the printout. Make certain that any abbreviations are clearly understood. Charts and graphs, available on most programs, often make data interpretation easier and are appropriately used with many client populations.

Interpretation of data is a key issue. Clients may attach importance to computer-generated information, even though they have been told of its limitations. The potential for misinterpretation is great. To reduce the incidence of misinterpretation, printouts should bear a statement of their limitations as well as the name, address, and phone number of the health professional who generated the reports, and to whom questions should be directed.[6,7]

Preprogrammed text should be checked to establish accuracy. A common feature is the matching of computed data against program standards and recommendations. Written interpretations are then printed by the program. For example, if vitamin C is consumed at 125% of the RDA, how is this interpreted by the program? Some programs, using a strict cutoff point (100% of the RDA), might advise the user to reduce the intake of vitamin C. If text does not accompany the printout figures, it would be worth considering how clients might interpret the information without written explanations. Recommendations for apparent deficiencies are also problematic, especially if the number of missing values is substantial.

Finally, determine if the amount of information to be printed for an analysis can be chosen by the user. Programs can generate a large amount of data, some of which might not be useful for a particular client. Having the ability to save an analysis on disk for later review is also an important feature. This feature allows for a subsequent review of a list of foods without having to reenter the list.

► COMPUTERIZED FITNESS ASSESSMENTS

Besides computerized nutrient-analysis programs, fitness planning and assessment programs are available for both home and office use. The types of programs available within the fitness/wellness area include body-composition assessment, fitness assessment (including, strength, flexibility, heart rate, blood pressure, aerobic fitness), health-risk appraisals, exercise monitoring (including determination of energy expenditure) and planning, and managerial programs for health clubs and spas. Programs that monitor and/or determine fitness level and body composition and that help in assessing energy expenditure will be most helpful to the dietitian working in the area of nutrition and exercise. However, as with nutrient analysis programs, these programs must be carefully critiqued before purchasing to assure that the results generated are both accurate and useful. The following questions will help in evaluating these commercially available programs.

What is the database source? Any software program that produces an assessment or health-risk appraisal profile, must first be evaluated for its database. What formula and database are used to generate the assessment value and client profile? What are the norms against which a client's profile is compared? Is the database representative of the client population with which you are working? For example, if the program is calculating percentage body fat based on skinfold measurements, is the formula given? Was the formula developed for the type of client population currently measured in your facility?

Is the program well documented? A program that does not have a complete bibliography (that documents norms and formulas used to calculate assessment values or cutoff criteria) is useless. Without these data it is impossible to track errors or determine if the program is representative of your client population. In addition, without documentation there is no background information to explain how the criteria and norms were developed. Therefore, this part of the program is very important, and it should be thoroughly examined before purchasing the software.

Can the program be customized to meet special needs? Many software programs are written for the widest possible audience or client profile. However, if you are working with a special population, you may want to customize the program to meet your needs. Therefore, programs that offer flexibility for altering client norms, modifying standardized formulas, or customized the client printout are desirable.

Is the program updated on a regular basis?   All fitness- and wellness-assessment programs use research data to generate population norms against which client data are compared. In addition, research data are used to generate the formulas and predict a client's value (for example, predicting resting metabolic rate base on weight, fat-free mass). The research literature is constantly changing, with better population norms and prediction formulas being developed regularly. Therefore, it is imperative that the program database be updated regularly. In addition, regular program updates will eliminate the constant pressure to stay current with the most recent formulas and population norms. Finally, each program update should include a complete reference source that specifically outlines new changes.

Is the program user friendly? Is the output easy for the client to understand?   In our fast-paced world, anything that saves time also saves money. Therefore, choose a program that is easy to use and for which customer support is readily available. This will save valuable hours of start-up time and reduce frustration. In addition, examine the client printout for ease of understanding. If the client can easily understand the printout, less time will be needed to explain the results. Easy-to-read printouts will also make it simpler for clients to review recommendations when the dietitian is not available.

Can the program store client data and compare data over time?   Many clients return for follow-up visits to determine if specified dietary, weight, and fitness goals have been met. A program that allows tracking of client data over time makes client monitoring easier. In addition, graphic presentations of changes in dietary intakes (and so on) help clients see the progress they have made and may motivate them to continue working toward specified goals. If summary and aggregate reports are necessary or desired, ask if the data can be transferred to ASCII files for transfer to data-analysis programs (eg, SAS, SPSSX) or data-management programs (eg, Lotus III, Quattro Pro). This feature is essential to follow a group for an extended period or create summary reports.

REFERENCES

1. Eck LH, Klesges RC, Hanson CL, Baranowski T, Henske J. A comparison of four commonly used nutrient database programs. *J Am Diet Assoc.* 1988;88:602-604.
2. Nieman DC, Nieman CN. A comparative study of two microcomputer nutrient data bases with the USDA Nutrient Data Base for Standard Reference. *J Am Diet Assoc.* 1987;87:930-932.
3. Nieman DC, Butterworth DE, Nieman CN, Lee KE, Lee RD. Comparison of six microcomputer dietary analysis systems with the USDA Nutrient Data Base for Standard Reference. *J Am Diet Assoc.* 1992;92:48-56.
4. Taylor ML, Kozlowski BW, Baer MT. Energy and nutrient values from different computerized data bases. *J Am Diet Assoc.* 1985;85:1136-1138.
5. Schakel SF, Sievert YA, Buzzard IM. Sources of data for developing and maintaining a nutrient database. *J Am Diet Assoc.* 1988;88:1268-1271.
6. Byrd-Bredbenner C. Computer nutrient analysis software packages: considerations for selection. *Nutr Today.* Sept/Oct 1988:13-21.
7. Frank GC, Pelican S. Guidelines for selecting a dietary analysis system. *J Am Diet Assoc.* 1986;86:72-75.
8. Ralston CE, Matthews ME. Software selection: can a demonstration computer package help? *J Am Diet Assoc.* 1988;88:1087-1089.
9. Penfield MP, Costello CA. Microcomputer programs for diet analysis: a comparative evaluation. *J Am Diet Assoc.* 1988;88:209-211.
10. Kris-Etherton P, ed. *Cardiovascular Disease: Nutrition for Prevention and Treatment.* Chicago, Ill: The American Dietetic Association; 1990.

III

Conditions Requiring Special Consideration

Mitchell Kanter, Editor

The pursuit of fitness is no longer the domain of the young and healthy. People of all ages and abilities are embarking on fitness programs. However, as more and more people with diverse backgrounds and diverse levels of fitness and health become involved in physical exercise, it is increasingly important for the health professional to have knowledge of the physiological and health-related changes that occur as people age. Knowing how these factors affect physical performance and nutritional needs can help the professional design the most effective care plan for a client. The following section contains pertinent information regarding nutritional and physiological concerns during various stages of the life cycle, and under a variety of disease states.

Pregnancy and Lactation

Sheri L. Riel and Barbara A. Bowman

► EFFECTS OF EXERCISE DURING PREGNANCY

Exercise has beneficial effects for most pregnant women. Years ago, women were told to remain sedentary during pregnancy. The consensus now is that active women who become pregnant may continue their exercise programs after gaining the approval of their doctors. Women with sedentary life-styles who become pregnant and wish to exercise should begin at very low levels of intensity and increase their activity levels slowly.[1] Recent studies have demonstrated several benefits of exercise during pregnancy; these benefits have been comprehensively reviewed elsewhere.[2-6]

Psychological Benefits

Exercise brings many people a psychological lift. According to studies using the Rosenberg self-esteem scale, exercising women have a more positive self-image and experience less tension during pregnancy than pregnant women who do not exercise.[2,7]

Maternal Weight Gain

Appropriate amounts of exercise during pregnancy may help to promote a more optimal weight gain. Wolfe and colleagues[3] suggested that excess weight gain may lead to postpartum obesity. However, excessive physical activity and inadequate energy intakes could lead to suboptimal maternal weight gain and growth retardation of the fetus.[2,3] Obviously, fine-tuning the amount of exercise that may be accomplished during pregnancy requires a delicate balancing act. More studies are needed to determine whether the composition and pattern of weight gained, particularly fat deposition, are altered in exercising pregnant women.

Maternal Aerobic Fitness

During normal pregnancy, maximum oxygen consumption ($\dot{V}O_2max$), expressed as a function of body weight (mL/kg) declines. Studies demonstrate that $\dot{V}O_2max$ can be maintained or even increased during pregnancy with weight-bearing exercises such as jogging and aerobics. However, swimming and biking are not considered weight-bearing exercises and do not have the same effect on $\dot{V}O_2max$ in pregnant women.[3,4]

Cardiac output increases during pregnancy, and is further increased by exercise. Heart rate and stroke volume are the components of the cardiac output. Heart rate increases during pregnancy and so does stroke volume, but during the third trimester stroke volume begins to decrease and continues to decrease until term. The effects of exercise on heart rate and stroke volume during pregnancy are difficult to measure; further studies are needed. It has been demonstrated, however, that aerobic exercise performed 3 days per week for 15 to 30 minutes per session can help lower blood pressure and enhance maternal work capacity in pregnant women.[3,4]

▶ EFFECTS OF EXERCISE ON LABOR AND FETAL OUTCOME

Fewer Complications in Exercising Women

Pregnant women who exercise have more vaginal deliveries and fewer surgical interventions.[3,8] Some (but not all) studies have also documented fewer preterm births and shorter (but not before term) pregnancies in exercising women. The facilitation of labor could be the result of the enhanced tone of muscles used during labor and an increased work capacity.[3,8] Several studies have demonstrated a significantly decreased use of epidural anesthesia, a reduction in labor stimulation, and decreased use of forceps in exercising women.[8,9]

Shorter Duration of Labor

The duration of labor is often used as an index of the difficulty of labor. In a recent study, exercising women were found to have a shorter active stage of labor than the nonexercising controls.[10] Other studies have shown all stages of labor to be shorter in exercising women.[8] Generally, women who exercise during pregnancy have shorter labors and quicker, easier deliveries.[2]

Lower Birth Weight

Studies examining obstetric outcomes, particularly infant birth weight, of exercising and nonexercising pregnant women have obtained diverse results. More recent studies have shown that the birth weights of babies of exercising women are significantly lower than those of babies of nonexercising controls. However, the lower birth weights observed were still within the normal range in all of the studies. In one study, infants of mothers in the exercising group had significantly lower birth weights and lower percentages of body fat than infants of sedentary control subjects.[11] However, numerous studies have found no difference in birth weight between infants of exercising women and nonexercising controls.[7,10]

Apgar Score

One useful measurement of neonatal outcome is the Apgar score. The Apgar score is assigned by a delivery room nurse or a physician in attendance, who rates the baby on a scale of 0 to 2, using five criteria. The baby gets a score of 0, 1, or 2 points for each criterion, as shown in *Table 3.1.*

In some studies, the Apgar scores of infants born to exercising mothers have been significantly higher statistically than the scores of infants born to sedentary controls.[7,11] In other studies, however, maternal exercise did not affect Apgar scores.[10]

TABLE 3.1   Apgar Score Criteria

Sign	0	1	2
Heart rate	Absent	Slow, <100	100 or above
Respiratory effort	Absent	Weak cry, hypoventilation	Crying lustily
Muscle tone	Flaccid	Some flexion, extremities	Well-flexed
Reflex irritability	No response	Some motion	Cry
Color	Blue, pale	Blue hands and feet	Entirely pink

From Graef JW, Cone TE, eds. *Manual of Pediatric Therapeutics.* Boston, Mass: Little Brown and Co; 1980:94. Used by permission.

▶ WHO SHOULD NOT EXERCISE?

Table 3.2 lists conditions that are absolute contraindications for exercise during pregnancy. Other moderate contraindications are anemia, essential hypertension, thyrotoxicosis, preeclampsia, cervical bleeding, multiple pregnancy, obesity, and diabetes.[2,4,5]

▶ COMMON PRECAUTIONS FOR EXERCISE DURING PREGNANCY

A pregnant woman should consult her physician before participating in any exercise program. Even with this consultation, certain activities are not recommended under any circumstance[2,3,6,12]:

- ▶ Board diving
- ▶ Scuba diving (a hyperbaric activity)
- ▶ Water skiing
- ▶ Contact sports
- ▶ Exercise done at high elevation
- ▶ Exercise in hot and humid environments
- ▶ Exercise in the supine position

The American College of Obstetricians and Gynecologists[1] has set the following exercise guidelines for pregnant women:

Pregnancy and Postpartum
1. Regular exercise (at least three times per week) is preferable to intermittent activity. Competitive activities should be discouraged.
2. Vigorous exercise should not be performed in hot, humid weather or during a period of febrile illness.
3. Ballistic movements (jerky, bouncy motions) should be avoided. Exercise should be done on a wooden floor or on a tightly carpeted surface to reduce shock and provide a sure footing.

TABLE 3.2   Absolute Contraindications for Exercising During Pregnancy

Factors Predisposing to Prematurity
    Incompetent cervix
    Multiple gestations
    History of premature labor
    Placental previa
    Ruptured membranes

Decreased Uterine/Placental Oxygenation
    Cyanotic cardiac disease and any disease that lowers cardiac output
    Pregnancy-induced hypertension
    Smoking

Data from Sady SP, Carpenter MW. Aerobic exercise during pregnancy. *Sports Med.* 1989;7:357-375.

4. Deep flexion or extension of joints should be avoided because of connective tissue laxity. Activities that require jumping, jarring motions, or rapid changes in direction should be avoided because of joint instability.
5. Vigorous exercise should be preceded by a 5-minute period of muscle warm-up. This can be accomplished by slow walking or stationary cycling with a low resistance.
6. Vigorous exercise should be followed by a period of gradually declining activity that includes gentle stationary stretching. Because connective tissue laxity increases the risk of joint injury, stretches should not be taken to the point of maximum resistance.
7. Heart rate should be measured at times of peak activity. Target heart rates and limits (established in consultation with the physician) should not be exceeded.
8. Care should be taken to rise from the floor gradually to avoid orthostatic hypotension. Some form of activity involving the legs should be continued for a brief period.
9. Liquids should be taken liberally before and after exercise to prevent dehydration. If necessary, activity should be interrupted to replenish fluids.
10. Women who have had sedentary life-styles should begin with physical activity of very low intensity and advance their activity levels very gradually.
11. Activity should be stopped and the physician consulted if any unusual symptoms appear.

Pregnancy Only
1. Maternal heart rate should not exceed 140 beats per minute.
2. Strenuous activities should not exceed 15 minutes in duration.
3. No exercise should be performed in the supine position after the fourth month of gestation is completed.
4. Exercises that employ the Valsalva maneuver (prolonged breath holding that may lead to a blackout, commonly associated with lifting heavy weights) should be avoided.
5. Caloric intake should be adequate to meet not only the extra energy needs of pregnancy, but also the needs of the exercise performed.
6. Maternal core temperature should not exceed 38°C (100.4°F).

▶ EFFECTS OF EXERCISE DURING LACTATION

Few studies have examined the effect of exercise on lactation, and those that have been conducted generally used animals as subjects. However, most of the studies on animals and humans have shown that exercise does not affect milk production or macronutrient composition. A study by Lovelady demonstrated that, although exercising lactating women had significantly lower percentages of body fat and higher levels of energy expenditure than nonexercising controls, the exercising subjects produced a greater volume of milk (although the increase was not significant).[13]

In a recent double-blind study, Wallace and colleagues reported that infant acceptance of breast milk collected prior to exercise was significantly higher than that of milk collected at 10 and 30 minutes after intensive exercise.[14] This effect may be attributable to the higher lactate concentration of breast milk following maximal exercise, because lactate causes a sour taste. Based on these results, the authors recommend that lactating women consider nursing or collecting milk for later feedings before exercising. Because the concentration of lactate may remain elevated for 90 minutes or longer, an optimal time to nurse after exercise could not be identified. Additional research is needed to determine whether milk lactate concentrations and milk acceptance also change significantly after moderate exercise, and to examine the relationship between blood and milk concentrations of lactate.

The increased nutritional demands of lactation can be met by adding 1 cup of milk and an additional serving from the bread and cereal group to the foods recommended during pregnancy. The recommended energy intake for lactating women is 2700 kcal, 500 kcal higher than that for nonpregnant women. For women who are experiencing low gestational weight gain, or for those whose weight falls below standards of height and weight during lactation, the recommendation is for an additional 650 kcal per day. The additional caloric needs of lactating women who exercise can be estimated by adding the energy needs of lactation and exercise to the basal needs.

The American College of Obstetricians and Gynecologists recommends liberal intake of liquids before and during exercise.[1] Lactation itself increases fluid needs by approximately three additional glasses of fluid daily. Consequently, lactating exercising women should be extremely vigilant of their fluid intakes, and should make adjustments accordingly as the quantity of exercise in which they participate increases.

REFERENCES

1. *Exercise During Pregnancy and the Postnatal Period.* Washington, DC: American College of Obstetricians and Gynecologists; 1985.
2. Jarski RW, Trippett DL. The risks and benefits of exercise during pregnancy. *J Fam Pract.* 1990;30:185-189.
3. Wolfe LA, Hall P, Webb KA, Goodman L, Monga M, McGrath MJ. Prescription of aerobic exercise during pregnancy. *Sports Med.* 1989;8:273-301.
4. Sady SP, Carpenter MW. Aerobic exercise during pregnancy. *Sports Med.* 1989;7:357-375.
5. Fishbein EG, Phillips M. How safe is exercise during pregnancy? *J Obstet Gynecol Neonatal Nurs.* 1990;19:45-49.
6. Huch R, Erkkola R. Pregnancy and exercise-exercise and pregnancy: a short review. *Br J Obstet Gynaecol.* 1990;97:208-214.
7. Hall DC, Kaufmann DA. Effects of aerobic and strength conditioning on pregnancy outcomes. *Amer J Obstet Gynecol.* 1987;157:1199-1203.
8. Clapp JF. The course of labor after endurance exercise during pregnancy. *Am J Obstet Gynecol.* 1990;163:1799-1805.
9. Beckman CRB. Effect of a structured antepartum exercise program on pregnancy and labor outcome in primiparas. *J Reprod Med.* 1990;35(7):704-709.
10. Kulpa PJ. Aerobic exercise in pregnancy. *Am J Obstet Gynecol.* 1987;156:1395-1403.
11. Clapp JF. Neonatal morphometries after endurance exercise during pregnancy. *Am J Obstet Gynecol.* 1990;163:1805-1811.
12. Pirie L, Curtis L. *Pregnancy and Sports Fitness.* Tucson, Ariz: Fisher Books; 1987:66-70.
13. Lovelady CA, Lonnerdal B, Dewey KG. Lactation performance of exercising women. *Am J Clin Nutr.* 1990;52:103-109.
14. Wallace JP, Inbar G, Ernsthausen K. Infant acceptance of postexercise breast milk. *Pediatrics.* 1992;89:1245-1247.

Childhood

Peggy H. Paul

▶ BODY WEIGHT CONSIDERATIONS

If it is determined that a child needs to lose weight, weight monitoring, caloric intake stabilization, and increased physical activity are recommended over drastic, restricted-calorie programs. This conservative approach to weight control is particularly important for prepubescent children, who require a nutritionally sound diet to support optimal growth and development. It must be remembered that, proportionately, children require higher amounts of nutrients than adults.[1] The 1989 Recommended Dietary Allowances (RDAs) provide a guideline for intake of vitamins and minerals.

A gradual gain or loss of no more than 1 or 2 lb per week, combined with a supervised exercise program, is suggested. Identifiable cases of anorexia nervosa and bulimia should be referred immediately to a registered dietitian or to a specialist trained in counseling individuals with these conditions. With respect to a child's participation in organized sport, consideration must be given to the young athlete's level of physical maturity to minimize the risk of injury. Awareness of the child's attitude toward exercise and competition should be considered as well.

▶ FLUID REQUIREMENTS

The function of water in an exercising person, regardless of age, is to mediate energy reactions, serve as a transport medium for circulating body substances, and to regulate body temperature. Water content in the body is predominantly controlled by sweat rate, urine output, and thirst. Frequently, however, the thirst mechanism is not an adequate gauge of fluid needs. Factors associated with competition, such as event preparation and anxiety, can distract an athlete of any age from responding to the body's thirst signal. Activities such as hiking, biking, jogging, and outdoor team sports, especially when undertaken in hot, humid weather, will place participants at risk of dehydration. Thus, regularly planned fluid intake is necessary.

Fluid replacement is a special concern for the prepubescent athlete; however, information regarding the thermoregulatory capacity of the exercising child is lacking. There are, in part, ethical considerations for this paucity of information. In most studies on thermoregulation, subjects are exposed to "hostile" environments, such as extreme heat, high humidity, and cold. Oftentimes, subjects are required to dehydrate themselves. Scientists, for obvious reasons, have been reluctant to expose children to such extreme conditions.[2]

It is well established, however, that their greater relative surface area and lower sweating capacity make children more susceptible than adults to extremes in environmental temperature. During exercise, children produce more heat than adults, yet have a more limited ability to transfer this heat from the muscles to the skin.[3] Furthermore, the young athlete generally takes longer to acclimatize to exercise under warm weather conditions. Parents and coaches should be cognizant of these facts, and should ensure that scheduled fluid breaks are adhered to. Training periods should be gradual, to allow the child adequate time to adjust to elevated environmental temperatures.

The electrolyte concentration and osmolality of prepubescent children's sweat tends to be lower than that of the pubescent child or the adult. The reason for this is not clear; it may represent a more economical way of preserving body salt. Nonetheless, these differences should be considered when planning fluid and electrolyte replenishment for child athletes.[3]

In conclusion, the child's responses to exercise under varying environmental conditions are often characterized by the following[2,3]:

▶ A lower sweat rate as compared with those of postpubescents and adults.
▶ A lower tolerance and decreased ability to dissipate heat under extreme environmental conditions (eg, >45°C or 113°F).
▶ Dizziness, faintness, and nausea when exercising in the heat. These symptoms may be related to the child's inability to maintain arterial blood pressure, possibly as a result of a lower cardiac output than that of an adult (see *Table 3.3*).
▶ A slower rate of acclimatization.

TABLE 3.3 Heat Index Chart

Relative Humidity	Temperature (F°)										
	70°	75°	80°	85°	90°	95°	100°	105°	110°	115°	120°
	Apparent temperature*										
0%	64°	69°	73°	78°	83°	87°	91°	95°	99°	103°	107°
10%	65°	70°	75°	80°	85°	90°	95°	100°	105°	111°	116°
20%	66°	72°	77°	82°	87°	93°	99°	105°	112°	120°	130°
30%	67°	73°	78°	84°	90°	96°	104°	113°	123°	135°	148°
40%	68°	74°	79°	86°	93°	101°	110°	123°	137°	151°	
50%	69°	75°	81°	88°	96°	107°	120°	135°	150°		
60%	70°	76°	82°	90°	100°	114°	132°	149°			
70%	70°	77°	85°	93°	106°	124°	144°				
80%	71°	78°	86°	97°	113°	136°					
90%	71°	79°	88°	102°	122°						
100%	72°	80°	91°	108°							

*Combined index of heat and humidity . . . what it "feels like" to the body.

How to use heat index:

1. Across top locate temperature
2. Down left side locate relative humidity
3. Follow across and down to find apparent temperature
4. Determine Heat Stress Risk on chart at right

Apparent Temperature	Heat Stress Risk with Physical Activity and/or Prolonged Exposure
90°–105°	Heat cramps or heat exhaustion *possible*
105°–130°	Heat cramps or heat exhaustion *likely* Heatstroke *possible*
130° and up	Heatstroke *highly likely*

Note: This heat index chart is designed to provide general guidelines for assessing the potential severity of heat stress. Individual reactions to heat will vary. In addition, studies indicate that susceptibility to heat disorders tends to increase with age. Exposure to full sunshine can increase heat index values by up to 15°F.

From Team Weight Chart. © 1990, Gatorade. Data from National Oceanic and Atmospheric Administration.

Based on children's responses to exercise in hot climates, the American Academy of Pediatrics suggests the following[4]:

▶ In activities lasting 30 minutes or more, the intensity of exercise should be reduced whenever relative humidity and air temperature are above critical levels. (*Table 3.4* summarizes the energy expenditure of different activities.)

▶ At the beginning of a strenuous exercise program, or after traveling to a warmer climate, the intensity and duration of exercise should be restrained initially and then gradually increased over a period of 10 to 14 days to ensure more effective acclimatization.

▶ Clothing should be lightweight and limited to one layer of absorbent material to facilitate the evaporation of sweat. Sweat-saturated garments should be replaced by dry ones.

▶ Rubberized sweat suits should never be used by children to produce weight loss. They greatly increase sweat loss, and may produce severe heat-related illness.

General hydration recommendations are as follows: Before prolonged physical activity, the child should be fully hydrated. Drinking 14 to 20 oz of fluid 15 minutes before exercise is generally recommended as a prehydration regimen. During exercise, consumption of 4 to 10 oz of fluid every 15 minutes will help to maintain a euhydrated condition.

▶ ENERGY REQUIREMENTS

The RDA for children provides a starting point to estimate a child's energy requirement. Children aged 4 to 10 years require approximately 80 kcal per day per kilogram (36 kcal/lb) of ideal body weight. Young males aged 11 to 14 years require 55 kcal per day per kilogram (25 kcal/lb); their female counterparts of the same age require 47 kcal per day per kilogram (21 kcal/lb). As a comparison, adults need only 30 to 37 kcal per day per kilogram (14 to 17 kcal/lb), depending on their age and gender.[5] It must be remembered, however, that these estimates were determined for individuals who are only mildly active.

TABLE 3.4 Sports Activities of Children by Relative Level of Energy Expenditure

Low Energy Output	Moderate Energy Output	High Energy Output
Baseball	Basketball	Cycling (>14 mph)
Cycling (up to 9 mph)	Cycling (10-13 mph)	Calisthenics
Bowling	Football (touch)	(timed vigorous)
Calisthenics (light)	Hiking with pack (3 mph)	Judo
Football (moderate)	Ice hockey	Karate
Gymnastics	Horseback riding	Running (<6 mph)
Horseback riding	(posting and gallop)	
(sitting to trot)	Mountain climbing	
Table tennis	Roller skating	
Tennis (doubles,	Running 10 min/mile	
recreational)	(<6 mph)	
Walking (up to 4 mph)	Ice skating (9 mph)	

The relative energy expenditure rate of the 3 categories are:

Low energy < 4 kcal/min; 240 additional kcal per hour = 390 kcal use per hour

Moderate energy = 4-7 kcal/min (5 1/2 kcal/min average); 330 additional kcal per hour = 480 kcal use per hour

High energy > 7 kcal/min; 420 additional kcal per hour = 570 kcal use per hour

Adapted from Williams MH. *Nutrition for Fitness and Sport*. Dubuque, Iowa: Wm C Brown & Co; 1983. Reprinted with permission.

A child athlete would have a significantly higher energy need than a sedentary child, although total caloric requirement would vary with the duration and intensity of activity.

Recommended energy intakes for individuals of various ages, heights, and weights have been published. Table 3.4 can be used to estimate the caloric expenditures for children engaged in various sports activities.

Data from several studies have demonstrated that children use more energy than adults pursuing similar activities. In a study involving 47 preschool children (17 to 45 months old), energy expenditure on a kcal/kg per minute basis was two times greater for the children than for the adults during sedentary activity, and 1.2 times greater during moderate activity.[5] Further, research with 6- and 7-year-old children demonstrated the following[6]:

▶ Boys expended 12% to 16% more calories than girls during treadmill exercise at three different speeds.
▶ Children (at all levels of activity) expended more energy than adults.
▶ The relationship between energy cost and speed of movement was higher and followed a curvilinear path in children, compared with a linear pattern in adults (ie, as a child increases speed, he or she burns increasingly more calories than an adult).

Similarly, Freedson and colleagues demonstrated that energy expenditure was higher in prepubescent males than in older male children.[5] Thus, it is apparent that an inverse relationship exists between age and energy expenditure. Application of this relationship begins in the preschool years and continues throughout the life cycle. For example, it is estimated that a 75-lb child needs as many calories as a 150-lb adult.

In general, the best way to judge whether a child's food and fluid intakes are adequate is to observe the child's performance, growth, and weight fluctuations. Involuntary weight loss is almost always the result of food-energy intakes that are inadequate to satisfy the body's needs, and is inevitably associated with a deterioration in athletic performance.[6] Food and water intakes should immediately be increased to meet the needs of the active child if performance begins to deteriorate and weight begins to taper.

A healthful, high-performance diet for children is based on their energy needs. A young athlete should eat a carbohydrate-rich (60% to 65% of calories), low-fat (<30% of calories) diet with an adequate amount of protein (12% to 15% of calories). The diet should be varied, with an emphasis on breads and cereals, fruits, vegetables, and legumes. Further, a diet rich in carbohydrate will more adequately replace muscle glycogen stores following exercise than will a high-fat, high-protein diet.

▶ STRENGTH AND MUSCLE DEVELOPMENT

The practice of resistance strength training by young children is controversial. It has not been fully elucidated whether children can make significant gains in strength and muscle mass with weight training, or if they are more susceptible to injury than adolescents or adults.

On the basis of the few studies that have been done, it is apparent that children can increase strength and athletic performance with strength training.[7-9] Increases in muscle mass, however, are not as readily apparent.[10] Although the lack of hypertrophy in strength-trained, prepubescent boys has been attributed to low serum testosterone levels, young women (who also possess low testosterone levels) are clearly able to increase muscle mass with resistance training.[9,11] Therefore, other, as yet undiscovered mechanisms may be responsible for the apparent lack of muscle mass increases in prepubescent children who strength train.

Finally, no definitive studies indicate that prepubescent children are more susceptible to injury during resistive training than are adolescents or adults. Nonetheless, young children should never embark on a resistance-training program without proper supervision, and they should avoid high-risk exercises, such as single maximal lifts, overhead lifts, and ballistic efforts against inertia. *Tables 3.5* and *3.6* include the "Fitnessgram" reference standards for girls and boys as a guide to the fitness evaluation of children.

TABLE 3.5   Fitnessgram for girls

Age (y)	1 Mile Run/Walk* (min:s)	Body Composition		Sit and Reach (in)†	Sit-ups (in 1 min)	Pull-ups	Flexed Arm Hang (s)
		Percentage Fat	Body Mass Index				
5	17:00	32%	20	10:0	20	1	5
6	16:00	32%	20	10:0	20	1	5
7	15:00	32%	20	10:0	20	1	5
8	14:00	32%	20	10:0	25	1	8
9	13:00	32%	20	10:0	25	1	8
10	12:00	32%	21	10:0	30	1	8
11	12:00	32%	21	10:0	30	1	8
12	12:00	32%	22	10:0	30	1	8
13	11:30	32%	23	10:0	30	1	12
14	10:30	32%	24	10:0	35	1	12
15	10:30	32%	24	10:0	35	1	12
16	10:30	32%	24	10:0	35	1	12
16+	10:30	32%	25	10:0	35	1	12

*Lower scores indicate better performance.

†10 in is at the toes.

TABLE 3.6   Fitnessgram for boys

Age (y)	1 Mile Run/Walk* (min:s)	Body Composition		Sit and Reach (in)†	Sit-ups (in 1 min)	Pull-ups	Flexed Arm Hang (s)
		Percentage Fat	Body Mass Index				
5	16:00	25%	20	10:0	20	1	5
6	15:00	25%	20	10:0	20	1	5
7	14:00	25%	20	10:0	20	1	5
8	13:00	25%	20	10:0	25	1	10
9	12:00	25%	20	10:0	25	1	10
10	11:00	25%	21	10:0	30	1	10
11	11:00	25%	21	10:0	30	1	10
12	10:00	25%	22	10:0	35	1	10
13	9:30	25%	23	10:0	35	2	10
14	8:30	25%	24	10:0	40	3	15
15	8:30	25%	24	10:0	40	5	25
16	8:30	25%	25	10:0	40	5	25
16+	8:30	25%	26	10:0	40	5	25

*Lower scores indicate better performance.

†10 in is at the toes.

REFERENCES

1. National Research Council. *Recommended Dietary Allowances.* 10th ed. Washington, DC: National Academy Press; 1989.
2. Bar-Or O. Temperature regulation during exercise in children and adolescents. In: *Perspectives in Exercise Science and Sports Medicine.* Indianapolis, Ind: Benchmark Press; 1989;2.
3. Saris WHM, Browns F. Nutritional concerns for the young athlete. In: *Children and Exercise XII.* Champaign, Ill: Human Kinetics; 1986.
4. Cotterman S. Children and sports. *Sports Nutrition News.* 1984;3(2):3.
5. Freedson PS, Katch VL, Gilliam TB, MacConnie S. Energy expenditure in prepubescent children: influence of sex and age. *Am J Clin Nutr.* 1981;34:1827-1830.
6. Smith NJ. *Common Problems in Pediatric Sports Medicine.* Chicago, Ill: Year Book Medical Publishers Inc; 1989.
7. Sewall L, Micheli LJ. Strength training for children. *J Pediatr Orthop.* 1986;6:143.
8. Steban RE, Steben AH. The validity of the strength shortening cycle in selected jumping events. *J Sports Med Phys Fitness.* 1981;21:28.
9. Vrigena J. Muscle strength development in the pre- and postpubescent age. *Med Sci Sports Exerc.* 1978;11:152.
10. Weltman A, Janney C, Rians CB, et al. The effects of hydraulic resistance strength training in prepubescent males. *Med Sci Sports Exerc.* 1986;18:629.
11. Sale DG. Strength training in children. In: *Perspectives in Exercise Science and Sports Medicine.* Indianapolis, Ind: Benchmark Press; 1989;2.

Adolescence

Josephine Connolly Schoonen

▶ BODY COMPOSITION AND ENERGY BALANCE

Achieving weight and body-composition goals is of primary importance to adolescent athletes seeking to enhance competitiveness as well as social acceptance. Health-care professionals should help the adolescent athlete determine safe, realistic weight and body-composition goals based on objective data. Weight, height, and body-composition data should be measured and compared with normative data, such as body fat levels in male and female athletes participating in various sports.[1,2] In addition, the performance and training requirements of the sport should be considered. Although there is some subjectivity in the interpretation of these data, quantitative feedback is often superior to much of the information adolescents receive from the media and their peers. In addition, these methods separate health and performance issues from appearance and social issues. These latter issues often lead adolescent athletes to adopt unrealistic goals regarding weight loss and weight gain.

Athletes striving for the leanest body composition, such as wrestlers, gymnasts, dancers, and swimmers, are at the greatest risk for nutritional deficiencies. These athletes often restrict their energy intake severely, but do not have enough nutrition knowledge to plan their food intakes and meet their nutrition requirements. Studies suggest that adolescent gymnasts and young dancers consume diets that are not only low in kilocalories, but also low in nutrient density.[3] The combination of high nutrient and energy requirements to support growth and training and dietary self-restriction justifies monitoring these athletes for signs of dietary deficiencies and related health problems.[4] Furthermore, the training regimen for many of these athletes is primarily anaerobic, and involves repeated episodes of high-intensity, short-duration activities with alternating rest periods. Although this type of sport-specific skill or power training is effective in improving performance, it generally does not maximize energy expenditure for prolonged periods.

Adding aerobic exercise, such as 20- to 30-minute team running exercises, to the training program of the adolescent athlete engaged in power-type activities would facilitate maintenance of moderate to low body fat stores without excessive calorie restriction. Educating these athletes on the benefits of a high-carbohydrate, low-fat, nutrient-dense diet would also help to alleviate some of the observed nutrition-related problems.

Athletes participating in sports in which precompetition weigh-ins are required (wrestling, boxing, judo, weight lifting, lightweight rowers) commonly use methods that induce rapid, short-term weight loss, which may be dangerous.

113

Wrestlers' weight-loss techniques and eating behaviors have been studied extensively.[5-10] Methods of weight reduction usually include a combination of food and fluid restriction, as well as thermal- and exercise-induced dehydration.[5] Young wrestlers who use these extreme methods are typically lean, with body fat measurements ranging from 1.6% to 15.1% of their body weight; most wrestlers have less than 8% body fat.[5] Wrestlers typically fall into a weekly cycle of losing weight 2 to 4 days prior to a competition, and regaining weight beginning on the competition day and the following 2 to 4 days. This pattern has been called weight cycling.[11] Because the rapid weight loss associated with weight cycling is likely to cause a loss of lean tissue, the athlete's basal metabolic rate (BMR) is likely to decrease over time. This combination of lean tissue loss and lower BMR will make it more difficult for the athlete to maintain desirable weight with a normal intake of energy.

The medical community has warned against rapid weight loss resulting from food and fluid restriction and dehydration because of the potentially adverse physiological consequences.[5] These include:

▶ Impairment of thermoregulatory function
▶ Lower plasma and blood volumes
▶ Reduction in cardiac function during submaximal work conditions (associated with higher heart rates)
▶ Smaller stroke volumes
▶ Reduced cardiac output
▶ Loss of electrolytes
▶ Decreased renal blood flow
▶ Depletion of liver glycogen stores
▶ Decrease in work performance
▶ Decrease in muscular strength

Further, the potential for growth retardation exists, particularly when drastic food restriction coincides with the athlete's rapid growth periods. In spite of the multitude of problems that result from weight cycling, however, recommendations from health professionals have largely been ignored because many wrestlers do not believe that these physiological changes affect performance or long-term health.

While research advances in this area, health-care professionals should educate athletes who are self-restricting their dietary intake and striving to minimize body fat. Initially, educational messages should be directed at making the best food choices within self-imposed calorie limits so as not to alienate these athletes. Nutrient-dense, readily available foods should be emphasized so that adolescent athletes can meet their micronutrient requirements. For athletes on low-calorie diets, a multivitamin/mineral supplement with 50% to 100% of the RDAs may be warranted.

Information concerning appropriate weight goals based on body composition—and the caloric intake necessary to achieve and maintain those goals—should be gradually incorporated as the educator-athlete relationship develops. For males, the recommended minimum body fat level is 5% of total body weight, while the recommended minimum for females is 12% of total body weight.[1,5]

The energy RDAs for adolescent males and females, which do not account for extra energy expenditure resulting from training and competition, should be considered the minimum caloric intake to recommend for adolescent athletes. Ideally, health practitioners could predict adolescent athletes' energy requirements from resting energy expenditure (REE) equations and activity formulas to enhance the accuracy of the caloric requirement. Coaches and health-care professionals should encourage athletes who need to lose weight to begin weight-reduction programs before the season begins, or very early in the training season. A gradual weight change is desirable. The goal during the competitive season should be weight maintenance, not weight loss.

▶ IRON STATUS IN ADOLESCENT ATHLETES

Iron requirements are based on estimated storage levels, daily losses, and bioavailability of dietary iron. During adolescence, iron requirements also need to account for the increased demands for iron associated with rapid growth, such as expanding red cell mass, myoglobin deposits in enlarging muscle mass, increased iron losses associated with exercise (mainly via sweat and feces), and increased iron losses associated with menstruation in postpubescent females.[12] The first two demands tend to be greater in adolescent males than in females, and result in adolescent male requirements 2 mg higher than adult male requirements. Menstrual losses vary, but the female RDA of 15 mg iron is believed sufficient to meet the demands of growth and to replace menstrual losses.[12]

The body's total iron level can be divided into two categories[12]:

1. A functional iron pool in which iron is associated with hemoglobin, myoglobin, cytochromes, and other iron-containing structures.
2. A storage iron pool that makes up approximately 30% of the body's iron and is associated with ferritin and hemosiderin (mainly in the spleen, liver, and bone marrow), as well as with the transport protein, transferrin, found in the blood.

Iron deficiency is a progressive phenomenon, involving iron depletion, iron-deficient erythropoiesis, and iron-deficiency anemia. During the iron-depletion stage, iron stores in the liver and bone marrow decrease. Hemoglobin synthesis may not suffer if absorption of exogenous iron equals or exceeds iron losses, and reserves are not needed. If, however, iron losses exceed absorption of dietary iron, the individual enters the iron-deficient erythropoiesis stage. During this stage there is decreased hemoglobin production associated with increased free protoporphyrin, and decreased transferrin saturation. If not corrected, iron-deficiency anemia develops, and erythrocytes become microcytic and hypochromic.[13]

A variety of parameters are used to measure an individual's iron status. Indexes used to assess storage and transport iron include: serum ferritin, serum iron, percentage transferrin saturation, total iron-binding capacity (TIBC), and free erythrocyte protoporphyrin (FEP). Indexes used to assess functional iron status include: hemoglobin, hematocrit, packed cell volume (PCV), and mean corpuscular volume (MCV). The sensitivity and specificity of each of these measurements is limited by random and systematic error, as well as possible physiological conditions. Therefore, multiple measures suggesting a particular stage of iron-deficiency status allows for a stronger conclusion regarding iron status than one or two measures.

Iron losses in athletes may be greater than in sedentary people due to losses associated with the following[14]:

▶ Increased hemolysis due to increased mechanical intravascular red cell destruction (eg, foot-strike hemolysis)
▶ Increased sweating
▶ Increased gastrointestinal and urinary iron losses

Therefore, adolescents involved in contact sports or sports involving frequent impact with hard surfaces (running and gymnastics), as well as those frequently enduring severe dehydration (eg, wrestlers), may experience rather large iron losses. If these athletes also follow weight-loss diets, their risk of iron depletion is greatly increased.

Iron-deficiency anemia affects performance by limiting the delivery of oxygen to working tissues. At rest this may be compensated for by increased cardiac output. However, with the extra demands of exercise, it becomes increasingly difficult to compensate for the suboptimal oxygen-carrying capacity of the blood by simply increasing cardiac output. This is especially true with exercise in hot, humid environments, and with exercise in a dehydrated state. Earlier stages of iron deficiency may exert an independent effect on performance by impairing processes governed by iron-containing oxidative enzymes, such as adenosine triphosphate (ATP) production at the cellular level. The precise degree of iron depletion at which these effects may occur is presently unknown.[15,16]

Sports anemia is a vague term that has been used to describe hemoglobin concentrations less than those that are optimal for oxygen delivery in athletes. Unfortunately, an optimal hemoglobin level to maximize oxygen delivery during exercise has not been agreed upon, and is muddled by such factors as hematocrit levels and blood viscosity changes. Sports anemia is not synonymous with clinical anemia, because hemoglobin values may be normal, and the erythrocytes may be normocytic and normochromic. In addition, hemoglobin values may fall in response to sudden, large increases in training intensity or duration, and then normalize after an adaptation period.[17]

Dietary, exercise, and weight-management habits of adolescents (in combination with their increased iron requirement) warrants surveillance of dietary iron intake and iron status. Athletes restricting their calorie intake or obtaining a high percentage of their calories from low-nutrient-dense foods are at an increased risk for iron depletion or iron deficiency. The RDA for iron intake for females 11 to 50 years of age was reduced from 18 to 15 mg per day by the National Research Council.[12] Research to date indicates that 15 mg per day is sufficient to replace menstrual losses for most women, and that those with high menstrual losses appear to compensate for those losses with improved absorption of dietary iron. The RDA for adolescent males aged 11 to 18 years remains at 12 mg per day. In a study conducted from 1982 to 1989, daily intakes of iron were estimated for females and males aged 14 to 16 years. It was estimated that, on average, females in this group consumed 11.0 mg per day and males 18.1 mg per day of iron.[18] Iron deficiency (serum ferritin less than 12 g/dL) has been reported in 20% to 24% of adolescent females and 12% of adolescent males.[19] Many athletes do not become deficient until well into the competitive season, demonstrating the need for periodic testing.[20]

Iron supplements will improve iron nutriture in athletes with iron deficiency, and thereby can improve their exercise performance.[21,22] Dietary intakes of protein, vitamin B_{12}, and folic acid should also be assessed, since these nutrients are required for hemoglobin synthesis. If iron supplements are used for prevention of iron deficiency, RDA levels are recommended. All athletes should be encouraged to eat foods high in vitamin C (such as citrus fruits or juice, tomatoes, and peppers) with meals, and to avoid coffee or tea consumption with meals to maximize the absorption of nonheme iron found in plant foods.

► WATER

For any athlete, the primary nutrient requiring replacement before, during, or after exercise is water. The adolescent athlete does not differ from athletes of other ages in this respect. The key to achieving adequate hydration is *planned water intake*. The following schedule of fluid intake is recommended[23]:

- ► Two hours before the event, drink 16 oz water or a nonfat, noncarbonated beverage, such as Gatorade* or Exceed.†
- ► During the half hour before the event, drink 8 to 12 oz fluid.
- ► During the event, drink 4 to 8 oz of fluid every 15 to 20 minutes.
- ► After the event, the athlete should drink additional fluids to replace those lost during the event. The general guide is 16 oz (1 pint) of fluid for every 1-lb loss of body weight.
- ► Some substances, including caffeine- and alcohol-containing beverages, have a dehydrating effect and should be avoided.

Appropriate fluid replacement before, during, and after exercise is the primary prevention step an athlete can take to reduce the risk of heat injury during training and competition. For this reason, health professionals should make appropriate fluid consumption a major topic of conversation during educational opportunities with athletes.

► PROTEIN

Athletes do require more dietary protein than nonathletes to maintain positive nitrogen balance. This increased requirement may be due to changes in amino acid metabolism, or to insufficient energy intake that necessitates the use of amino acids for energy rather than synthesis of proteins. Increased protein requirements have been documented for individuals beginning a training program and for experienced endurance athletes.[24,25] For those beginning a training program, the increased protein requirement is thought to be necessary to minimize loss of blood proteins. In the experienced athlete, it is thought to be necessary as an energy substrate or for muscle repair.[26] If an athlete is not meeting the energy requirement through adequate consumption of carbohydrates and fats, protein requirements are further increased.[27]

Recommendations for dietary protein intake for adolescent athletes range from 1.2 to 2.0 g/kg body weight, as compared with 0.8 to 1.0 g/kg body weight listed in the RDA for adolescents.[23,28] The approximate breakdown of protein needs (based on 1.2 g protein per kilogram body weight) for a 70-kg (154-lb) male adolescent athlete is as follows:

28.7 g	Replacement of obligatory nitrogen loss in urine, feces, skin, and other sites (assuming largest loss)
8.6 g	Allowance for individual variation (30%)
4.8 g	Allowance for growth (assuming most rapid growth)
7.5 g	Replacement of nitrogen lost in sweat during 4 hours of vigorous exercise
6.3 g	Allowance for increased muscle mass, as during some kinds of training
8.6 g	Allowance for use of low biological value protein (nonanimal sources)
19.8 g	Allowance for use of protein for energy during vigorous exercise.
84.3 g	**Total estimated protein requirement = 1.2 g/kg per day**

---

*Quaker Oats Co, Chicago, IL 60654.

†Ross Laboratories, Columbus, OH 43216.

This amount of protein is easily obtained by an athlete eating a typically high-protein American diet. The recommended caloric intake for athletes ranges from 45 to 70 kcal/kg body weight.

The following example shows protein requirement calculations for a 70-kg athlete consuming 45 kcal/kg or 3150 kcal per day, with 12% to 15% of total calories as the lower and upper limits for protein intake:

1. *Lower limit of calories derived from protein* = 12% of total calories = 0.12 × 3150 = 378 kcal
   Upper limit of calories derived from protein = 15% of total calories = 0.15 × 3150 = 472.5 kcal
2. *Lower limit of daily protein requirement in grams* = 378/4 = 94.5 g protein needed to supply 378 kcal
   Upper limit of protein requirement in grams = 472.5/4 = 118.1 g protein needed to supply 472.5 kcal
3. *Lower limit of protein in grams required per kilogram of body weight for a 70-kg athlete* = 94.5/70 = 1.35 g
   Upper limit of protein in grams required per kilogram of body weight for a 70-kg athlete = 118.1/70 = 1.7 g
4. The protein requirement for a 70-kg athlete consuming 45 kcal/kg, using 12% to 15% of total calories as a guide, is 1.35 to 1.7 g protein per kilogram per day.

To relate these figures to actual food intake, consider the food items in *Table 3.7*, which total 198.9 g protein and 2777 kcal. When complemented with fruits, vegetables, other carbohydrates and condiments, these foods would contribute to a high-calorie, high-protein meal plan. This meal plan would more than satisfy the needs of any athlete with protein requirements at the higher range of recommended levels due to rapid growth and a rigorous training schedule.

For those adolescent athletes not consuming sufficient calories, the appropriate distribution of calories among protein, carbohydrates, and fats—or the appropriate absolute amount of protein—remains questionable. A high-carbohydrate, energy-restricted diet with moderate amounts of protein (0.8 g protein per kilogram body weight) may be associated with negative nitrogen balance. This indicates that protein is being used as an energy substrate, and the ability to increase (or even maintain) muscle mass would be impaired. On the other hand, a low-carbohydrate, energy-restricted diet with high amounts of protein (1.6 g per kilogram body weight) has been associated with a positive nitrogen balance but reduced muscular endurance.[27] Therefore, athletes not consuming enough calories are likely to impair muscle growth and

TABLE 3.7   Selected Food Items Totaling 198.9 g Protein and 2777 kcal

	Protein, g
5 glasses 1% milk	32.1
2 cups Life* cereal	16.2
2 slices whole wheat toast	4.8
2 tuna sandwiches	59.0
20 french fries	3.5
1 bagel and 2 tbsp peanut butter	15.1
6 oz chicken	52.8
1.5 cups rice	6.0
1 cup broccoli	4.6
1 cup ice cream	4.8
Total protein, g	198.9

*Quaker Oats Co, Chicago, Ill 60654.

maintenance, or muscular endurance. In either case, performance would be negatively affected.

In summary, when educating adolescent athletes about protein consumption, the following points should be emphasized:

▶ Athletes must plan their meals to ensure that they are eating enough calories.

▶ Consuming enough protein is easily achieved from foods commonly available.

▶ Excess dietary protein is stored as fat, and may decrease muscular endurance if high-carbohydrate foods are not consumed.

▶ When consuming large amounts of protein, maintaining a proper hydration state is critically important.

▶ It is important to compare the protein content of foods with the protein content of protein and amino acid supplements because many adolescent athletes do not realize that a glass of milk or a can of tuna has more protein than most supplements.

▶ A high-carbohydrate diet can prevent the excessive breakdown of protein for use as an energy source, and it allows protein to function as it was intended to—as an anabolic nutrient.

▶ VITAMINS AND MINERALS

To date, there is no documented advantage to athletes whose vitamins and mineral intake exceeds the RDAs.[28] The same is generally true for electrolytes (sodium, potassium, magnesium and chloride), which are essential minerals. The amount of electrolytes young athletes lose in sweat can usually be replenished by consuming a well-balanced diet. Long-duration activity, however, can greatly increase the loss of various electrolytes, particularly sodium. For example, sweat contains about 45 mEq sodium per liter. Assuming an hourly sweat loss of 1.5 L, an athlete can lose upward of 200 mEq sodium in 3 hours of exercise. When coupled with normal urinary sodium losses, an athlete can lose in excess of 10 to 12 g sodium per day.

Young athletes with marginal nutrient stores may benefit from increased dietary intake of nutrients, but this is a result of improving the deficiency state, not an independent, beneficial effect on performance. Due to the close relationship between caloric intake and vitamin and mineral intake, the major group of athletes at risk for inadequate micronutrient intakes is made up of athletes who are limiting their caloric intake. Athletes avoiding a whole food group, such as milk products or meats, may also be at risk. If, after receiving nutrition education, these athletes still fail to consume a well-balanced diet with adequate calories, a multivitamin/mineral supplement providing less than or equal to RDA levels for essential nutrients may be appropriate to ensure adequate nutriture.[29]

▶ EXERCISE AND MENSTRUAL ABNORMALITIES

The influence of exercise on the menstrual cycle of female athletes is difficult to assess since several variables associated with this life-style (such as dietary intake, calorie balance, type of exercise, and intensity of exercise) may affect endocrine function.[30] Some female athletes may menstruate regularly, but have reduced progesterone secretion and a short luteal phase. It is not clear if this hormonal pattern affects an athlete's fertility or her susceptibility to osteoporosis or cancer.[30] New experimental protocols and statistical methods for analyzing pulsatile hormonal secretions are being applied to the questions surrounding menstrual irregularities in athletes. Female athletes should be aware that, despite amenorrhea, ovulation may occur and pregnancy is possible.[11]

▶ OTHER FACTORS INFLUENCING THE ADOLESCENT ATHLETE'S DIET

Nutrition knowledge, food practices, food or diet fads, time management, and availability of preferred food choices are other factors that influence the adolescent athlete's diet. With active participation in sports, especially for intense training in one or two sports, time for meals and snacks may be competing with practice, competition, and regular classroom time. Meals and snacks may be skipped or abbreviated because of time pressures. Thus, for the dietitian or coach working with young athletes, it may be particularly helpful to explore ways of achieving healthful food choices "on the run." Athletes need to be encouraged to bring snacks with them to school, since the food choices generally available from vending machines or concession stands may not add to the overall nutrient quality of their diet. Bagels, pretzels, dry cereal, fruit, dried fruit, fruit juice, or nuts eaten between classes or after school will add to the overall nutrient quality of the young athlete's diet. In addition, these foods can be easily assembled the night before, and do not require refrigeration.

Monitoring an adolescent's interest in a diet or nutrition fad, and a diplomatic discussion of the fad, will be pertinent in some situations. Consider these additional factors when counseling the adolescent:

▶ Family income or food-budget limitations
▶ Family schedule (who purchases or prepares food at home?)
▶ Location of meals and snacks (home, school, or restaurant)

The professional counselor should also consider these factors occurring during adolescence:

▶ Growth, sexual maturation, and psychosocial development
▶ Increase in sports participation through increased variety and/or intensity of activities pursued
▶ Exposure to an increasingly demanding school and social schedule
▶ Peer influence
▶ Transition to adulthood

REFERENCES

1. McArdle WD, Katch FI, Katch VL. *Exercise Physiology, Energy, Nutrition, and Human Performance.* 2nd ed. Philadelphia, Pa: Lea & Febiger; 1986:488.
2. Wilmore JH. In: *Sports Medicine for Children and Youth: Report of 10th Ross Roundtable on Approaches to Common Pediatric Problems.* Columbus, Ohio: Ross Laboratories; 1979.
3. Calabrese LH. Nutritional and medical aspects of gymnastics. *Clin Sports Med.* 1985;4(1):23.
4. Benardot D, Czerwinski C. Selected body composition and growth measures of junior elite gymnasts. *J Am Diet Assoc.* 1991;91:29-33.
5. American College of Sports Medicine. Position stand on weight loss in wrestlers. *Med Sci Sports Exerc.* 1976;8:11-13.
6. Houston ME, Marrin DA, Green HJ, Thomson JA. The effect of rapid weight loss on physiological functions in wrestlers. *Phys Sports Med.* 1981;9:73-78.
7. Klinzing JE, Karpowicz W. The effects of rapid weight loss and rehydration on a wrestling performance test. *J Sports Med Phys Fitness.* 1986;26:149-156.

8. Morgan WP. Psychological effect of weight reduction in the college wrestler. *Med Sci Sports Exerc.* 1970;2:24-27.

9. Serfass RC, Stull GA, Alexander JF, Weing JL. The effects of rapid weight loss and attempted rehydration on strength and endurance of the handgripping muscle in college wrestlers. *Res Quar.* 1984;55:46-52.

10. Tipton CM. Commentary: physicians should advise wrestlers about weight loss. *Phys Sports Med.* 1987;15:160.

11. Smith NJ. Some health care needs of young athletes. *Adv Pediatr.* 1981;28:187.

12. National Research Council. *Recommended Dietary Allowances.* 10th ed. Washington, DC: National Academy Press; 1989:195-205.

13. Hillman RS, Finch CA. *Red Cell Manual.* 5th ed. Philadelphia, Pa: FA Davis; 1985.

14. Hallberg L, Magnusson B. The etiology of anemia. *Acta Med Scand.* 1984;216:145.

15. Newhouse IJ, Clement DB, Taunton JE, McKenzie DC. The effects of prelatent/latent iron deficiency on physical work capacity. *Med Sci Sports Exerc.* 1989;21:263.

16. Van Swearingen J. Iron deficiency in athletes: consequences or adaptation in strenuous activity. *J Orthop Sports Phys Ther.* 1986;7:192.

17. Puhl J. Iron and exercise interactions. *Contemp Nutr.* 1987;12:1.

18. Pennington JAT, Young BE. Total diet study nutritional elements, 1982 - 1989. *J Am Diet Assoc.* 1991;91:179.

19. Rowland TW, Block SA, Kelleher JF. Iron deficiency in adolescent endurance athletes. *J Adolesc Health Care.* 1987;8:322-326.

20. Risser WL, Lee EJ, et al. Iron deficiency in female athletes: its prevalence and impact on performance. *Med Sci Sports Exerc.* 1988;20:116-121.

21. Haymes EM. Nutritional concerns: need for iron. *Med Sci Sports Exerc.* 1987;19:S197-S200.

22. Sherman AR, Kramer B. Iron nutrition and exercise. In: Hickson JE, Wolisky, eds. *Nutrition in Exercise and Sports.* Boca Raton, Fla: CRC Press, Inc; 1989:291-300.

23. Williams MH. *Nutrition for Fitness and Sport.* 3rd ed. Dubuque, Iowa: Wm C Brown Publishers; 1992.

24. Butterfield GE. Whole-body protein utilization in humans. *Med Sci Sports Exerc.* 1987;19(suppl 5):S157-S165.

25. Tarnopolsky MA, MacDougall JD, Atkinson SA. Influence of protein intake and training status on nitrogen balance and lean mass. *J Appl Physiol.* 1988;64:187-193.

26. Lemon PWR. Nutrition for muscular development of young athletes. In: Gisolfi CV, Lamb DR, eds. *Perspectives in Exercise Science and Sports Medicine.* Indianapolis, Ind: Benchmark Press; 1989;2.

27. Walberg JL, Leidy MK, Sturgill DJ, Hinkle DE, Ritchey SJ, Sebolt DR. Macronutrient content of a hypoenergy diet affects nitrogen retention and muscle function in weight lifters. *Int J Sports Med.* 1988;9:261-266.

28. The American Dietetic Association. Nutrition for physical fitness and athletic performance for adults: technical support paper. *J Am Diet Assoc.* 1987;87:932.

29. Belko AZ. Vitamins and exercise: an update. *Med Sci Sports Exerc.* 1987;19:S191.

30. Loucks AB. Effects of exercise training on the menstrual cycle: existence and mechanisms. *Med Sci Sports Exerc.* 1990;22(3):275-280.

Adult Years

Connie Mueller

▶ MIDDLE-AGED ADULTS

Most physiologic standards of fitness and performance tend to peak between the late teens and 30 years of age.[1] After age 30, various markers of metabolic and cardiorespiratory fitness begin to decline (see *Figures 3.1* and *3.2*). This does not imply, however, that adults who undertake an exercise training program after age 30 cannot make significant performance gains. On the contrary, it is well established that, regardless of age, chronic physical activity can produce significant, measurable improvements in fitness.[2] What is still debatable, however, is whether habitual exercise can slow the rate of decline in physiologic function that routinely occurs with advancing age. More long-term research studies are required before this question can be answered with any degree of certainty.

The adult who exercises will enjoy a variety of benefits in addition to the previously alluded to physiologic benefits (greater flexibility, increased muscle strength and endurance, improved cardiovascular fitness). In general, exercising adults can expect to be able to:

▶ eat more and weigh less,
▶ maintain a greater lean body mass,
▶ improve their serum lipid profile (eg, increase HDL, decrease total cholesterol), and
▶ improve or maintain bone density.[3]

With respect to dietary needs, the high-carbohydrate, low-fat, moderate-protein diet that is recommended for athletes may be particularly important for the exercising adult. The third edition of the *Dietary Guidelines for Americans* recommends this type of diet to enhance health maintenance.[4,5]

The adult years are a time when preventive measures, including sound dietary practices, may delay the onset of chronic health problems such as coronary artery disease, hypertension, diabetes, obesity, and cancer. New evidence suggests that a comprehensive life-style change, one that incorporates moderate exercise and a low-fat diet (as well as smoking cessation and stress management), may actually produce regression of atherosclerotic plaque and decrease the risk of heart attack.[6] A study conducted by Ornish and colleagues incorporated a diet high in complex carbohydrates (70% to 75% of calories), low in fat (10% of calories), and moderate in protein (15% to 20% of calories).[7] Calories were not restricted. The study found a decline in plaque formation. The large number of variables that were manipulated makes it difficult to ascertain the relative importance of any single dietary or life-style change. Nonetheless, this study does demonstrate that the adoption of a more healthful

FIGURE 3.1   Decline in various human functional capacities with increasing age.

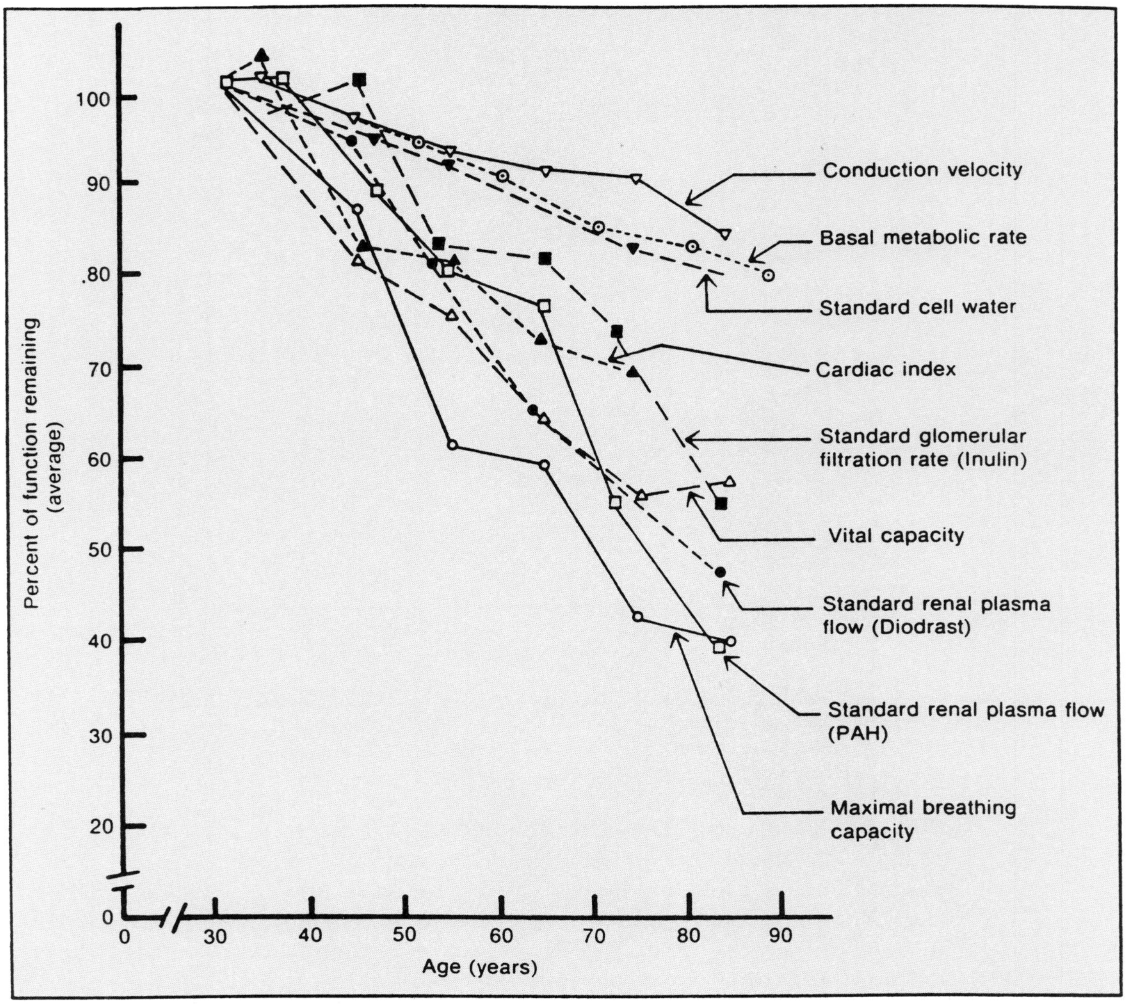

Values are adjusted so that the value at age 30 equals 100%. Adapted by permission of the publisher from Shock NW. Physical activity and the rate of aging. *Can Med Assoc J.* 1967;96:836.

life-style during the adult years has the potential to decrease disease risk.

Promotion of positive life-style changes should be a primary role of the sports nutritionist. Exercise and a healthful diet are, obviously, two important life-style changes that should be stressed. One word of caution: The American College of Sports Medicine suggests that adults over the age of 35 should undergo a medical evaluation, which preferably includes a stress test, before beginning an exercise program.[6] Health professionals should keep this recommendation in mind when working with adult clients.

► OLDER ADULTS

Sports participation can be an important and healthful part of the adult years. The beneficial effects of exercise for adults include cardiovascular fitness, increased flexibility, muscular strength, endurance, and a heightened sense of well-being. Although many adults enjoy exercise as a means of staying fit, others resort to exercise only after a catastrophic illness has forced them to consider their past life-style. An increased life expectancy has resulted in a

FIGURE 3.2   Body composition changes as a function of age.

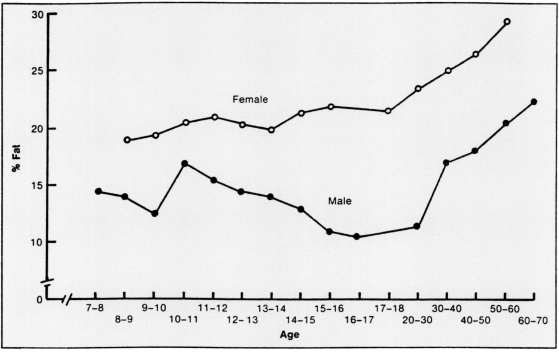

From Parizkova J. Body composition and exercise during growth and development. In: Rarick GL, ed. *Physical Activity: Human Growth and Development.* New York, NY: Academic Press; 1974. Used by permission.

rapid growth of population over the age of 75.[1] Exercise may be one of the strategies to prevent very old people from becoming "frail elderly."[2]

Little nutrition information is available for adult athletes aged 60 years and older. The nutritional requirements of the middle-aged athlete (below age 50) can be estimated by using the Recommended Dietary Allowances (RDAs). Recommendations for older persons, however, can be made only by extrapolation from the RDA data. The heterogeneity of this population has hampered the establishment of a separate RDA. Not only are degrees of mobility, activity level, and general health remarkably varied among older individuals, but 80% of the population aged 65 and older are estimated to have one or more diagnosed diseases. Added to that, the elderly population takes twice as many drugs as the general population.[4]

For the healthy adult, a high-carbohydrate, low-fat, moderate-protein diet similar to the US Department of Agriculture Dietary Guidelines will meet most nutrient requirements. It is important when counseling the older adult, however, to take into consideration the predisposition to, or presence of, any chronic disease conditions. Conditions such as adult-onset diabetes, hypertension, heart disease, arteriosclerosis, obesity, and back problems frequently manifest themselves during later years and can affect nutrient requirements. Further alterations in diet may be necessary to accommodate the physical stress and changes in metabolism that occur during exercise or as a result of exercise.

With aging, there are unavoidable changes in body composition and function. There is a reduction in lean body mass and an increase in body fat. Aging also appears to be associated with a greater atrophy of type II muscle fibers, than of type I muscle fibers.[6] This suggests that the strength of muscles involved in high-intensity movements tends to decrease, while the strength of muscles associated with maintaining posture and most low-intensity activities is more closely maintained.[8]

It is theorized that with aging, lean body mass may be replaced, in part, by metabolically inactive tissue.[9] Basal metabolic rate and strength tend to decrease as the proportion of lean body mass decreases.[10] Neural function and nerve conduction diminish. Aging affects the ability to detect a stimulus and process information; however, active older adults tend to maintain better neural response times than their sedentary counterparts. In this respect, exercise apparently slows the rate of decline that naturally occurs with age.

The energy requirements of the adult athlete will decrease over time due to the loss of lean body mass, even though the energy requirements for exercise do not change. Exercise training in the elderly has no apparent effect on age-related decreases in BMR.[11] As with younger active people, the energy needs for the active elderly should be determined with consideration given to age, type of activity, and time spent engaged in the activity.

Exercise in conjunction with weight loss is beneficial in lowering serum cholesterol, LDL cholesterol, and triglycerides, and in raising serum HDL-cholesterol levels.[12] In this respect, elderly people do not differ significantly from their younger counterparts. Exercise training has been shown to produce a more favorable lipid profile in elderly clients who participate in an exercise program.[13]

The well-nourished exercising adult generally will not require additional nutrients, except during exercise sessions of long duration and during exercise in hot weather.[14] Older adults exercising in endurance activities may benefit from a modified carbohydrate-loading regimen, unless certain disease-specific conditions exist.

Protein needs of elderly people may be higher than the RDA of 0.8 g protein per kilogram per day, but probably do not exceed average dietary intake.[15] The _____ on the protein needs of elderly people is unknown. Endurance ____ ages may have an increased requirement for some or all of the essential amino acids.[16] During and immediately following endurance exercise, hormonal changes may favor amino acid uptake by skeletal muscle.[17] However, more research is required before definitive protein guidelines for the active elderly are established.

Dehydration and heat-related injuries are a greater risk for the elderly than for younger individuals. Lowered renal function and a decreased ability to concentrate urine contribute to the increased incidence of dehydration. This leads to an impaired ability to maintain body temperature during exercise in hot, humid conditions.[18] Therefore, additional fluid replacement will be required before, during, and after exercise in hot weather. Since the sense of thirst may also decrease with aging, particular attention to hydration status during and after exercise is necessary.

More than 60% of Americans over the age of 65 have high blood pressure, and about 30% have heart disease.[15] Individuals who are taking diuretics or vasodilators for treatment of hypertension or cardiovascular conditions are at increased risk for dehydration.[19] In this regard, it should be remembered that a 3% loss of plasma volume can interfere with performance, a 5% loss will cause signs of heat exhaustion, a 7% loss may cause hallucinations, and a 10% loss may result in heat stroke and death.

Exercise increases insulin sensitivity and improves glucose tolerance.[20] Regular exercise may prevent age-related changes in insulin resistance and glucose tolerance.[21] Individuals with diabetes mellitus may require adjustment in the composition and timing of their meals and insulin to account for metabolic changes induced by exercise.[22] Most important, individuals with diabetes should always have a source of easily digested carbohydrate readily available in case hypoglycemia occurs.

Rheumatic disease prevents many people from participating in sports or exercise. These individuals should be encouraged to remain as active as possible to maintain flexibility and strength. During acute flare-ups of arthritis or rheumatic conditions, exercise should be mild or avoided until pain and swelling subside. For this population, weight control is especially important, because excess weight places an unnecessary burden on the weight-bearing joints. Swimming may be a good exercise modality for people with rheumatic conditions.

A decreased appetite and the tendency of elderly people to avoid dairy products (due to an inability to tolerate lactose) contribute to low calcium intakes.[23] Further compromising calcium status are the kidneys' reduced synthesis of calcitriol (the active form of vitamin D) and the decreased calcium absorption in the intestine, both of which are associated with aging.[15] Although controversial, the 1989 RDA for calcium was retained at 800 mg for postmenopausal women.[5] For women over age 50 with risk of osteoporosis, higher levels of calcium, as well as estrogen therapy, may be prescribed. For individuals ingesting a calcium supplement, calcium carbonate—the most common calcium supplement—should be taken at least 2 hours before or after other drug administrations, or at least 2 hours before or after consuming a meal with a high mineral content.[24] When calcium supplements are used, fluid intake of at least 2 L of water per day should be encouraged to decrease the potential for constipation.[14,15] For those taking supplements in excess of 600 mg per day, other side effects may include abnormal heart contractions, kidney stones, and altered absorption of iron and zinc.[14] Ideally, foods should be selected to provide sufficient calcium so that supplements are not necessary. An adequate intake of calcium coupled with a regular exercise program can reduce the risk of bone disease.

Vitamin requirements do not appear to change with aging, although some studies indicate that many elderly populations do not ingest adequate amounts of vitamins and minerals.[25,26] Little is known about the effects of physical activity on metabolism or the RDA for various vitamins in the elderly; however, the expectation is that a balanced diet should be adequate to cover any increased needs associated with exercise.[27] Further, active people tend to get more exposure to sun, thus enhancing vitamin D synthesis.[28] Drug therapy for many chronic diseases can also alter the absorption, digestion, and metabolism of certain vitamins.

When a diet history reveals a caloric intake of less than 1500 kcal per day or a diet low in overall nutrient content, a multivitamin supplement may be indicated. The older athlete should avoid taking unprescribed doses of any vitamin or mineral higher than the RDA, however, due to the possible toxic effects of a food or drug interaction.

Exercise increases the rate of blood flow and consequently the level of muscle and organ perfusion. Special attention should be given to persons who are new to exercise, or have just started drug therapy, or both. The metabolism and therapeutic effect of the drug may be altered due to changes in organ perfusion and subsequent clearance of the drug.[29]

Although the biological effects of aging change the body's response to exercise, regular vigorous physical activity produces physiologic improvement regardless of one's age. Therefore, exercise participation by the elderly should be encouraged. However, proper medical screening is strongly advised before an elderly individual embarks on a physical exercise program.

REFERENCES

1. National Center for Health Statistics. *Health, United States, 1987*. Washington, DC: US Govt Printing Office; 1988. US Dept of Health and Human Services publication (PHS) 88-1232.
2. Fiatarone MA, Marks EC, Ryan NC, et al. High-intensity strength training in nonagenarians: effects on skeletal muscle. *JAMA*. 1990;263:3029.
3. Blair SN, Clark DG, Cureton KJ, Powell KE. Exercise and fitness in childhood: implications for a lifetime of health. In: Gisolfi CV, Lamb DR, eds. *Perspectives in Exercise Science and Sports Medicine*. Indianapolis, Ind: Benchmark Press; 1989;2.
4. Hegsted DM. Recommended dietary intakes of elderly subjects. *Am J Clin Nutr*. 1989;50:1190.
5. National Research Council, Food and Nutrition Board. *Recommended Dietary Allowances*. 10th ed. Washington, DC: National Academy Press; 1989.
6. Evans WJ, Meredith CN. Exercise and nutrition in the elderly. In: Munro HN, Danford DE, eds. *Nutrition, Aging, and the Elderly*. New York, NY: Plenum Publishing Corp; 1989.
7. Ornish D, Brown SE, Scherwitz LW, et al. Can lifestyle changes reverse coronary heart disease? The lifestyle heart trial. *Lancet*. 1990;336:129.
8. Larsson L. Histochemical characteristics of human skeletal muscle during aging. *Acta Physiol Scand*. 1983;117:469.
9. Mayre LG, et al. A forty-year study of lean body mass in aging man. *Fed Proc*. 1985;44:620.
10. Tzankoff SP, Norris AH. Effect of muscle mass decrease on age-related BMR changes. *J Appl Physiol*. 1977;32:1001.
11. Lundholm K, Holm G, Lindmark B, Larsson B, Sjostrom L, Bjorntorp P. Thermogenic effect of food in physically well-trained elderly men. *Eur J Appl Physiol*. 1986;55:486.
12. Tran ZV, Weltman A. Differential effects of exercise on serum lipid and lipoprotein levels seen with changes in body weight: a meta-analysis. *JAMA*. 1985;254:919.
13. Reaven PD, McPhillips JB, Barrett-Connor EL, Criqui MH. Leisure time exercise and lipid and lipoprotein levels in an older population. *J Am Geriatr Soc*. 1990;38:847.
14. Williams MH. *Nutrition for Fitness and Sport*. 3rd ed. Dubuque, Iowa: Wm C Brown Publishers; 1992.
15. US Dept of Health and Human Services, Public Health Service. *The Surgeon General's Report on Nutrition and Health*. Washington, DC: US Govt Printing Office; 1988. DHHS publication (PHS) 88-50210.
16. Evans WJ, Fisher EC, Hoerr RA, Young VR. Protein metabolism and endurance exercise. *Phys Sports Med*. 1983;11:64.
17. Zorzano A, Balon T, Garetto LP, Goodman MN, Ruderman NB. Muscle alpha-aminoisobutyric acid transport after exercise: enhanced stimulation by insulin. *Am J Physiol*. 1985;248:E546.
18. Philips PA, Rolls BJ, Ledingham JG, et al. Reduced thirst after water deprivation in healthy elderly men. *N Engl J Med*. 1984;311:754.
19. Nadel ER. Recent advances in temperature regulation during exercise in humans. *Fed Proc*. 1985;44(7):2286.
20. Holloszy JO, Skinner S, Toro G, Cureton TK. Effects of a six-month program of endurance exercise on the serum lipids of middle-aged men. *Am J Cardiol*. 1964;14:753.
21. Rosenthal M, Haskell WL, Solomon R, Widstrom A, Reaven GM. Demonstration of a relationship between level of physical training and insulin-stimulated glucose utilization in normal humans. *Diabetes*. 1983;32:408.
22. Barnard RJ, Massey MR, Cherny S, O'Brien LT, Pritikin N. Long-term use of high-complex-carbohydrate, high-fiber, low-fat diet and exercise in the treatment of NIDDM patients. *Diabetes Care*. 1983;6:268-273.
23. Sellery SB. New product opportunities: diet food for older Americans. *J Nutr Elderly*. 1984;4:31.
24. Murray JJ, Healy MD. Drug mineral interactions: a new responsibility for the hospital dietitian. *J Am Diet Assoc*. 1991;91(1):66.
25. Garry PJ, Goodwin JS, Hunt WC, Gilbert BS. Nutritional status in a healthy elderly population: vitamin C. *Am J Clin Nutr*. 1982;36:332.

26. Bren M, Bauernfund JC. Vitamin needs of the elderly. *Postgrad Med.* 1978;633:155.
27. Williams MH. Vitamin and mineral supplements to athletes: do they help? *Clin Sports Med.* 1984;3:623.
28. Nelson ME, Meredith CN, Dawson-Hughes B, Evans WJ. Hormone and bone mineral status in endurance-trained and sedentary postmenopausal women. *J Clin Endocrinol Metab.* 1988;66:927.
29. Greenblatt DJ, Sellers EM, Shader RI. Drug disposition in old age. *N Engl J Med.* 1982;306:1081.

Cardiovascular Disease*

Meg Binnie Molloy

Although the incidence of coronary heart disease (CHD) has decreased since the late 1960s, CHD remains the leading cause of death in the United States. The prevalence and economic cost of CHD are enormous, with almost 66 million Americans affected. The American Heart Association estimates that the cost of heart disease in 1989 was $88.2 billion.[1]

▶ RISK FACTORS

A risk factor for CHD is defined as a trait that increases the probability that some form of cardiovascular disease (CVD) will develop.[2] The identified risk factors are:

▶ Statistical correlates of CHD
▶ Modifiable and unmodifiable factors that cause CHD
▶ Personal characteristics that predispose a person to CHD

Well-established risk factors for CVD include[3]:

▶ Cigarette smoking
▶ High blood pressure
▶ High blood cholesterol
▶ Diabetes mellitus

Other, less well-established risk factors for CVD include[3]:

▶ Physical inactivity
▶ Obesity
▶ Stress
▶ Certain drugs

Risk factors can be classified as modifiable or unmodifiable. Unmodifiable risk factors include:

▶ Family history
▶ Gender
▶ Hormonal factors that are genetically prescribed
▶ Age

Modifiable risk factors include:

---

*Information for this section is derived mainly from the ADA publication *Cardiovascular Disease: Nutrition for Prevention and Treatment.* Kris-Etherton PM, ed. Chicago, Ill: The American Dietetic Association; 1990. For a more in-depth treatment of the issues regarding cardiovascular disease, the reader is advised to consult that publication.

129

▶ Blood lipids
▶ Blood pressure
▶ Weight
▶ Diabetes
▶ Cigarette smoking
▶ Physical activity
▶ Stress
▶ Personality profile
▶ Oral contraceptive use

Dietitians and other health professionals can play an important role in helping clients to alter their modifiable risk factors in a positive manner.

▶ PREVENTION AND TREATMENT OF CVD BY DIET

The dietitian can do much to help people understand how to eat to promote health and reduce the risk of CHD. Dietary modifications can do much to reduce serum cholesterol, thereby reducing the risk of morbidity and mortality from CHD. Dietary recommendations for the prevention of CHD were released by the American Heart Association in 1986.[4] These recommendations, which follow, are intended to reduce blood lipids and hypertension:

1. Dietary saturated fatty acids should be less than 10% of total calories.
2. Total fat should be less than 30% of calories.
3. Cholesterol intake should be less than 100 mg per 1000 kcal, not to exceed 300 mg per day.
4. Protein should contribute approximately 15% of calories.
5. Carbohydrate should contribute 50% to 55% or more of calories, with an emphasis on complex carbohydrates.
6. The sodium intake should be reduced to 1 g per 1000 kcal, not to exceed 3 g per day.
7. If alcoholic beverages are consumed, intake should be limited to 15% of total calories, not to exceed 50 mL of ethanol per day.
8. Total calories should be sufficient to maintain a desirable body weight.
9. A variety of foods is recommended.

The National Research Council's Committee on Diet and Health recently proposed dietary guidelines for maintaining health and reducing chronic disease risk (including risk of CHD). These guidelines are based on a critical review of the scientific evidence, and are similar to the guidelines put forward by the American Heart Association. The committee's guidelines follow:

▶ Reduce total fat intake to 30% or less of calories. Reduce saturated-fatty-acid intake to less than 10% of calories and the intake of cholesterol to less than 300 mg daily. The intake of fat and cholesterol can be reduced by substituting fish, poultry without skin, lean meats, and low-fat or nonfat dairy products for fatty meats and whole-milk dairy products; by choosing more vegetables, fruits, cereals, and legumes; and by limiting oils, fats, egg yolks, fried foods, and other fatty foods.
▶ Every day eat five or more servings of a combination of vegetables and fruits, especially green and yellow vegetables and citrus fruits. Also, increase intake of starches and other complex carbohydrates by eating six or more daily servings of a combination of breads, cereals, and legumes.
▶ Maintain protein intake at moderate levels.

▶ Balance food intake and physical activity to maintain appropriate body weight.

▶ The committee does not recommend alcohol consumption. For those who drink alcoholic beverages, the committee recommends limiting consumption to the equivalent of less than 1 oz of pure alcohol in a single day. This is the equivalent of two cans of beer, two small glasses of wine, or two average cocktails. Pregnant women should avoid alcoholic beverages.

▶ Limit total daily intake of salt (sodium chloride) to 6 g or less. Limit the use of salt in cooking and avoid adding it to food at the table. Salty, highly processed, salt-preserved, and salt-pickled foods should be consumed sparingly.

▶ Maintain adequate calcium intake.

▶ Avoid taking dietary supplements in excess of the RDA in any one day.

▶ Maintain an optimal intake of fluoride, particularly during the years of primary and secondary tooth formation and growth.

The average US diet contains approximately 13% of calories from saturated fatty acids (SFA).[5] Reducing SFA intake to the goal of 10% of total calories should have a measurable impact on total cholesterol and low-density lipoprotein (LDL) levels. A reduction of total fat intake is an effective strategy for reducing plasma lipid levels. Achieving a total fat reduction reduces saturated fats and also lowers the intake of the most concentrated form of calories. This latter dietary modification will lower body weight, which also is related to lowered blood lipids.

Substitution of dietary fat with complex carbohydrates is the centerpiece of the recommended diet. People who consume 60% to 70% of total calories from complex carbohydrates have a lower prevalence of atherosclerosis, and they also tend to weigh less. Added benefits to consuming a low-fat, high-carbohydrate diet are that it has a higher nutrient density than the traditional US diet, and is also high in soluble fiber, which tends to lower serum cholesterol levels.[6]

Sodium

Although the minimum daily requirement of sodium for healthy persons is 0.5 g, most Americans consume foods that have a sodium content of 4 to 5 g. The recommended sodium intake is 1 g per 1000 kcal, up to a maximum of 3 g daily. Limiting sodium intake to this level helps to prevent the development of hypertension in individuals who are sodium-sensitive. It should be remembered, however, that athletes who exercise habitually, particularly in hot, humid environments, may require more sodium than the average, sedentary person.

Alcohol

The incidence of high blood pressure increases significantly with the consumption of three to four alcoholic drinks per day.[7] Because of this finding it is recommended that, for those who consume alcohol, the intake should not exceed two 4-oz glasses of wine, or two 12-oz bottles of beer per day.

There is some evidence that alcohol increases plasma triglyceride and HDL-cholesterol levels, and some epidemiologic studies suggest that alcohol consumption is a negative risk factor for CHD. However, alcohol is easily abused, and its consumption may cause social, physiologic, and psychological problems. Therefore, alcohol consumption should not be encouraged. If alcohol is consumed, moderate consumption should be the recommendation.

Excess Calories

Excessive caloric intake is a dietary risk factor for CHD because it often leads to a higher body fat level, higher blood pressure, higher serum cholesterol, and diabetes mellitus. Maintenance of ideal body weight is an important means of reducing CHD risk. In overweight people, weight reduction lowers LDL-cholesterol and triglyceride levels, and may raise HDL-cholesterol levels. Exercise is an important factor in losing and controlling weight, and it favorably affects plasma lipid levels by decreasing serum triglycerides, increasing HDL cholesterol, and (occasionally) lowering LDL cholesterol.

▶ TREATMENT OF CORONARY HEART DISEASE

Diet is the primary treatment for elevated blood cholesterol levels. The minimum goal of therapy is to lower LDL-cholesterol levels to below 160 mg/dL, or below 130 mg/dL if CHD or two other CHD risk factors are present (see *Figure 3.3*). The Step One Diet to reduce blood cholesterol appears in *Table 3.8*.

FIGURE 3.3   Classifications and treatment decisions for LDL-cholesterol levels.

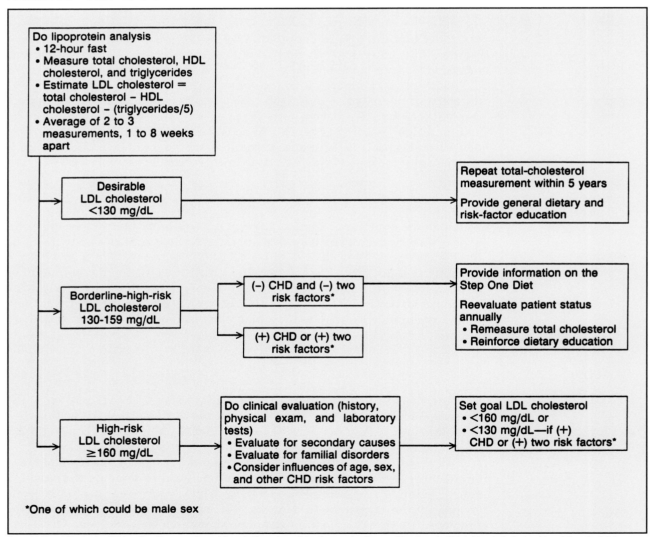

From National Cholesterol Education Program Expert Panel. Report on detection, evaluation, and treatment of high blood cholesterol in adults. *Arch Intern Med.* 1988;148:36.

TABLE 3.8 Recommended Diet Modifications to Lower Blood Cholesterol: The Step One Diet

Food Group	Choose	Decrease
Fish, chicken, turkey, and lean meats	Fish; white-meat poultry without skin; lean cuts of beef, lamb, pork or veal; shellfish	Fatty cuts of beef, lamb, pork; spare ribs; organ meats; regular cold cuts; sausage; hot dogs; bacon; sardines; roe
Skim and low-fat milk, cheese, yogurt, and dairy substitutes	Skim or 1% fat milk (liquid, powdered, evaporated); buttermilk; substitute 1 cup skim milk alone or with up to 1 cup nonfat dry-milk powder added instead of whole milk (for consistency in cooking) For acceptable whipped topping: combine ⅓ cup ice water, 1 tbsp lemon juice, ¾ tsp vanilla, and ⅓ cup nonfat dry-milk powder; beat 10 min or until stiff; add 2 tbsp sugar Nonfat (0% fat) or low-fat yogurt Low-fat cottage cheese (1% or 2% fat) Low-fat farmer, or pot cheeses (all of these should be labeled no more than 2-6 g fat/oz) Sherbet, sorbet	Whole milk (4% fat): regular, evaporated, condensed; cream; half and half; 2% milk; imitation milk products; most nondairy creamers; whipped toppings Whole-milk yogurt Whole-milk cottage cheese (4% fat) All natural cheeses (eg, blue, Roquefort, Camembert, cheddar, Swiss) Low-fat or "diet" cream cheese, low-fat or "diet" sour cream Cream cheese, sour cream Ice cream
Eggs	Egg whites (2 whites = 1 whole egg in recipes), or mix together 1 egg white, 2 tsp nonfat milk powder, and 2 tsp acceptable oil*; cholesterol-free egg substitutes	Egg yolks
Fruits and vegetables	Fresh, frozen, canned or dried fruits and vegetables	Vegetables prepared in butter, cream, or other sauces
Breads and cereals	Homemade baked goods using unsaturated oils sparingly, angelfood cake, low-fat crackers, low-fat cookies Rice, pasta, barley, bulgur, legumes Whole-grain breads and cereals (oatmeal, whole wheat, rye, bran, multigrain, etc)	Commercial baked goods; pies, cakes, doughnuts, croissants, pastries, muffins, biscuits, high-fat crackers, high-fat cookies Egg noodles Breads in which eggs are a major ingredient, cereals with coconut oil or palm oil or palm kernel oil
Fats and oils	Acceptable unsaturated vegetable oils* Margarine or shortening made from one of the acceptable unsaturated oils Reduced-fat margarine Mayonnaise, salad dressings made with acceptable unsaturated oils Low-fat dressings Seeds and nuts, nonhydrogenated, old-fashioned-style peanut butter (100% peanuts)	Butter, coconut oil, palm oil, palm kernel oil, bacon fat, hydrogenated vegetable shortening Dressings made with egg yolk Coconut, hydrogenated peanut butter

*Acceptable oils include canola, corn, cottonseed, olive, safflower, sesame, soybean, and sunflower.
From National Cholesterol Education Program Expert Panel. Report on detection, evaluation, and treatment of high blood cholesterol in adults. *Arch Intern Med.* 1988;148:36.

A two-step diet-therapy approach for cholesterol lowering is recommended by both the American Heart Association and the National Cholesterol Education Program (NCEP). The goal of the recommended dietary therapy is to provide a nutritionally adequate intake while progressively lowering saturated fatty acids and cholesterol, and to promote weight loss when indicated. The Step One Diet and the Step Two Diet are described in *Table 3.9*. The Step One Diet recommends a total fat intake of less than 30% of calories, saturated fats less than 10% of calories, and cholesterol less than 300 mg per day. The Step Two Diet reduces saturated fats to less than 7% of calories, and cholesterol to less than 200 mg per day. Because of the more dramatic drop in fat and cholesterol in the Step Two Diet, this diet is more difficult for most people to follow.

Total Fat

In both the Step One and Step Two Diets, total fat should not exceed 30% of calories. This represents a drop of about 7% in fat intake (the average US diet is 37% calories from fat). The goal of this reduction is to help in lowering the saturated fat intake level and promoting weight reduction.

Saturated Fats

Saturated fats are the most hypercholesterolemic dietary components, and some saturated fatty acids (especially lauric, myristic, and palmitic fatty acids) have a greater hypercholesterolemic effect than others. Stearic acid, one of the fatty acids found in meat, does not appear to have hypercholesterolemic properties. To achieve the greatest reduction in hypercholesterolemic potential, foods consumed should be low in saturated fats, including animal fats, palm oil, palm kernel oil, and coconut oil. (See appendix 1 for a list of commonly consumed foods and their predominant fatty acid contents.)

Polyunsaturated Fatty Acids

About 7% of the calories consumed by Americans comes from polyunsaturated fatty acids (PUFAs). It is recommended that diets contain at least this amount, and preferably more (up to and not exceeding 10% of calories). Consumption of this level of PUFAs aids in lowering plasma total cholesterol and LDL-cholesterol levels. However, if provided in amounts higher than the recommended level, certain PUFAs, particularly the omega-6 fatty acids, may have the undesirable effect of lowering the plasma HDL-cholesterol level.

The major categories of PUFAs are omega-6 fatty acids (from safflower oil, sunflower seed oil, soybean oil, corn oil, and other vegetable oils), and omega-3 fatty acids (from fish oils). Large doses of the omega-3 fatty acids (mainly eicosapentenaenoic [EPA] and docosahexaenoic [DHA] fatty acids) have been shown to lower plasma triglycerides consistently, but do not consistently lower plasma total-cholesterol levels. Consumption of more fish (at least two fish

TABLE 3.9 Dietary Therapy for High Blood Cholesterol

	Recommended Intake	
Nutrient	*Step One Diet*	*Step Two Diet*
Total fat	Less than 30% of total calories	Less than 30% of total calories
Saturated fatty acids	Less than 10% of total calories	Less than 7% of total calories
Polyunsaturated fatty acids	Up to 10% of total calories	Up to 10% of total calories
Monounsaturated fatty acids	10% to 15% of total calories	10% to 15% of total calories
Carbohydrates	50% to 60% of total calories	50% to 60% of total calories
Protein	10% to 20% of total calories	10% to 20% of total calories
Cholesterol	Less than 300 mg/d	Less than 200 mg/d
Total calories	To achieve and maintain desirable weight	To achieve and maintain desirable weight

From National Cholesterol Education Program Expert Panel. Report on detection, evaluation, and treatment of high blood cholesterol in adults. *Arch Intern Med.* 1988;148:36.

meals per week) as a replacement for meats and cheese is recommended as a means of increasing omega-3 fatty acid intake. Consumption of omega-3 fatty acid (fish oil) supplements is not recommended.

Monounsaturated Fats

Monounsaturated fatty acids should provide 10% to 15% of calories in both the Step One and Step Two diets. Americans presently consume 14% to 16% of calories as monounsaturated fatty acids (mainly oleic acid), but much of this intake comes from animal products that are also high in saturated fatty acids. Non-animal-product sources of monounsaturated fatty acids include olive oil, rapeseed (canola) oil, and high-oleic-acid sunflower seed and safflower oil.

It has recently been shown that monounsaturated fatty acids are effective at reducing plasma total cholesterol and LDL cholesterol. However, unlike omega-6 fatty acids (polyunsaturated fats), monounsaturated fatty acids do not lower HDL cholesterol when eaten in abundance. This finding makes monounsaturated fatty acids a more attractive lipid-lowering fat than omega-6 fatty acids.

Dietary Cholesterol

Dietary cholesterol is hypercholesterolemic and elevates both plasma total cholesterol and LDL-cholesterol levels. For this reason, it is desirable to limit the intake of dietary cholesterol to no more than 300 mg per day. Those at high risk for CHD should further restrict their intake to no more than 200 mg per day (as recommended in the Step Two diet).

▶ EXERCISE INTERVENTION FOR CHD

Plasma lipid/lipoprotein profiles are consistent with lowered CHD risk in those who participate in regular, vigorous, endurance activities. The improvement in risk profile is demonstrated by lower plasma triglycerides, and higher HDL cholesterol levels than those seen in matched inactive controls. Regular exercise also is shown to improve (increase) blood coagulation time and reduce platelet aggregation.[8-11] Platelets are involved in the atherosclerotic process, and thrombosis of coronary arteries is a mechanism of myocardial infarction. A recent study confirms that low levels of physical activity are associated with a higher risk of CHD in men, independent of other conventional risk factors.[12]

Plasma Total Cholesterol

Some longitudinal studies of endurance-trained athletes have shown that exercise reduces plasma total cholesterol.[13-16] However, other well-designed studies have shown that no significant change in plasma total cholesterol occurs.[13,17] The relationship between exercise and plasma total cholesterol is not well understood. It is speculated that an increase in the cholesterol content of one lipoprotein may be counterbalanced by a decrease in the cholesterol content of other lipoproteins, with the result that total cholesterol is not changed.[13] Consequently, it is important to measure subfractions of cholesterol when attempting to assess CVD risk. Total cholesterol levels alone may not tell the entire story.

Low-Density-Lipoprotein Cholesterol

The effect of exercise on LDL-cholesterol levels generally has been small and highly variable in both cross-sectional comparisons of active and inactive subjects, and in longitudinal training studies.[13,18,19] A number of training studies have found that LDL cholesterol is lower following training,[13,14,16,18] while others have shown no effect from either high- or low-intensity training.[13,19] In those studies that have reported a decrease in LDL cholesterol, exercise intensity has been moderate (60% to 85% of $\dot{V}O_2$max), and exercise frequency ranged from daily to three times weekly with 30- to 60-minute sessions. Reductions in LDL cholesterol were more frequent when the exercise was associated with weight loss, but LDL-cholesterol reduction also occurred in exercising subjects who did not lose weight. If LDL cholesterol is elevated prior to the initialization of an exercise regimen, it is more likely to decrease with a regular exercise program.[13]

High-Density-Lipoprotein Cholesterol

The average HDL-cholesterol values are 45 mg/dL for young men and 55 mg/dL for young women in the United States and Canada.[20] The difference between values for endurance athletes and sedentary controls is approximately 12 to 20 mg/dL (20% to 35%).[13,20] In contrast, HDL-cholesterol levels in trained weight lifters are comparable to those of nonathletes.[21] Nevertheless, physical activity with an endurance component is consistently associated with higher plasma HDL-cholesterol levels.[13,17,20,22] Elevations in HDL cholesterol have been reported for long-distance runners, cross-country skiers, speed skaters, soccer players, and tennis players.[13,18,22,23]

People who are generally active on the job or during leisure time, but who are not involved in endurance-type activity or sports, typically have higher concentrations of HDL cholesterol than their less-active counterparts. While these differences are statistically significant, the magnitude of difference is small (generally less than 5 mg/dL).[13]

HDL Cholesterol and Exercise Training

Prospective studies that have looked at the relationship between HDL cholesterol and exercise training report conflicting findings. About 50% of the studies with clinically healthy men who have engaged in endurance training have reported significant or near-significant increases in HDL cholesterol,[13-16,18,24,25] while other studies have found no change or a decrease.[13,14,19,26] When HDL cholesterol is raised, the increase typically ranges from 3 to 8 mg/dL (5% to 16%).[13,27]

HDL Cholesterol and Power Sports

Heavy-resistance exercise is not typically associated with increased HDL cholesterol.[13] However, bodybuilders have been shown to have higher HDL-cholesterol levels than powerlifters,[17] and weight training has been shown to change lipid and lipoprotein levels favorably in previously sedentary men and women.[14]

Gender Differences, Exercise, and HDL Cholesterol

The observation that exercise training increases HDL-cholesterol levels in men more frequently than in women suggests a gender-related difference in response to exercise.[14,28,29] Changes in endogenous testosterone and estrogen levels may account for the increase in HDL cholesterol in men.[28] However, HDL cholesterol has also been shown to increase in women running an average of 12 miles per week.[30] It has been suggested that sedentary women may need more frequent, more intensive, and longer training programs than men to increase HDL-cholesterol levels[26] and that higher initial levels of HDL cholesterol in women may be the result of a greater lipoprotein lipase (LPL) activity in women.[31]

Energy Expenditure From Exercise and HDL Cholesterol

A minimum beneficial threshold of 1000 kcal per week in energy expenditure has been recommended to increase HDL cholesterol.[13] In addition, it has been suggested that there is a dose-response relationship between the level of physical activity and HDL-cholesterol levels, with increased HDL cholesterol correlating with increases in energy expenditure up to about 4500 kcal per week.[13,17] Therefore, running mileage and length of training have also been positively correlated with HDL cholesterol.[16,25] However, regardless of this dose-response relationship, the greatest increase in HDL-cholesterol levels appears to occur when sedentary men become more active, particularly if they have low HDL-cholesterol levels before training.[13,32]

Exercise and Plasma Triglycerides

Physically active people and endurance-trained athletes usually have lower plasma concentrations of very low-density lipoprotein (VLDL) cholesterol and triglyceride than inactive controls.[13,19,33] Compared with the general population, lower plasma triglyceride levels have been reported for long-distance runners, cross-country skiers, and tennis players,[13] but no difference from controls has also been reported.[18]

Plasma triglyceride levels of athletes involved in power or speed-type training are similar to those observed in inactive people. Lower plasma triglyceride values have been reported for people who are more active on the job or during leisure time in selected populations, but not in others.[13,22] However, both short- and long-term increases in aerobic exercise have been shown to cause decreases in plasma triglycerides, except for those who already have low normal levels.[13,23]

REFERENCES

1. *1989 Heart Facts.* Dallas, Tex: American Heart Association; 1989.
2. Kannel WB, Shatzkin A. Risk-factor analysis. *Prog Cardiovasc Dis.* 1984;26:309.
3. *Dietary Treatment of Hypercholesterolemia: A Handbook for Counselors.* Dallas, Tex: American Heart Association; 1988.
4. Horg J, Gregg RE, Brewer HB Jr. Special communication: an approach to the management of hyperlipoproteinemia. *JAMA.* 1986;225:512.
5. Carroll MD, Abraham CS, Dresser CM. *Dietary Intake Source Data: United States, 1976-80.* Washington, DC: US Govt Printing Office; 1983. US Dept of Health and Human Services publication PHS 83-1681. Vital and Health Statistics series 11-231.
6. Rosenthal MD, Barnard RJ, Rose DP, et al. Effects of a high-complex-carbohydrate, low-fat, low-cholesterol diet on levels of serum lipids and estradiol. *Am J Med.* 1985;78:23.
7. Hennekens CH. Alcohol. In: Kaplan NM, Stamler JS, eds. *Prevention of Coronary Heart Disease.* Philadelphia, Pa: WB Saunders Co; 1983:130.

8. Kopitsky RG, Switzer ME, Williams RS, et al. The basis for the increase in factor VIII procoagulant activity during exercise. *Thromb Haemost*. 1983;49:53.

9. Williams RS, Logue EE, Lewis JL, et al. Physical conditioning augments the fibrinolytic response to venous occlusion in healthy adults. *N Engl J Med*. 1980;302:987.

10. Rauramaa R, Salonen JT, Seppanen K, et al. Inhibition of platelet aggregability by moderate-intensity physical exercise: a randomized clinical trial in overweight men. *Circulation*. 1986;74:939.

11. Rauramaa R, Salonen JT, Kukkonen-Harjula K, et al. Effects of mild physical exercise on serum lipoproteins and metabolites of arachidonic acid. *Br Med J*. 1984;288:603.

12. Eklund LG, Haskell WL, Johnson JL, et al. Physical fitness as a predictor of cardiovascular mortality in asymptomatic North American men. *N Engl J Med*. 1988;319:1379.

13. Haskell WL. Exercise-induced changes in plasma lipids and lipoproteins. *Prev Med*. 1984;13:23.

14. Goldberg L, Elliot DL, Schutz RW, et al. Changes in lipid and lipoprotein levels after weight training. *JAMA*. 1984;252:504.

15. Kiens B, Jorgensen I, Lewis S, et al. Increased plasma HDL cholesterol and apo A-1 in sedentary middle-aged men after physical conditioning. *Eur J Clin Invest*. 1980;10:203.

16. Wood PD, Haskell WL, Blair SN, et al. Increased exercise level and plasma lipoprotein concentrations: one-year, randomized, controlled study in sedentary, middle-aged men. *Metabolism*. 1983;32:31.

17. Hurley BF, Seals DR, Hagberg JM, et al. High-density lipoprotein cholesterol in bodybuilders v powerlifters: negative effects of androgen use. *JAMA*. 1984;254:507.

18. Huttunen JK, Lansimies E, Voutilainen E, et al. Effect of moderate physical exercise on serum lipids: controlled clinical trial with special reference to serum high-density lipoproteins. *Circulation*. 1979;60:1220.

19. Gaesser GA, Rich RG. Effects of high- and low-intensity exercise training on aerobic capacity and blood lipids. *Med Sci Sports Exerc*. 1984;16:269.

20. Deshaies Y, Allard C. Serum high-density lipoprotein cholesterol in male and female Olympic athletes. *Med Sci Sports Exerc*. 1982;14:207.

21. Farrell PA, Maksud MG, Pollock ML, et al. A comparison of plasma cholesterol, triglycerides, and high-density lipoprotein cholesterol in speed skaters, weight-lifters and nonathletes. *Eur J Appl Physiol*. 1982;48:77.

22. Vodak PA, Wood PD, Haskell WL, et al. HDL cholesterol and other plasma lipid and lipoprotein concentrations in middle-aged male and female tennis players. *Metabolism*. 1980;29:745-752.

23. Herbert PN, Bernier DN, Cullinane EM, et al. High-density lipoprotein metabolism in runners and sedentary men. *JAMA*. 1984;252:1034.

24. Cook TC, Laporte RE, Washburn RA, et al. Chronic low-level physical activity as a determinant of high-density lipoprotein cholesterol and subfractions. *Med Sci Sports Exerc*. 1986;18:653.

25. Williams PT, Wood PD, Haskell WL, et al. The effects of running mileage and duration on plasma lipoprotein levels. *JAMA*. 1982;247:2674.

26. Frey MAB, Doerr BM, Laubach LL, et al. Exercise does not change high-density lipoprotein cholesterol in women after ten weeks of training. *Metabolism*. 1982;31:1142.

27. Thompson PD, Cullinane EM, Sady SP, et al. Modest changes in high-density lipoprotein concentration and metabolism with prolonged exercise training. *Circulation*. 1988;78:25.

28. Frey MAB, Doerr BM, Srivastava LS, et al. Exercise training, sex hormones, and lipoprotein relationships in men. *J Appl Physiol*. 1983;54:757.

29. Brownell KD, Bachorik PS, Ayerle RS. Changes in plasma lipid and lipoprotein levels in men and women after a program of moderate exercise. *Circulation*. 1982;65:477.

30. Moore CE, Hartung H, Mitchell RE, et al. The relationship of exercise and diet on high-density lipoprotein cholesterol levels in women. *Metabolism*. 1983;32:189.

31. Levy RI, Rifkind BM. The structure, function, and metabolism of high-density lipoproteins: a status report. *Circulation*. 1980;62(suppl 4):4.

32. Goldberg L, Elliot DL. The effect of physical activity on lipid and lipoprotein levels. *Med Clin North Am.* 1985;69:41.
33. Curfman GD, Thomas GS, Paffenbarger RS. Physical activity and primary prevention of cardiovascular disease. *Cardiol Clin.* 1985;3:203.

Hypertension

Josephine Connolly Schoonen

Hypertension is one of the primary risk factors associated with the development of cardiovascular disease. The upper limit of normal blood pressure is considered to be 140/90 mm Hg by most clinicians. The risk of cardiovascular complications increases with increasing levels of both systolic and diastolic blood pressure.[1]

The effectiveness of antihypertensive drugs in reducing blood pressure is well documented. However, side effects of these drugs (malaise, fatigue, depression, decreased libido, episodes of weakness, and increased serum cholesterol) are also well documented. Fortunately, some of the drugs used more recently to control hypertension (eg, calcium channel blockers and angiotensin-converting enzyme inhibitors) have fewer adverse side effects.[2] The decision to treat clients pharmacologically depends on the severity of the blood pressure elevation and the presence of other cardiovascular risk factors or cardiovascular disease. Nonpharmacologic approaches are used both as definitive intervention and in conjunction with pharmacologic therapy. When used in conjunction with drugs, alternative therapies can permit maintenance of blood pressure with less medication, fewer side effects, enhanced compliance to therapy, and reduced expense.[1] Alternative therapies used in the treatment of hypertension include weight reduction, sodium restriction, mineral supplementation, alcohol and tobacco reduction, and increased physical activity. Various therapeutic modalities are briefly assessed below.

▶ WEIGHT REDUCTION

Obesity and blood pressure have been directly associated in worldwide epidemiologic studies.[1] The incidence of hypertension is greater in overweight people and in those who have recently gained weight. Studies have shown that weight loss produces a significant reduction in blood pressure, even if ideal body weight is not achieved and sodium intake is not reduced.[3] Therefore, people who are obese and hypertensive should participate in a weight-reduction program and strive to maintain a weight within 15% of their ideal body weight.[1]

▶ SODIUM RESTRICTION

A high sodium intake appears to play a role in maintaining the elevated blood pressure of some hypertensive clients, and in limiting the effectiveness of certain antihypertensive drugs.[1] Unfortunately, it is difficult to identify clients who would benefit from sodium restriction. For those who are salt-sensitive, restricting sodium intake to 70 to 100 mEq per day (1610 to 2300 mg) has been shown to decrease blood pressure.[4] This degree of restriction is generally achievable if an individual becomes proficient in label reading and low-salt cooking techniques. Hypertensive clients are typically placed on a sodium-restricted diet to determine if their blood pressure responds favorably. For those who prove to be resistant to salt reduction, a more favorable result may be achieved with weight loss.

▶ ROLE OF OTHER CATIONS

Potassium

Low potassium intake has been associated with high blood pressure.[5] In addition, a high potassium intake (>80 mEq or 3 to 4 g per day) has been demonstrated to produce a modest blood-pressure-lowering effect.[6] More research is necessary, however, before recommendations regarding potassium intake are warranted. Increased potassium intake would only be appropriate for individuals with normal renal function, and those who are not taking drugs known to increase serum potassium levels (eg, potassium-sparing diuretics and angiotensin-converting enzyme inhibitors).[1]

Calcium

Some studies have demonstrated an inverse relationship between serum calcium levels and blood pressure,[7] and others have documented decreased blood pressure in individuals with increased calcium intake.[8] Since the risk for renal calculi development increases with increased dietary calcium, however, more research is necessary before increased intake of calcium is recommended as a means of controlling blood pressure.

Magnesium and Zinc

Magnesium and zinc are other cations being studied as potential blood-pressure-lowering agents. However, recommendations suggesting increased dietary intake of these minerals are not justified at this time.[1]

It is becoming increasingly clear that the control and regulation of blood pressure is an intricate process that involves the integrated effects of many anions and cations. The levels of these minerals in the body may influence how the body handles excess dietary sodium.[9]

▶ ALCOHOL RESTRICTION

Alcohol consumption of more than four drinks per day (50 g alcohol) has been related to elevated blood pressure levels. Population studies have shown that the higher the daily intake of alcohol, the greater the prevalence of hypertension and the higher the average blood pressure.[10] In addition, excess alcohol intake leads to poor adherence to antihypertensive therapy, and possibly leads to refractory hypertension.[11] Hypertensive clients who consume alcohol are recommended to do so in moderation, limiting themselves to 1 oz of ethanol per day (ie, 2 oz of 100-proof whiskey, approximately 8 oz of wine, or 24 oz of beer).[5]

▶ MODIFICATION OF DIETARY FATS

Results of studies concerning the effects of low-saturated-fat, high-polyunsaturated-fat diets on blood pressure have been inconsistent. Since eating a diet low in total fat and saturated fat is consistent with recommendations for minimizing the risk for coronary artery disease, it is an appropriate recommendation for the hypertensive client as well.[1]

▶ TOBACCO RESTRICTION

Nicotine increases arterial blood pressure acutely. However, prolonged use of tobacco is not associated with an increased prevalence of hypertension.[1] Smokers do appear to have a higher frequency of malignant hypertension[12] and, overall, more than double the risk of coronary artery disease and sudden death.[13,14]

Smoking also affects the efficacy of antihypertensive drugs. Smoking interacts with propranolol hydrochloride in such a way that smokers require larger doses of this drug to achieve reductions in blood pressure similar to those seen in nonsmokers.[1] In addition, risk reduction induced by antihypertensive therapy may not be as great in smokers as in nonsmokers.[15] Hypertensives who smoke should be involved in group or individual counseling to help them stop smoking.[16]

▶ EXERCISE

Regular aerobic exercise (eg, walking, swimming, jogging, or bicycling) promotes weight loss and may help reduce blood pressure.[1] The potential benefits of exercise on blood pressure modification are:

- ▶ Reduction in systolic and diastolic blood pressure at rest
- ▶ Reduction in blood pressure at a given submaximal workload after exercise training
- ▶ Reduction of circulating catecholamines at rest and during exercise.

These changes are thought to decrease the stress on the arterial wall, decrease the rate of atheroma formation, and decrease myocardial oxygen demand.[9]

Strengthening exercises have been routinely discounted for all hypertensive clients. However, since many everyday or job-related activities require muscular strength, this issue is being reconsidered. The magnitude of a blood pressure response to a strength-related activity is proportional to the percentage of a client's maximum voluntary contraction (ie, maximum strength output for a single contraction). Therefore, by increasing a client's strength, everyday or work-related activities will require a lower percentage of the client's maximum voluntary contraction, and the blood pressure response to these activities will tend to decrease. Therefore, some hypertensives would benefit from muscular strength and endurance exercises using light to moderate weight loads. However, this does not include clients with poor left ventricular function or with a blood pressure reading above 200/90 mm Hg.

Initially, clients should be closely monitored, and they should be trained in proper breathing and lifting techniques.[2] Hypertensive clients should be encouraged to embark on some type of physical exercise program gradually, only after appropriate medical evaluation.[1]

▶ BIOFEEDBACK AND RELAXATION

Behavioral approaches to hypertension management, such as biofeedback, transcendental meditation, yoga, and other relaxation techniques produce modest long-term reductions in blood pressure in select groups.[1] Studies have shown that individuals who can elicit a relaxation response may circulate higher norepinephrine levels after exposure to stress without a subsequent rise in blood pressure and pulse, implying a decreased end-organ responsiveness to adrenergic stimulation.[4] Such regimens are most useful in controlling mild hypertension, and may also be used in combination with pharmacologic therapy. However, these regimens should not be considered as definitive treatment until they are subject to more rigorous clinical trial evaluation.

All the suggestions that can be gleaned from the above findings (decreasing body weight, restricting processed foods and other high-sodium foods, eating more fruits and vegetables that are high in calcium or potassium, increasing the polyunsaturated-fat to saturated-fat ratio, moderate alcohol consumption, and smoking cessation) are in line with positive life-style changes that can help prevent debilitating diseases and improve the quality of life. All individuals (hypertensive and nonhypertensive alike) could benefit by adopting more of these dietary and life-style recommendations.

REFERENCES

1. US Dept of Health and Human Services, Joint National Committee on Detection, Evaluation, and Treatment of High Blood Pressure. *The 1988 Report.* Bethesda, Md; National Heart, Lung, and Blood Institute; 1988. NIH publication 88-1088.
2. American Association of Cardiovascular and Pulmonary Rehabilitation. *Guidelines for Cardiac Rehabilitation Programs.* Champaign, Ill: Human Kinetics Books; 1991:10-11.
3. Frohlich ED, Grim C, Labarthe DR, et al. Recommendations for human blood pressure determination by sphygmomanometers: report of a special task force appointed by the steering committee, American Heart Association. *Hypertension.* 1988;11:209A-222A.
4. Kaplan N. Use of non-drug therapy in treating hypertension. *Am J Med.* 1984;3:273.
5. Kihara M, Fujikawa J, Ohtaka M, et al. Interrelationships between blood pressure, sodium, potassium, serum cholesterol, and protein intake in Japan. *Hypertension.* 1984;6:736-742.
6. MacGregor GA, Smith SJ, Markandu ND, et al. Moderate potassium supplementation in essential hypertension. *Lancet.* 1982;2:567-570.
7. Kesteloot H, Geboers J, Van Hoof R. Epidemiological study of the relationship between calcium and blood pressure. *Hypertension.* 1983;5(suppl 11):52-56.
8. McCarron DA, Morris CD. Blood pressure response to oral calcium in persons with mild to moderate hypertension: a randomized, double-blind, placebo-controlled, crossover trial. *Ann Intern Med.* 1985;103(pt 6):825-831.
9. McCarron DA. A consensus approach to electrolytes and blood pressure. *Hypertension.* 1991;17(suppl 1):170-172.
10. Dyer A, et al. Alcohol consumption, cardiovascular risk factors, and mortality in two Chicago epidemiologic studies. *Circulation.* 1977;56:1067.
11. Madiano BW, Norton RN. Alcohol and hypertension: suggestions for prevention and treatment. *Ann Intern Med.* 1986;105:124-125.
12. Isles C, Brown JJ, Cumming AMM, et al. Excess smoking in malignant-phase hypertension. *Br Med J.* 1979;1:579-581.
13. Dawber TR. *The Framingham Study: The Epidemiology of Atherosclerotic Disease.* Cambridge, Mass: Harvard University Press; 1980:172-189.
14. Management Committee of the Australian National Blood Pressure Study. Prognostic factors in the treatment of mild hypertension. *Circulation.* 1984;69:668-676.

15. Greenberg G, Thompson SG, Brennan PJ. The relationship between smoking and the response to antihypertensive treatment in mild hypertensives in the Medical Research Council's trial treatment. *Int J Epidemiol.* 1987;16:25-30.

16. Working Group on Physician Behaviors to Reduce Smoking Amongst Hypertensive Patients, National High Blood Pressure Education Program. *The Physician's Guide: How to Help Your Hypertensive Patients Stop Smoking.* Bethesda, Md: National Heart, Lung, and Blood Institute; 1985. NIH publication 84-1271.

Diabetes

Sara Hinkle

Both type I (insulin-dependent) and type II (non-insulin-dependent) diabetes are characterized by resistance to insulin action. Complications of diabetes include hyperlipidemia, as well as neural, renal, and ophthalmic lesions, which are thought to occur as a result of prolonged hyperglycemia.[1] Dietary control and insulin therapy are the two principal modes of treatment for diabetes mellitus. Exercise training is often recommended as a therapeutic modality for the client with diabetes, because exercise can increase insulin sensitivity, improve cardiovascular function and the serum lipid profile, and decrease body fat. It must be remembered, however, that exercise is not a panacea; it is doubtful that it will improve glycemic control, particularly in the client with type I diabetes.[2] Consequently, clients with diabetes should be encouraged to seek the advice of a qualified health professional before commencing an exercise program. Nonetheless, physical exercise can promote many physiologic and psychological benefits, and the client with diabetes who wishes to exercise should be encouraged to do so.

Blood glucose levels may change unpredictably when a client with diabetes begins an exercise program or exercises sporadically. Individuals who exercise more frequently tend to have fewer glucose-management problems. Therefore, exercise training (particularly for people with type I diabetes) requires much discipline.

A regular schedule of exercise, food intake, and insulin administration will decrease fluctuations in blood glucose concentration. Another key to ensuring stability of blood glucose levels is to do blood glucose self-testing before, during, and after exercise. Records should be kept of test results, time of exercise, length of time since the last meal, what foods were consumed, the type of exercise done, and for how long it was performed. These records provide health professionals with valuable information to help clients develop guidelines for adjusting the frequency and amount of food intake and insulin injections.[1,2]

► TYPE I DIABETES

Because exercise improves the blood glucose-lowering effect of injected insulin, it is important to be aware of the peak action times of insulin and to allow for the lowering effects that exercise can cause at these times. For example, one must be cognizant of the fact that vigorous exercise can lead to postexercise late-onset hypoglycemia 3 to 15 hours after exercise.

Additional food intake secondary to exercise may be necessary for clients with diabetes (see *Table 3.10*). Extra food should be consumed prior to exercise and during long periods of activity. The additional food should not be subtracted from the daily meal plan. Individuals who are well trained and who exercise regularly usually require less food than those who exercise occasionally.

TABLE 3.10 General Guidelines for Making Food Adjustments for Exercise

Type of Exercise and Examples	If Blood Sugar Is:	Increase Food Intake By:	Suggestions of Food to Use
Exercise of short duration and of low to moderate intensity Examples: Walking a half mile or leisurely bicycling for less than 30 min.	<80 mg ≥80 mg	10–15 g carbohydrate per h Not necessary to increase food	1 fruit or 1 bread exchange
Exercise of moderate intensity Examples: Tennis, swimming, jogging, leisurely bicycling, gardening, golfing or vacuuming for one hour	<80 mg 80–170 mg 180–300 mg ≥300mg	25–50 g carbohydrate before exercise, then 10–15 g per h of exercise 10–15 g carbohydrate per h of exercise Not necessary to increase food Don't begin exercise until blood glucose is under better control.	½ meat sandwich with a milk or fruit exchange 1 fruit or 1 bread exchange
Strenuous activity or exercise Examples: Football, hockey, racquetball, or basketball games, strenuous bicycling or swimming, shoveling heavy snow	<80 mg 80–170 mg 180–300 mg	50 g carbohydrate; monitor blood glucose carefully 25–50 mg carbohydrate depending on intensity and duration 10–15 g carbohydrate per h of exercise	1 meat sandwich of 2 slices of bread with a milk and fruit exchange ½ meat sandwich with a milk or fruit exchange 1 fruit or 1 bread exchange

Adapted from Franz M. *Diabetes and Exercise: Guidelines for Safe and Enjoyable Activity.* Minneapolis, Minn: International Diabetes Center; 1985. Reprinted with permission.

▶ INSULIN ADJUSTMENTS FOR EXTENDED EXERCISE

During long periods of exercise, it may be difficult to avoid low blood glucose levels by increasing caloric intake alone. In these cases, it may be necessary to lower the insulin dosage administered prior to exercise. Exercise tends to have an insulin-like effect, which, in conjunction with food, can serve to maintain blood glucose levels within the normal range. The following guidelines may be helpful in adjusting insulin dosage prior to long-duration (>1 hour) exercise:

Example: To decrease insulin dosage prior to activity by 10%.[1,2]

If the usual insulin dose is 4 regular, 24 isophane insulin suspension (NPH) before breakfast, and 2 regular, 6 NPH before evening meal, the total dose is 6 regular and 30 NPH, 36 units. A 10% reduction is 3.6, which rounds to 4 units.

Rapid-acting insulin peaks during the morning hours. For cross-country skiing all morning, decrease the morning regular dose by 10% of the total insulin dose. The morning insulin would therefore be 0 regular (4 minus 4) and 24 NPH.

Intermediate-acting insulin taken before breakfast will peak during the afternoon hours. For canoeing all afternoon, the morning insulin would be 4 regular and 20 NPH (24 minus 4).

For activity lasting all day (eg, downhill skiing), both the regular and NPH dosages would be decreased: morning insulin would be 0 regular (4 minus 4) and 20 NPH (24 minus 4).

Blood glucose monitoring should be performed before and after activity to ensure proper adjustments of these general recommendations. In addition, it is important to be aware of the signs of an approaching insulin reaction. Individuals with diabetes should always carry a fast-acting glucose food (such as a small tube of cake frosting) or a commercial glucose gel during and after exercise. Ultralente, regular insulin, and the use of insulin pumps have become more popular in recent years as well. It is also important for insulin-dependent athletes to inform their teammates, coaches, and partners how to react if help is required. While adjusting their insulin and food intakes, people with diabetes should never exercise alone.

► TYPE II DIABETES

Individuals with type II diabetes generally need to lose weight to improve their insulin sensitivity. Regular exercise in conjunction with a weight-loss program is often sufficient to control type II diabetes. In some cases, the dosage of insulin or oral agent can be reduced or curtailed as a result of a regular exercise and weight-maintenance program. Blood glucose levels are generally not as unstable in people with type II diabetes as they are in people with type I diabetes, because people with type II diabetes are still producing some insulin.

General exercise guidelines for people with type II diabetes, as outlined in a position statement by the American Diabetes Association, follow[1,2]:

► Aerobic exercise at 50% to 70% of the individual's maximum oxygen uptake
► Twenty to 45 minutes of activity, to be repeated at least 3 days per week
► A low-intensity warm-up and cool-down period
► The activity should be appropriate to the person's general physical condition and life-style

The American Diabetes Association further recommends that all individuals with diabetes who exercise should:

1. use proper footwear, and, if appropriate, other protective equipment;
2. avoid exercise in extreme heat or cold;
3. inspect feet daily after exercise; and
4. avoid exercise during periods of poor metabolic control (ie, blood sugar above the goal level).

REFERENCES

1. Staten MA. Managing diabetes in older adults: how exercise can help. *Phys Sports Med*. 1991;19(3):66.
2. Franz M. *Diabetes and Exercise: How to Get Started*. Minneapolis, Minn: Park Nicollet Medical Foundation; 1984.

Osteoporosis

Jane Kerstetter, with Elizabeth Markley

Osteoporosis is an age-related bone disorder characterized by a decrease in bone mass accompanied by an increase in susceptibility to bone fracture.[1] Most fractures occur in the proximal femur, vertebrae, and radius. Hip fractures are associated with a 12% to 20% increase in mortality.[2] Osteoporosis is a major public health problem that accounts for 1.2 million fractures annually in the United States.[3] Approximately $7 billion is spent annually to treat this disease; by the year 2020, we may be spending up to $60 billion.[4] With rising medical costs, the increasing number of older persons, and the limitations of current treatment regimes for osteoporosis, the focus has turned to maximizing bone deposition during youth and preventing bone loss in older age.

Bone is heterogenous tissue. All bone is composed, to various degrees, of trabecular (spongy, cancellous) and cortical (compact) bone. Vertebrae and the distal forearm are primarily trabecular, while the hip and long bone shafts are primarily cortical. Approximately 80% of the total skeleton is cortical bone, which has a slower turnover rate than trabecular bone. Because of trabecular bone's greater surface area and higher rate of turnover, it is more sensitive to hormonal changes.[5]

After the attainment of peak bone mass in the third decade of life, cortical and trabecular bone are lost slowly (0.3% to 0.5% loss per year) well into old age. Slow bone loss is responsible for type II (senile) osteoporosis that occurs in both men and women older than 70 years. Superimposed on the natural bone loss is a 10-year period of accelerated loss (1% to 3% loss per year) that women experience following menopause. Disproportionately more trabecular bone than cortical bone is lost, resulting in vertebral crush fractures ("dowager's hump") and Colles' fractures. This type of osteoporosis is known as type I (or postmenopausal) osteoporosis.[5]

▶ HORMONES

Estrogen deficiency clearly is an important contributor to osteoporosis, although its action mechanism is unknown. It is equally clear that estrogen-replacement therapy is the single most effective means of preventing bone loss under estrogen-deficient conditions such as menopause.[6] Clinical trials show that, in oophorectomized women, estrogen-replacement therapy retards bone loss for up to 10 years and prevents fractures.[6,7] Estrogen-replacement therapy may cause a 50% reduction in lifetime risk for hip fracture.[8] Estrogen may have its positive effect on bone by stimulating calcitonin synthesis, which in turn reduces calcium resorption from bone and decreases serum calcium levels. Lower serum calcium levels in turn stimulate production of parathyroid hormone (which increases 1,25-dihydroxyvitamin D_3 activation), resulting in increased calcium absorption and improved calcium balance.[4,9] Women receiving estrogen therapy have a slightly increased risk for certain cancers. Regularly performed breast examinations, mammograms, and pelvic examinations help ensure early detection should cancer develop.

▶ NUTRITION

Calcium is the major constituent of bone hydroxyapatite and is required for bone development and maintenance. Theoretically, a low-calcium diet results in low bone density and premature fractures. However, research on the effects of dietary calcium on bone density is extremely controversial. Many conflicting research results exist because of these technical difficulties: measuring relatively small changes in bone, the heterogeneity of bone loss, the inherent difficulties in measuring dietary calcium (past and present), the lack of control for estrogen status or physical activity, the small sample sizes, and the lack of epidemiologic and statistical expertise by researchers.[10]

Even though results conflict, trends do emerge. In general, calcium may slow bone loss in cortical, but not trabecular bone.[11] Cumming recently performed a metaanalysis of 37 published research studies on calcium intake and bone mass in adult women.[10] In early postmenopausal women, supplemented calcium (1000 mg in tablet form) appeared to prevent an approximately 1% bone loss from all bones studied (except vertebrae). Although 1% may appear insignificant, it is enough to alter fracture risk over a 10-year period.[10]

Heaney suggests that calcium has a permissive role, rather than a causative role, in the development of osteoporosis.[12] That is, adequate calcium needs to be present if hormone-replacement therapy or weight-bearing exercise is to have maximal effects on bone density.

Increasing dietary calcium to recommended levels remains a reasonable and safe method of preventing osteoporosis; however, it should not be relied on as the sole treatment. The current RDA for adults over the age of 19 years who are not pregnant or lactating is 800 mg per day. The adequacy of this level for postmenopausal women and for elderly men and women is questionable.[13] The Consensus Conference on Osteoporosis conducted by the National Institutes of Health recommended 1000 mg per day for men and premenopausal women, and 1500 mg per day for estrogen-deficient women.[14]

Vitamin D deficiency is common in older persons, and it contributes to poor calcium absorption from the gastrointestinal tract. Clinical trials using vitamin D to treat osteoporosis have yielded conflicting and disappointing results. Toxicity resulting in hypercalcemia, hypercalciuria, nephrocalcinosis, and soft tissue calcification are reported problems. However, treatment with synthetic vitamin D analogs are most promising. They may normalize calcium absorption, improve calcium balance, prevent bone loss, and reduce fracture rates.[4]

Fluoride stimulates bone formation and increases bone mass; however, there have been serious questions regarding the strength of the newly formed bone. Most recently, Riggs and colleagues published the results of a 4-year prospective, randomized, double-blind, placebo-controlled clinical trial in postmenopausal osteoporotic patients.[15,16] Indeed, fluoride-treated subjects increased bone mineral density at trabecular sites, but they demonstrated a decreased density at cortical bone sites. This resulted in a slight decrease in vertebral fractures but a significantly higher fracture rate in cortical bone. Fluoride treatment may increase skeletal fragility; therefore, its effectiveness and safety are questionable.

▶ MECHANICAL FORCES

Bone health is partially dependent on weight-bearing physical activity. Bone is a metabolically and structurally dynamic tissue that changes mass and architecture in response to load-bearing stimuli. Weightlessness, immobility, bed rest, or paralysis are associated with negative calcium balance and rapid loss of bone mass. During bed rest or space travel, bone loss of 1% to 2% weekly may occur. This far exceeds what was previously termed accelerated loss: 1% to 2% yearly seen in postmenopausal women. Disuse osteoporosis is manifested by an increase in bone resorption, resulting in net bone loss. Conversely, those athletes who regularly participate in weight-bearing or weight-training activities have up to 40% higher bone density than their nonexercising counterparts.[5] Mechanical stress stimulates bone deposition, resulting in elevated bone mass.

Physical activity, like calcium, is not a substitute for estrogen replacement in conditions of estrogen deficiency. Amenorrheic athletes suffer decreased lumbar bone mineral density, which suggests that exercise training cannot overcome the negative effects of estrogen loss.[5] Amenorrheic nonrunners had lumbar bone densities approximately 90% of normal, while eumenorrheic runners had lumbar bone density 110% of normal. Amenorrheic athletes may suffer trabecular bone loss rather than cortical loss. The shorter the episode of estrogen loss, the greater the chances of recovering lost bone density.[17] There is good evidence that anorexia nervosa, because of its association with amenorrhea, reduced nutrient intake, and lowered estrogen production, may increase the current risk of musculoskeletal problems and future risk of osteoporosis.[18-20]

Adequate calcium nutrition is probably needed for mechanical loading to have optimal positive effects on bone density. The work of Kanders and colleagues in premenopausal women supports this hypothesis.[21]

The following factors also are associated with increased risk of bone loss:

▶ Smoking
▶ Drug therapy involving chronic use of glucocorticosteroids, anticonvulsants, or heparin.[1]
▶ Alcoholism and associated factors, including reduced body weight, decreased physical exercise, poor nutrition, inadequate calcium and vitamin D intake, malabsorption from accompanying pancreatitis or liver disease, hypercalciuria, low circulating vitamin D, and overuse of antacids containing aluminum.[1]

▶ ASSESSING FRACTURE RISK

A decrease in bone mass results in a decrease in bone strength and an increased risk of fractures. In much the same way that serum cholesterol predicts heart disease, bone density predicts propensity to fracture.[7] Standard laboratory tests, appraisal of risk factors, clinical observation, and medical and family history are indirect ways of estimating fracture risk. There is no substitute for direct measurement of bone density—using single- or dual-photon absorptiometry, dual-energy x-ray absorptiometry, or quantitative computed tomography.[7]

▶ PREVENTING BONE LOSS

Several recommendations are provided for preventing bone loss or slowing the rate of loss. They are:

1. Maintenance of normal estrogen status at any age in women is critical for bone health. Postmenopausal women should be considered candidates for estrogen-replacement therapy with the aim of preventing bone loss.

2. Regular participation in a physical activity (running, jogging, weight training, aerobics, stair climbing, field sports, racquet sports, court sports, and dancing) of approximately 30 minutes per day is important. Walking, biking, and swimming are of questionable value.[22]

3. Adequate dietary calcium should be supplied from low-fat or nonfat dairy products. Intake should range from a minimum of 800 mg per day for an adult to 1000 to 1500 mg per day in older persons or persons with estrogen deficiency.

4. Encourage consumption of vitamin D-enriched dairy products and exposure to sunlight to maintain adequate vitamin D status in older persons. Vitamin D supplements should be considered if serum 25-hydroxyvitamin D_3 is low.

5. Investigational therapies (calcitonin, fluoride, biphosphonates, parathyroid hormone, etidronate, coherence therapy, androgens, vitamin D) may be considered on an individual basis.

6. Avoid smoking and excessive alcohol; possibly avoid caffeine ingestion.

The presence of risk factors (advanced age, thin body size, estrogen deficiency for any reason, white or Asian ethnicity, long-term glucocorticoid or anticonvulsant therapy, family history of osteoporosis, cigarette smoking, alcoholism, limited dietary calcium intake, immobilization or physical inactivity) warrants further investigation and potential treatment.[2,3]

REFERENCES

1. Schapira D. Prevention and treatment of osteoporosis. *Compr Ther*. 1990;16:27-33.
2. AMWA position statement on osteoporosis. *J Am Med Wom Assoc*. 1990;45:75-79.
3. Riggs BL, Melton LJ III. Involutional osteoporosis. *N Engl J Med*. 1986;314:1676-1686.
4. Gallagher JC. The pathogenesis of osteoporosis. *Bone Miner*. 1990;9:215-227.
5. Dalsky GP. Effect of exercise on bone: permissive influence of estrogen and calcium. *Med Sci Sports Exerc*. 1990;22:281-285.
6. Peck WA. Estrogen therapy (ET) after menopause. *J Am Med Wom Assoc*. 1990;45:87-90.
7. Melton LJ III, Eddy DM, Johnston CC. Screening for osteoporosis. *Ann Intern Med*. 1990;112:516-528.
8. Melton LJ III, Kan SH, Wahner HW, Riggs BL. Lifetime fracture risk: an approach to hip fracture risk assessment based on bone mineral density and age. *J Clin Epidemiol*. 1988;41:985-994.
9. Maclennan WJ. Osteoporosis. *Br Med Bull*. 1990;46:94-112.
10. Cumming RG. Calcium intake and bone mass: a quantitative review of the evidence. *Calcif Tissue Int*. 1990;47:194-201.
11. Amaud CD. Role of dietary calcium in osteoporosis. *Adv Intern Med*. 1990;35:93-106.
12. Heaney RP. Calcium, bone health, and osteoporosis. In: Pack WA, ed. *Bone and Mineral Research*. 4th ed. New York, NY: Elsevier Science Publishing Co; 1986:255-301.
13. Anderson JJB. Dietary calcium and bone mass through the lifecycle. *Nutr Today*. 1990;25:9-14.
14. Osteoporosis Consensus Conference. *JAMA*. 1984;252:799-802.
15. Riggs BL, Hodgson SF, O'Fallon WM, et al. Effect of fluoride treatment on the fracture rate in postmenopausal women with osteoporosis. *N Engl J Med*. 1990;322:802-809.
16. Riggs BL, Melton LJ III. Clinical heterogenisity of involution osteoporosis: implications for preventative therapy. *J Clin Endocrinol Metab*. 1990;27:1229-1232.
17. Wolman RL. Bone mineral density levels in elite female athletes. *Ann Rheum Dis*. 1990;49:1013-1016.

18. Barrow G, Saha S. Menstrual irregularity and stress fractures in collegiate female distance runners. *Am J Sports Med*. 1988;16:209-216.

19. Lloyd T, et al. Women athletes with menstrual irregularity have increased musculoskeletal injuries. *Med Sci Sports Exerc*. 1986;18:374-379.

20. Mansfield M, Emans S. Anorexia nervosa, athletics, and amenorrhea. *Pediatr Clin North Am*. 1989;36:533-549.

21. Kanders B, Dempster DW, Lindsay R. Interaction of calcium nutrition and physical activity on bone mass in young women. *J Bone Miner Res*. 1988;3:145-149.

22. Drinkwater BL. Physical exercise and bone health. *J Am Med Wom Assoc*. 1990;45:91-97.

Anorexia Nervosa and Bulimia

Lisa Dorfman

Eating disorders such as anorexia nervosa and bulimia are complex diseases characterized by gross disturbances in eating behaviors. The general prevalence of anorexia nervosa, found mainly in young adolescent females, is low (<1% of the general population), but is as high as 2% in college underclassmen. Bulimia has a higher prevalence than anorexia nervosa, with symptoms prevalent in 20% of college students and 2% to 3% of the general population.[1]

In the *Diagnostic and Statistical Manual* (*DSM III-R*) of the American Psychiatric Association, anorexia nervosa is described as the refusal to maintain a normal predicted body weight for height; intense fear of gaining weight or fat; a distorted body image; and amenorrhea.[2]

Bulimia, as a distinct entity, is an act of excessive eating followed by a method of purging; that is, self-induced vomiting or the use of cathartics. The typical bulimic is an 18- to 25-year-old female who is overly concerned about her appearance, although she is usually of normal weight. To maintain and preserve her perceived body image, she becomes entrapped in a vicious cycle: diet, starve, binge, guilt and shame, purge, relief, and diet.[3] Purging is the coping mechanism that alleviates the shame and guilt of the binge. As long as the outlet for relief is available and accessible, the potential exists for the bulimic to gorge secretly on her forbidden foods.[3]

The classic anorexic is an intelligent, high-achieving, well-organized adolescent female from a moderately affluent family. As a child, she was nondemanding, quiet, well behaved, and willing to please. She may have been slightly overweight initially, and on the subtle suggestion of her family or a friend, went on a diet.[4] The anorexic becomes enmeshed in rituals, including regular weigh-ins (sometimes two to five times a day), conscious denial of hunger, moving food with utensils without taking a bite, preparing and serving food to others, and a vigorous personalized exercise program. Researchers in psychology theorize that by regressing into a thin, nonmenstruating, childlike body, the anorexic can temporarily alleviate her fears about relating to the opposite sex, underachieving, losing control, and becoming obese.[5] The self-denial and the rituals become her means of coping with those fears.

A correlation between the mindset of the anorexic and that of the obsessive, habitual athlete has been suggested. There are, however, distinguishing features of the anorexic and, perhaps, the bulimic anorexic, which can make the diagnosis of these disturbances a bit easier.[6-8] These features include:

▶ Aimless physical activity
▶ Poor or decreasing exercise performance
▶ Poor muscular development
▶ Flawed body image
▶ Body fat level below normal range
▶ Electrolyte abnormalities

▶ Dry skin
▶ Cardiac arrhythmias
▶ Lanugo hair (hirsutism)
▶ Leukocyte dysfunction

Although each disorder is distinct in various signs and symptoms, anorexics and bulimics share the characteristics of low self-esteem, depression, isolation from friends and family, weight phobia, and malnutrition. The incidence of anorexia nervosa and bulimia in athletes is not statistically clear. Eating disorders have been associated with, but not limited to, runners, dancers, gymnasts, figure skaters, bodybuilders, divers, wrestlers, and boxers. Some athletes develop aversions to food and body fat in the belief that a lighter weight will increase their speed, vertical jump, or artistic interpretation. Some of these eating practices are transient; others are not. The athletes who continue to thrive on maladaptive eating behaviors are especially in need of individualized nutrition counseling.

Athletes with eating disorders are a particular concern and challenge to the sports nutritionist, due to their inability to recognize their disease despite a compulsive need to train harder and eat less than their sport demands. Initially they perform well, if not better than average, until the disease progresses to the point of substantial loss in body weight or muscle tissue. The athlete needs to be made aware of the unhealthy consequences of their eating habits, such as hypotension, cold intolerance, edema, epigastric distress, and disturbed sleep patterns. It is only then that the nutritionist will successfully be able to help these athletes improve their nutritional status.[6]

▶ TREATMENT GOALS

The dietitian treating an athlete with an eating disorder should set the following goals[3]:

▶ Educate the client about how the body digests, stores, and uses carbohydrate, fat, and protein during exercise and nonexercise states.
▶ Reassure the client that his or her body performs the same biochemical functions as other people's bodies.
▶ Dissolve the client's black-and-white, good-or-bad prejudices toward food and exercise by encouraging gradual additions to or deletions from the food and exercise repertoires.
▶ Identify and applaud evidences of moderation.

The dietitian should not be the sole therapist. The web that the anorexia or bulimic client weaves around himself or herself is best unraveled by a multidisciplinary team. Many psychotherapeutic treatments focus on alleviation of fears and the discovery of acceptable, nonmaladaptive coping mechanisms. In general, anorexic clients are coached in how to develop and maintain personal relationships. Bulimic clients are taught to work on their abilities to plan, organize, and sense control.[3,8]

Nutrition consultants and members of the therapeutic team need to approach nutrition education, counseling, meal planning, etc, with congruent philosophies. There must be regular communication among all involved for the client to progress.[8]

▶ INITIAL INTERVIEW

A 24-hour recall and 3-day food record is likely to show only a small part of the whole nutrition picture. Although an anorexic client's intake may be monotonously regular, he or she may overexaggerate portions consumed by describing the amount served instead of the amount actually eaten. A bulimic client may not be able to recall all the foods consumed or the number of times purging occurred. Sometimes clients with bulimia respond better to the listing of foods as "binge foods," "OK foods," or "forbidden foods." Do not assume portion sizes; ask specifically. To obtain a more complete evaluation of nutritional status, inquire about the consumption of alcohol, caffeine, supplements, laxatives, diuretics, and other medications (what kind, how much, how often, and when taken). These may represent cross-addictions, and the therapist should be aware of them.[2,9,10]

Inquire about the client's attitudes toward eating, the eating environment (eg, eating companions), where food is eaten (eg, car, bathroom, kitchen, basement), how quickly food is eaten, and how soon purging is induced. Obtain the details of physical exercise (type, frequency, duration, and intensity). Intensity can be described in terms of heart rate, ability to talk, and heavy or light breathing.

The measurement of body composition via skinfold thickness may be perceived as too invasive during the initial interview, but when attained, this information will certainly complement the nutrition report. The depletion of somatic protein stores can be estimated by applying the following equation:

$$MAMC = MAC - (3.14 \times TSF)$$
$$\text{where} \quad MAMC = \text{midarm muscle circumference in cm}$$
$$MAC = \text{midarm circumference in cm}$$
$$TSF = \text{triceps skinfold in cm}$$

The standard MAMC for adults is 23.2 cm for females and 25.3 cm for males. (See appendix 16 for age-related MAMC norms.) Interpretation of calculated values is as follows:

- ▶ *Mild depletion* of somatic protein is 90% of standard.
- ▶ *Moderate depletion* of somatic protein is 90% to 60% of standard.
- ▶ *Severe depletion* of somatic protein is 60% of standard.

▶ MEDICAL WORK-UP

Serum levels of albumin, transferrin, hemoglobin, and total lymphocyte count may be normal despite significant depletions in somatic protein reserves. The anorexic client displays caloric malnutrition rather than protein-energy malnutrition. Abnormal elevations in total cholesterol or blood urea nitrogen may be seen.[1] Clients with anorexia may experience cardiovascular abnormalities in the form of hypotension, bradycardia, decreased left ventricular mass, and/or abnormal ventricular response to exercise.[12] See *Table 3.11* for common physical signs suggestive of malnutrition.

Most physiologic changes seen in bulimic clients reflect the practices of vomiting and the abuse of laxatives and diuretics. Findings may include hypotension, abnormal ECGs, cardiac arrhythmias, low serum potassium levels, periodontal disease, esophagitis, and hiatal hernia.[12] The secondary amenorrhea frequently seen in anorexic and bulimic women may contribute to decreased bone density in these clients, despite participation in weight-bearing exercise.[13]

TABLE 3.11 Physical Signs Suggestive of Malnutrition

Body Area	Normal Appearance	Signs Associated With Malnutrition
Hair	Shiny; firm; not easily plucked	Lack of natural shine; hair dull and dry; thin and sparse; hair fine, silky and straight; color changes (flag sign); can be easily plucked
Face	Skin color uniform; smooth, pink, healthy appearance; not swollen	Skin color loss (depigmentation); skin dark over cheeks and under eyes (malar and supra-orbital pigmentation); lumpiness or flakiness of skin of nose and mouth; swollen face; enlarged parotid glands; scaling of skin around nostrils (nasolabial seborrhea)
Eyes	Bright, clear, shiny; no sores at corners of eyelids; membranes a healthy pink and are moist. No prominent blood vessels or mound of tissue or sclera	Eye membranes are pale (pale conjunctivae); redness of membranes (conjunctival injection); Bitot's spots; redness and fissuring of eyelid corners (angular palpebritis); dryness of eye membranes (conjunctival xerosis); cornea has dull appearance (corneal xerosis); cornea is soft (keratomalacia); scar on cornea; ring of the fine blood vessels around corner (circumcorneal injection)
Lips	Smooth, not chapped or swollen	Redness and swelling of mouth or lips (cheilosis); especially at corners of mouth (angular fissures and scars)
Tongue	Deep red in appearance; not swollen or smooth	Swelling; scarlet and raw tongue; magenta (purplish color) of tongue; smooth tongue; swollen sores; hyperemic and hypertrophic papillae; and atrophyic papillae
Teeth	No cavities; no pain; bright	May be missing or erupting abnormally; gray or black spots (fluorosis); cavities (caries)
Gums	Healthy; red; do not bleed; not swollen	"Spongy" and bleed easily; recession of gums
Glands	Face not swollen	Thyroid enlargement (front of neck); parotid enlargement (cheeks become swollen)
Skin	No signs of rashes, swellings, dark or light spots	Dryness of skin (xerosis); sandpaper feel of skin (follicular hyperkeratosis); flakiness of skin; skin swollen and dark; red swollen pigmentation of exposed areas (pellagrous dermatosis); excessive lightness or darkness of skin (dyspigmentation); black and blue marks due to skin bleeding (petechiae); lack of fat under skin
Nails	Firm, pink	Nails are spoon-shape (koilonychia); brittle, ridged nails
Muscular and skeletal systems	Good muscle tone; some fat under skin; can walk or run without pain	Muscles have "wasted" appearance; baby's skull bones are thin and soft (craniotabes); round swelling of front and side of head (frontal and parietal bossing); swelling of ends of bones (epiphyseal enlargement); small bumps on both sides of chest wall (on ribs)–beading of ribs; baby's soft spot on head does not harden at proper time (persistently open anterior fontanelle); knock-knees or bow-legs; bleeding into muscle (musculoskeletal hemorrhages); person cannot get up or walk properly
Internal systems		
Cardiovascular	Normal heart rate and rhythm; no murmurs or abnormal rhythms; normal blood pressure for age	Rapid heart rate (above 100 tachycardia); enlarged heart; abnormal rhythm; elevated blood pressure
Gastrointestinal	No palpable organs or masses (in children, however, liver edge may be palpable)	Liver enlargement; enlargement of spleen (usually indicates other associated diseases)
Nervous	Psychological stability; normal reflexes	Mental irritability and confusion; burning and tingling of hands and feet (paresthesia); loss of position and vibratory sense; weakness and tenderness of muscles (may result in inability to walk); decrease and loss of ankle and knee reflexes

From Christakis G, ed. Nutritional assessment in health programs. *Am J Public Health.* November 1973;63(suppl 1). Used by permission.

▶ NUTRITIONAL THERAPY

For the underweight client, the most important goals are to establish 95% of normal body weight and to overcome the medical complications of malnutrition. Although these disorders typically take several months or years to develop, and generally as long to correct, the medical consequences require immediate attention and care through an adequate nutrition program. The initial program for the anorexic client should include approximately 800 to 1200 kcal per day, or about 400 kcal within the predicted basal energy expenditure (BEE) at the time of presentation. There is some evidence that bulimics require less than the BEE prediction for energy.[14]

The nutrition plan should consist of approximately 30% of total calories as fat, and provide about 1.5 to 2 g protein per kilogram body weight. The meal plan should include five to six small meals that are low in fat to avoid gastric distress and anxiety caused by large meals. This is particularly important when working with a purging individual. Diet foods and drinks should be avoided because they tend to keep the client entrenched in a dieting mode.

Specific meal guidelines should be provided to avoid the anxiety of selecting foods. It is important to take into consideration the food preferences of clients, and provide support for their self-selected individualized diet plans (eg, vegetarianism), as long as their choices are generally healthful in nature. High-calorie supplements should be used only when the client has an extremely low body weight or is extremely anxious about eating six meals daily. Support should be given regarding fear-of-fatness issues, and clients should be reassured that the program will help them achieve their personal health goals.

After the first week of the program, increments of 200 kcal each week can be added in conjunction with a supervised exercise program to achieve a weight gain of 0.5 to 3 lb per week. Bizarre food practices previously followed may be discussed at this time. It is important to express to clients that they will not feel any better about themselves, nor will they benefit from their newly adopted healthful eating habits, if they continue abusing their bodies with laxatives, diuretics, diet pills, or using recreational substances (such as alcohol, marijuana, and cocaine) to avoid feelings and food issues.

A food, mood, and activity diary may help clients with eating disorders feel like active participants in their treatment. Tools such as the computerized dietary analysis, percentage-body-fat analysis, and blood examinations can give clients additional feedback on their progress. Positive support and education from the nutritionist is a must for nutritional success.

Nutrition treatment for the bulimic who is of normal weight is similar to that for the low-body-weight anorexic; the principal exception is the lack of need to achieve ideal weight through a 1200 kcal diet. Avoidance of binge foods is suggested initially; the client can gradually progress to eating these foods in a controlled environment, with the nutritionist present. For clients with bulimia, behavioral changes in eating habits are as important as restoring normal metabolism. It is important to encourage bulimic clients to avoid excessive hunger by eating at least three meals per day. These clients should be encouraged to eat in the presence of others, because more often than not, these individuals tend to eat most of their meals alone.

Constipation and fluctuations in weight are a common side effect after bulimic clients eliminate laxatives and diuretics from their daily routine. These potential problems should be discussed with the client.

Exercise can be a healthy tool for achieving a better body image, fitness, and ideal body size; but it can be detrimental if it becomes another compulsion to replace the vomiting and other purgative agents. The food, mood, and activity diary may help to open conversation regarding this potential problem.

During each session, it is important to remember that anorexic and bulimic clients are experts in deception and manipulation. If they sense the dietitian or other therapist is vulnerable or inexperienced, they might attempt to exploit a perceived weakness by lying, creating a feeling of inadequacy in the dietitian, or by trying to arouse conflict between professional consultants. A confident attitude on the part of the dietitian can be helpful in the treatment of the client.

In conclusion, both anorexia nervosa and bulimia have a nutritional component that cannot be ignored when a therapeutic plan is devised. The nutritionist will be able to offer very useful information to both clients and the medical team to assist in the recovery of these special people.

REFERENCES

1. Williams MH *Nutrition for Fitness and Sport*. 3rd ed. Dubuque, Iowa: Wm C Brown Publishers; 1992.
2. *Diagnostic and Statistical Manual of Mental Disorders*. 3rd ed, rev. Washington, DC: American Psychiatric Association; 1987.
3. Gross M. Bulimia. In: Gross M, ed. *Anorexia Nervosa*. Lexington, Mass: DC Heath Co; 1982.
4. Rosen JC, Leitenberg H. Bulimia nervosa: treatment with exposure and response prevention. *Behav Res Ther*. 1982;13:117.
5. Garkinel PE, Garner DM. *Anorexia Nervosa: A Multidimensional Perspective*. New York, NY: Brunner/Mazel; 1982.
6. Smith NJ. Excessive weight loss and food aversion in athletes simulating anorexia nervosa. *Pediatrics*. 1980;66:139.
7. Blackburn GL, et al. Nutritional and metabolic assessment of the hospitalized patient. *J Enteral Parenter Nutr*. 1977;1:11.
8. Halmi KA. Anorexia and bulimia. *Psychomatics*. 1983;24:1111.
9. McSherry J. The diagnostic challenge of anorexia nervosa. *Am Fam Physician*. 1984;29:139-145.
10. Story M. Nutrition management and dietary treatment of bulimia. *J Am Diet Assoc*. 1986;86:517-519.
11. Kovach KM. The assessment of nutritional status in anorexia nervosa. In: Gross M, ed. *Anorexia Nervosa*. Lexington, Mass: DC Heath Co; 1982.
12. Moodie DS. Cardiac function in anorexia nervosa. In: Gross M, ed. *Anorexia Nervosa*. Lexington, Mass: DC Heath Co; 1982.
13. Drinkwater BL, Nilson K, et al. Bone mineral content of amenorrheic and eumenorrheic athletes. *N Engl J Med*. 1984;311:277.
14. Kaye W, Gwirtsman H, Obarzanek E, George T, Jimerson D, Ebert M. Caloric intake necessary for weight maintenance in anorexia nervosa: nonbulimics require greater caloric intake than bulimics. *Am J Clin Nutr*. 1986;44:435-443.

Physical and Mental Disabilities

Karen Hare

Nearly 4% of the total US population has some type of disability. Disabilities can be defined in terms of a limited ability to function, either physically or mentally, and may include motor as well as sensory limitations.

Essentially, disabled people face many of the same health issues as other people–nutrition problems, obesity, physical inactivity, alcohol and drug abuse, and stress-related disorders. Disabled people have at least as great a need for fitness as the able-bodied. From the perspective of health promotion and the prevention of secondary health problems, people with disabilities have even greater needs. They can experience accentuated benefits from involvement in sports and physical fitness programs. With proper application, fitness activities may help people with asthma improve their respiratory capabilities, help blind people better cope with the stress of living, help handicapped youngsters become able to work to their potential in a variety of life's activities, and help emotionally disturbed individuals gain self-esteem.

The range of disorders requiring special attention is considerable, and those who devise fitness and nutritional care programs must consider all aspects of the individual's health. Obesity is probably one of the greatest concerns regarding individuals with disabilities. Limited motivation to lose weight coupled with a sedentary life-style and lowered metabolism in individuals with disorders such as Down syndrome makes the development of fitness and nutrition programs for these clients especially challenging. Persons with emotional disturbances often must take medications that result in increased thirst and appetite. This encourages weight gain, making physical activity difficult. Many individuals have substantially reduced muscle mass, which must be considered when evaluating caloric and protein needs.

Clients with spinal cord injuries often lack temperature-control or sweating mechanisms and may experience hypothermia or hyperthermia with exertion. Adequate fluid replacement, as well as adequate clothing, is a critical part of their care.

With such a vast degree of challenges, it is essential that any nutrition care program be coordinated with other professionals working with the individual. A multidisciplinary approach should include the dietitian, physician, recreational or physical therapist, or special adapted physical educator, and counselor or psychologist. Nutrition guidelines for specific sports as outlined in other sections of this manual can be applied to disabled clients, providing consideration is made for those medications that might affect metabolism or fluid balance. Energy and protein requirements should be adjusted to reflect active muscle mass, depending on the specific disability.

Practical Considerations and Applications

June Alberici, Editor

As practitioners, dietitians and other health professionals must use information from a wide range of sources to solve real-world, real-time problems. They must provide practical solutions that a client can willingly integrate into his or her life-style. Without this focus on practical considerations and applications, all the available information for improving health and athletic performance would not be of much use to those who are in greatest need of it. The following section contains material that is aimed at helping practitioners reach clients with needed information.

Protocols for Developing Exercise Prescriptions

Josephine Connolly Schoonen and June Alberici

Optimal health requires reaching beyond a current disease-free state, because much of what we do today will affect our health in the future. Health professions must emphasize the importance of life-style factors, including:

▶ diet
▶ weight control
▶ exercise
▶ smoking cessation
▶ stress reduction

This section highlights the rationale for regular exercise and offers guidelines for exercise prescription.

It is often difficult to convince people that regular exercise is an important component of optimal health and, for many who are convinced, it is even more difficult to bring home the message that *moderate* exercise is essential for long-term health and well-being. Paffenbarger and colleagues[1] found that, among 17 000 Harvard University alumni, those who participated in activities (such as walking, stair climbing, and sports) that increased their energy expenditure by 2000 kcal or more per week, had mortality rates 25% to 33% lower than alumni who did not. For those who expended more than 3500 kcal per week through activities, death rates stabilized. This indicates that there is a maximum level of exercise, beyond which there appears to be no additional benefit derived.

Blair and colleagues monitored the cardiorespiratory capacity of 13 344 men and women and divided them into five groups ranging from sedentary individuals to those running 30 to 40 miles per week.[2] For men, the age-adjusted death rates per 10 000 person-years dropped from 64 among the least fit, to 25.5 in the group with the next (higher) level of fitness. However, the death rate among the extremely active men was only about 7 points lower than those who exercised just a little bit. Similar effects were reported for the smaller group of women in the study, although their death rates declined more steadily than the men's as exercise levels increased. Based on the results, it was concluded that a brisk walk 30 to 60 minutes per day is sufficient for individuals to decrease their risk of dying from heart disease, cancer, or other chronic ailment.

These benefits of moderate, aerobic exercise add to the long-known benefits of structured exercise programs designed to elicit measurable effects on maximum oxygen consumption. The benefits of these types of exercise programs include protection against:

▶ coronary heart disease
▶ hypertension
▶ obesity

▶ hypercholesterolemia
▶ hypertriglyceridemia
▶ osteoporosis

These types of structured exercise programs are also effective therapeutic tools in the treatment of angina pectoris, hypertension, type II diabetes mellitus, obesity, and peripheral vascular disease. It has also been documented that regular physical activity often enhances the quality of life and encourages a health consciousness that often results in a renewed attention to diet and, among smokers, a reduction in cigarette smoking.[3]

Any type of added activity in one's daily routine is beneficial. However, to promote measurable and predictable improvements in the cardiovascular system, an exercise program must safely and adequately *stress* the system. An exercise program meeting this criterion must include a warm-up phase, an aerobic phase, and a cool-down phase. Flexibility exercises and strengthening exercises are also important in promoting safe exercise and fitness.

Designing an exercise prescription requires that the health-care professional consider the individual's health goals, time constraints, sports and recreational interests, current exercise habits, medical history, and risk of injury or cardiovascular event. A medical examination is *always* desirable before an individual begins a new exercise regimen. However, an apparently healthy individual under the age of 45 can usually begin an exercise program safely if the program proceeds gradually, and the person knows these warning signs of exercise intolerance[4]:

▶ Pain or pressure in the center of the chest, the arm, or the throat during or immediately after exercise
▶ Substantial increase in shortness of breath with exercise
▶ Dizziness, light-headedness, sudden lack of coordination, confusion, or fainting
▶ Sudden burst of rapid heartbeats or a sudden slowing of a rapid pulse
▶ Nausea or vomiting during or after exercise
▶ Unexplained weight changes

Individuals at higher risk for complications during exercise include those with at least one major risk factor, and/or symptoms suggestive of cardiopulmonary disease or metabolic disease, such as diabetes mellitus. A medical examination and an exercise tolerance test are recommended for these individuals before they begin an exercise program, especially for those over the age of 45. Individuals at any age with known cardiovascular, pulmonary, or metabolic disease should have a medical examination and an exercise tolerance test before beginning an exercise program.[4] It is also important to consider a client's history of musculoskeletal problems, including those of the back, knee, hip, or ankle, which may limit certain types of physical activity.

Information from a monitored graded exercise test determines the limitations (related to intensity and duration) of the optimal exercise program. If the results of a graded exercise test are available, these should be reviewed prior to making a prescription. The following key issues should be considered when designing an exercise program[4]:

▶ mode of exercise
▶ warm-ups
▶ cool-downs
▶ frequency
▶ duration
▶ rate of progression
▶ intensity

▶ MODE OF EXERCISE

The American College of Sports Medicine (ACSM) advises us to follow both an aerobic and resistance training program.[5] Aerobic exercise involves large muscle groups in continuous, rhythmic activity, and should be pleasurable. Resistance training is strength training of a moderate intensity, sufficient to develop and maintain fat-free weight (FFW), and should be an integral part of an adult fitness program. A cross-training program, alternating the modes of exercise, is recommended for the following reasons. Cross-training:

- ▶ minimizes the danger of "overuse" injury,
- ▶ adds variety to the workout scheme,
- ▶ provides options in inclement weather, and
- ▶ furnishes a variety of workout alternatives during recovery days.

It is important for clients to be eased into an exercise program. The "no pain, no gain" mentality of exercise is wrong and should be discouraged. Clients should be informed that muscular stiffness, soreness, and continued fatigue 1 hour after an exercise session is a indication that the work load for the past exercise session was too high and should be reduced for the next session.

▶ WARM-UP AND COOL-DOWN

Warm-up and cool-down sessions are essential for all exercise programs. They should last, individually, 5 to 10 minutes, and consist of activities done during the aerobic phase of the session, but at a lower intensity, followed by stretching exercises. Stretching and strengthening exercises, especially those involving the abdominal and lower back muscles, are also recommended. If a shorter than usual workout is planned, it is essential to shorten the aerobic phase and not the warm-up or cool-down phase.[6] Following this recommendation should reduce the chance of injury during exercise.

▶ FREQUENCY OF EXERCISE

Exercising one day and resting on the next day is the recommended frequency of exercise for those starting a structured fitness program. ACSM recommends exercising aerobically 3 to 5 days per week, and recommends a 2-day-per-week resistance training program.[5] Exercising aerobically three to four times per week is sufficient to elicit cardiovascular benefits. Exercising more than 4 days per week may result in more dropouts and injuries in those people who were previously sedentary, and may be a psychological impediment to the exercise.[6]

It should be made clear to the client that *any amount of activity* greater than the amount undertaken previously, even if it is a 5-minute walk, is beneficial. Providing too much structure too fast (eg, a minimum of 30 minutes, three or four times per week) may turn a person away from the exercise program because it is too dramatic a change. Therefore, the amount of time spent exercising and the frequency of exercise should only be considered goals that clients can work up to at their own comfortable pace. The goals should *not* be considered minimums for gleaning cardiovascular benefit.

▶ DURATION OF EXERCISE

As a rule of thumb, once the client has adjusted to the exercise program, the duration of an exercise program should be sufficient to expend 300 kcal per session. This amount of exercise promotes significant fitness improvements over a relatively short period. However, the client's initial fitness and motivational level must be considered before this goal can be considered reasonable. The 300-kcal expenditure may be a long-range goal for some clients (see *Table 4.1*).

For resistance training, the recommended minimum is one set of 8 to 12 repetitions of eight to ten exercises that condition the major muscle groups performed at least 2 days per week. The duration of aerobic activity should be 20 to 60 minutes of continuous activity. Duration is dependent on the intensity of the activity, so lower-intensity activities should be conducted over a longer period. For a nonathletic adult, a low to moderate intensity activity of longer duration is recommended.

Research suggests that workouts as brief as 10 minutes, if done often enough, can promote fitness.[7] One group of men in the study jogged at moderate intensity (reaching 65% to 75% of their maximal heart rates) for 10

TABLE 4.1 Summary of Measured Energy Cost of Various Physical Activities

| Activity | kcal (kg*min) | kcal/h | | |
		50 kg	70 kg	90 kg
Basketball	0.050-0.200	150-600	210-840	270-1080
Canoeing, rowing, kayaking	0.050-0.133	150-400	210-560	270-720
Cycling	0.050-0.133+	150-400	210-560	270-720
Dancing (social)	0.050-0.117	150-350	210-490	270-630
Dancing (aerobic)	0.066-0.167	200-500	280-700	360-900
Golf (power cart)	0.033-0.050	100-150	140-210	180-270
Golf (pull/carry)	0.066-0.117	200-350	280-490	360-630
Jogging/running				
4 mph	1.78 per (kg*mile)			
5 mph	1.73 per (kg*mile)			
6 mph	1.69 per (kg*mile)			
7 mph	1.68 per (kg*mile)			
8 mph	1.66 per (kg*mile)			
9 mph	1.64 per (kg*mile)			
10 mph	1.63 per (kg*mile)			
Paddle/racquetball	0.133-0.200	400-600	560-840	720-1080
Rope jumping	0.150-0.200	450-600	630-840	810-1080
Skating (ice/roller)	0.083-0.133	250-400	350-560	450-720
Skiing (downhill)	0.083-0.133	250-400	350-560	450-720
Skiing (x-country)	0.100-0.200	300-600	420-840	450-1080
Soccer	0.083-0.200	250-600	250-840	450-1080
Swimming (crawl)				
Women				
Skilled	260 kcal/mile			
Average	300 kcal/mile			
Unskilled	360 kcal/mile			
Men				
Skilled	360 kcal/mile			
Average	440 kcal/mile			
Unskilled	560 kcal/mile			
Tennis	0.066-0.150	200-450	280-630	360-810
Volleyball (recreational)	0.050-0.100	150-300	210-420	270-540

Adapted from *Anthropometric Standardization Reference Manual* (p 160) by T.G. Lohman, A.F. Roche, and R. Martorell (eds), 1988, Champaign, IL: Human Kinetics. Copyright 1988 by Timothy G. Lohman, Alex F. Roche, and Reynaldo Martorell. Reprinted by permission.

minutes three times daily for 8 weeks. During this same period, another group jogged continuously at the same intensity for 30 minutes a day. The group that jogged continuously experienced greater improvements in cardiovascular endurance, but both lost significant amounts of weight. The men in both groups lost similar amounts of weight (average loss of 4 lb during the 8 weeks). This should be especially encouraging news for people with tight work and family schedules.

▶ PROGRESSION OF EXERCISE

Clients should exercise at a level that does not result in continued fatigue and soreness 1 hour after the exercise session. It is important for them to understand that gradual progression to their desired exercise goal is an important key to fitness. To assist them and to reinforce this point, health professionals should encourage clients to record their *distance* or *work load* (eg, miles, repetitions, level on an exercise machine) and *duration* of exercise. When clients can easily walk 4 or 5 miles briskly without stopping and their goal is to improve fitness further, they can slowly incorporate short intervals of jogging if no medical contraindications exist. The ratio between walking and jogging can gradually change until the client can jog 3 miles continuously.[6] This concept of interval training is also appropriate for exercise machines. When clients are comfortable with a low work level, they can incorporate short intervals of exercise at a higher work load until they are able to work continuously at the higher work load.

▶ INTENSITY OF EXERCISE

Intensity is the variable in an exercise program that can most easily precipitate injuries and untoward cardiac events. When recommending an exercise intensity, it is best to err on the conservative side, monitor the client's response, and progress toward goals slowly. Ideally, exercise intensity is based on a percentage of measured maximum oxygen consumption or on the heart rate at which maximum oxygen consumption is known to occur during a graded exercise test. Since oxygen consumption is linearly related to heart rate, heart rate is often used to determine and monitor intensity during an exercise session. However, when maximum oxygen consumption and measured maximal heart rate are not available, the maximal heart rate can be estimated with the following equation:

Maximal heart rate = 220 – age in years

The American College of Sports Medicine has set a training heart rate guideline for healthy individuals at 60% to 90% of maximal heart rate, or 50% to 85% of maximum oxygen consumption (see *Table 4.2*). The intensity of exercise that provides an adequate stimulus for cardiorespiratory improvement varies with age and activity level. Most of the population can exercise safely and derive positive cardiovascular benefits when exercising at an intensity corresponding to *below* 70% to 85% of their maximal heart rate. The maximum target range for a training heart rate for a 40-year-old could be calculated as follows[6]:

(220 – 40) × 0.70 = 126 beats per minute

Table 4.2 shows the relationship between relative intensity based on percentage of maximal heart rate (HRmax), percentage of maximal oxygen

TABLE 4.2 Classification of Intensity of Exercise Based on
20 to 60 min of Endurance Training

Relative Intensity (%)		Rating of Perceived Exertion	Classification of Intensity
HRmax	$\dot{V}O_2$max* or *HRmax reserve		
<35%	<30%	<10	Very light
35-59%	30-49%	10-11	Light
60-79%	50-74%	12-13	Moderate (somewhat hard)
80-89%	75-84%	14-16	Heavy
≥90%	≥85%	>16	Very heavy

Table from Pollock ML, Wilmore JH. *Exercise in Health and Disease: Evaluation and Prescription for Prevention and Rehabilitation.* 2nd ed. Philadelphia, Pa: WB Saunders; 1990. Published with permission.

*HRmax = maximum heart rate. $\dot{V}O_2$max = maximum oxygen uptake.

consumption ($\dot{V}O_2$max) and the rating of perceived exertion (RPE). The use of RPE has become a valid tool in the monitoring of intensity of exercise training programs. It is generally considered adjunct to monitoring relative exercise intensity, but once the relationship between heart rate and RPE is known, RPE can be used in place of heart rate. This would not be the case in certain client populations in whom more precise knowledge of heart rate may be critical to the determination of the safety of the exercise program.

Clients with heart disease or those who are taking beta-blocker medications require a graded exercise test to determine their appropriate exercise intensity accurately. With older or very poorly conditioned individuals, it is appropriate to initiate a program at 50% of estimated maximal heart rate. This allows them to adjust physiologically and psychologically to exercise, as well as to demonstrate any signs or symptoms of heart disease before exercising at more strenuous intensities. Clients should be educated regarding signs and symptoms that require medical attention, and should be followed up with a physician before continuing an exercise program if any signs or symptoms have occurred during exercise.

When considering exercise intensity, duration, and frequency together, duration and frequency should be increased before progressing to a more intensive exercise. As a client's fitness level advances and maintenance levels are approached, games and modified sports may be added for variety and to maintain interest. In most games and sports the alternating higher and lower energy demands may be accompanied by heart rates 10% higher or 10% lower than the prescribed target heart rate. However, the exercise intervals should be of such duration that the heart rate over time averages out to the prescribed level.[4]

If a graded exercise test is available, heart rate, electrocardiographic tracings, and signs and symptoms in response to graded increases in work load are recorded. This information allows the exercise physiologist to determine a target heart rate range based on the actual maximal heart rate. It also allows the exercise specialist to evaluate the client's signs, symptoms, and ECG for indicators of cardiovascular disease or ischemia with the prescribed target heart rate range. This allows for a safer estimate of target heart rate. The variables of mode, duration, frequency, and progression would be addressed in a similar fashion as discussed above.[4]

The key to long-term adherence to any exercise regimen is *motivation*. The client must be willing to alter his or her current level of activity to promote the desired results. As with any dietary changes, modifications in exercise pattern should be individualized and should evolve gradually to maximize the potential for long-term adherence.

The following are suggested guidelines for implementing an exercise plan[8-11]:

▶ Obtain a health history on all clients before the initiation of an exercise program. This should include a list of medications currently and commonly taken, symptoms, and known contraindications. Physician approval is recommended for everyone.

▶ Begin at the client's current level of activity. Walking for several minutes a day may be a realistic starting point for a sedentary person.

▶ Encourage participation in aerobic activities that the client already enjoys, or help him or her learn the new activities he or she wishes to try.

▶ Encourage activity with a friend, coworker, or family member. Referral to a credible group exercise facility may be indicated if the client has no one to exercise with.

▶ When an activity other than walking is undertaken, it must be easily accessible and fit the client's life-style. For example, it is not practical to recommend swimming for someone who does not live near a pool or who cannot swim.

▶ Build in opportunities for frequent feedback sessions for praise and reinforcement of achievements. As much as possible, involve family and friends in this process.

▶ EXERCISE FOR WEIGHT LOSS

An exercise or physical fitness component should be included in all weight-loss programs when not medically contraindicated. Physiologically, exercise helps to balance calorie intake and expenditure, and to maintain muscle mass while decreasing body fat. Exercise also improves glucose tolerance, increases the HDL to LDL ratio, decreases triglycerides, lowers blood pressure, and improves cardiovascular fitness. Since most obese individuals' fitness levels quickly respond to small training stimuli, exercise also has psychological benefits by increasing the sense of success and self-control, and improving self-image.[12]

It is important to consider that changes in weight alone are not a viable indicator of improvement in fitness. A periodic medical examination and feedback from an exercise physiologist are recommended to obtain valid information on fitness parameters. By conducting baseline and follow-up fitness tests, concrete information can be documented and used for positive reinforcement. This information could include blood pressure, circumference measurements, body composition, resting heart rate, improvements in duration and work load of exercise tolerance, stamina, size, lean body mass to fat ratio, and blood pressure.

The amount of exercise needed to decrease body fat is most strongly related to duration and frequency of exercise. Low intensity, greater frequency, and longer duration of activities are recommended for maximizing fat loss and minimizing orthopedic complications.[4] Obese individuals use more energy and burn more body fat for the same amount of activity than nonobese individuals, because the energy cost of exercise is proportional to body weight. A rough guide to energy expenditure for walkers or joggers is 100 kcal/mile; slightly less for thin people or slower-paced walking or jogging; and slightly more for heavier people or faster-paced walking or jogging. It is recommended that obese individuals move toward an initial goal of expending at least 300 kcal per workout a *minimum* of three times per week to promote weight loss.

Special circumstances must be considered when obese individuals initiate exercise. Due to the insulating qualities of fat, obese clients often report excessive sweating and heat intolerance, even with minimum exertion. Proper ventilation and air-conditioning in warm weather are necessary. In addition, it is essential to emphasize adequate hydration. Special attention to body mechanics is critical with this population. It is important that they receive coaching on spine and knee alignment during exercise to reduce orthopedic problems. Finally, it is important to help obese people find a nonjudgmental atmosphere where they can exercise comfortably.

▶ FOOTWEAR FOR EXERCISE

Fancy equipment and the latest in fashion exercise-wear do not contribute to effective exercise, but good-fitting exercise shoes are essential for exercising safely and limiting injuries. Advise clients that selecting the right shoe for exercise is important. Tennis shoes do not make good running shoes. Encourage patients to frequent stores with knowledgeable staff, and to ask about the following components of an exercise shoe:

- ▶ length
- ▶ width
- ▶ heel counter
- ▶ heel height
- ▶ midfoot support
- ▶ sole flexibility
- ▶ balance
- ▶ quality of construction
- ▶ materials

REFERENCES

1. Paffenbarger RS Jr, Hyde RT, Wing AL, Hsich CC. Physical activity, all cause mortality, and longevity of college alumni. *N Engl J Med*. 1986;314:605.
2. Blair SN, Kohl HW III, Paffenbarger RS Jr, Clark DG, Cooper KH, Gibbons LW. Physical fitness and all cause mortality. *JAMA*. 1989;262:2395.
3. Thomas G, et al. *Exercise and Health: The Evidence and Implications*. Cambridge, Mass: Oelgeschlager Gunn and Hain Publishers Inc; 1979.
4. American College of Sports Medicine. *Guidelines for Exercise Testing and Prescription*. 4th ed. Philadelphia, Pa: Lea & Febiger; 1991.
5. American College of Sports Medicine. The recommended quantity and quality of exercise for developing and maintaining cardiorespiratory and muscular fitness in healthy adults. *Med Sci Sports Exerc*. 1990;22:265-274.
6. Howley ET, Franks BD. *Health/Fitness Instructors Handbook*. Champaign, Ill: Human Kinetics Publishers Inc; 1986.
7. De Busk RF, Stenestrand U, Sheehan M, Haskell W. Training effects of long versus short bouts of exercise in healthy subjects. *Am J Cardiol*. 1990;65:1010-1013.
8. Pollock ML, Wilmore JH, Fox SM. Prescribing exercise for the apparently healthy. In: *Exercise in Health and Disease: Evaluation and Prescription for Prevention and Rehabilitation*. Philadelphia, Pa: WB Saunders Co; 1984.
9. Crimmins C, Guggenheim F. Obesity management: a clinical approach. In: *Primary Care Medicine*. 2nd ed. Philadelphia, Pa: JB Lippincott Co; 1985.
10. Pollock ML, et al. Effects of frequency and duration of training on attrition and incidence of injury. *Med Sci Sports Exerc*. 1977;9:31.
11. Serfass RD, Gerberich SG. Exercise for optimal health: strategies and motivational considerations. *Prev Med*. 1984;13:79.
12. Harris J. Exercise considerations for obese women. *Sports Nutrition News*. 1987;5:5.

Protocols for Developing Dietary Prescriptions

Charlene Harkins, Ruth Carey, Nancy Clark, and Dan Benardot

Regular exercise has a positive effect on overall health by promoting increased cardiovascular performance, favorable body composition, and increased bone density. However, regular exercise does not negate the need for a well-balanced diet. Many exercise enthusiasts should be reminded that dietary saturated fat promotes increases in LDL-cholesterol levels, and excess dietary fat promotes increased storage of body fat and promotes some types of cancer, *regardless of the frequency, duration, and intensity of exercise.* When they complement each other, diet and exercise modifications are most effective in preventing or managing chronic diseases and obesity.

► TIPS FOR DIETARY COUNSELING OF ACTIVE PEOPLE[1]

- ► It helps to be an athlete or an active person yourself when counseling an active person on what to eat to enhance performance and fitness.
- ► Learn about your client's sport or activity.
- ► Ask specific questions about the training regimen, including type(s) of training, sleep patterns, and how much time is spent on training per day.
- ► Stress that proper nutrition does not take the place of talent, conditioning, skills training, and effort. Philosophically, poor nutrition should be considered a potential limiting factor in optimal performance by adversely affecting benefits from conditioning and training. In reality, virtually all athletes could improve nutrient intake. Therefore, an improvement in nutrition may well have real, discernable benefits in athletic performance.
- ► When working with a team-sport player, try to understand the coach's (or athletic trainer's) view of training and diet.
- ► Talk in practical and positive terms. For instance, rather than lecturing on the importance of avoiding high-fat foods, give examples of high-carbohydrate foods that are easy to obtain, provide ideas for what to select at a fast-food restaurant, or help college athletes select the best foods from the campus foodservice.
- ► Get an understanding of fluid-consumption patterns and practical sports limitations in consumption of fluids during practice or competition. Recommendations for fluid intake should be congruent with the limitations of the sport.
- ► Try to be involved with the physiologic evaluation of team members. This will help to make you a more valued and integral part of the sports medicine team and the athletic team.

▶ Begin with small goals. Just getting a wrestling team to consider eating breakfast or drinking a glass of water on the day of the meet may be a major breakthrough.

▶ When planning diets, focus on frequent meals, adequate hydration, adequate calories, and adequate protein. Predict daily caloric and protein needs for each individual, and help him or her understand what foods to eat to meet these needs.

▶ Reinforce your work (especially with young athletes) by helping parents understand what you are trying to achieve, and give them tools to help, such as recipes and food lists. Make them part of your team.

▶ Stress familiar foods the day before and the day of an event.

▶ Give enough food information so athletes are secure with the idea that they can obtain all the nutrients they require from food, without taking nutrient supplements. Take athletes, individually or in groups, on grocery shopping trips and, if possible, give them cooking classes. The activities can be fun and effective educational experiences.

▶ If meeting with a member of a team, do so in confidence and in a private space, not the locker room. Be careful never to breach the confidentiality of any information you may have on a player. Even acknowledging to the media that you are working with a particular player, without that player's permission, would be a breach of this special relationship.

▶ Be aware that you might elicit an angry response if you recommend something that is appropriate, but conflicts with coaching policy.

▶ Reinforce basic training principles. You cannot build muscle just by eating protein, and you cannot ski well by working out on a simulator. Training must be specific to the activity.

▶ Combat nutrition fraud by comparing products with easily available foods while trying not to put the athlete on the defensive.

▶ Do not try to cover everything in a single session. Have a small but clear goal for each session, and focus on that.

▶ Remember that the psychological aspect of food is powerful for many athletes. If an athlete is convinced in the power of a certain food, and it is not dangerous, do not attempt to change his or her mind about it.

▶ Spend most of the time listening. Ann Grandjean, an experienced sports nutritionist, recommends: "The secret to success when working with elite athletes is to listen 90% of the time and talk no more than 10%. The goal is to serve as a facilitator, not a lecturer. To facilitate, one must understand. To understand, one must listen."

▶ Stay positive. It takes a long time to change habits or behaviors that may be rooted in false information provided by other "professionals." Say the same thing over and over again in many different ways.

▶ GUIDE TO DIETARY PRESCRIPTION

1. Determine the individual's current health and nutrition status.
   a. Assessment of individual needs should begin with a physical examination. Blood work can help determine deficiencies and pinpoint possible disease states (eg, diabetes, high cholesterol) that will require diet modifications.
   b. Determine height, weight, height/weight ratio, and body composition, and compare these with age- and sex-adjusted norms. This is particularly important in children and adolescents.

2. Estimate actual dietary intake.
   a. Use a 24-hour food recall, food frequency questionnaire, or 3- to 5-day food record. A combination of any two of these yields reliable information.
   b. Conduct an interview to develop rapport and assess general meal patterns:

   ▶ Where are most meals eaten?
   ▶ Who prepares the food?
   ▶ What foods does the client avoid?
   ▶ What are the client's snacking patterns and snack choices?
   ▶ What are his or her cultural and ethnic practices?
   ▶ What are the client's perceptions of good nutrition?

3. Determine training and competition practices.
   a. Determine the amount and time spent in training as well as the intensity and duration; these will figure prominently into caloric needs.
   b. Ask specific questions with regard to competition.

   ▶ What time is the game or meet?
   ▶ When will the athlete eat or drink?
   ▶ What foods are available to eat?
   ▶ What sleeping patterns are followed?

4. Determine caloric needs using one of the following methods:
   a. Use information obtained from the food recall or diet assessment. If the active person is an adult maintaining his or her weight, this is the starting point.
   b. Use the current Recommended Dietary Allowances[2] as a starting point for adolescents. Adolescent males tend to overestimate their intake and females tend to underestimate their intake. For example, many young females consume only 1000 kcal, but the RDA for energy is 2200 kcal.
   c. Predict the resting energy expenditure (REE) plus the activity factor for an estimate of caloric requirement.
5. Determine protein needs.
   a. Use the RDA for protein.
   b. Increase protein needs above the RDA if the diet is entirely plant-based.
   c. The protein needs of athletes are typically within the range of 1 to 1.5 g/kg body weight.
   d. If using percentage contribution of protein to total calories (usually 12% to 15% of total calories), make certain the calculated amount does not exceed 2 g protein per kilogram weight.
6. Ensure adequate hydration.
   a. Encourage liberal use of water and, when appropriate, fluid-replacement beverages.
   b. Encourage athletes who work out for long periods in hot and/or humid environments to monitor their own weights. The difference in pre- and postexercise weight is equal to 1 pint of fluid (2 cups) for each pound lost.
   c. If there is a big difference between pre- and postexercise weights, athletes should be encouraged to:

   ▶ consume sufficient fluid so weight returns to normal before the next training session, and

▶ consume more fluid during training sessions to reduce the chance of dehydration.

d. If weight after a training session does not return to within a few pounds of the preexercise weight before the next training session, athletes should be encouraged to refrain from training until weight returns to a normal range.

7. Ensure correct energy substrate distribution.
   a. The recommended intake for athletes matches closely the recommendations in the *Dietary Guidelines for Americans*:

   ▶ Fifty-five to sixty percent of calories should come from carbohydrates, with less than 10% of this amount from refined carbohydrates (sugars).
   ▶ Fifteen percent of calories should come from proteins, not to exceed 2 g/kg body weight.
   ▶ Thirty percent (or less) of calories should come from fat, with an even distribution of saturated, polyunsaturated, and monounsaturated fat.

   b. If high-calorie diets are necessary to maintain weight (eg, for linemen on football teams and weightlifters), carbohydrates should constitute the primary source of calories.

8. Ensure that calcium intake, at a minimum, meets the RDA.
   a. For those athletes who do not like or cannot consume dairy products, alternative sources of calcium should be described.
   b. Young female athletes who are amenorrheic are at risk for long-term bone disease, so they should be encouraged to consume ample amounts of calcium-containing foods or, when necessary, supplements.

9. Ensure adequate iron intake.
   a. Because of iron's role in energy metabolic processes, adequate intake is essential for optimal athletic performance.
   b. Endurance athletes and menstruating athletes should pay special attention to iron status.

10. Discourage use of nutritional supplements.
    a. Supplements may give athletes a false sense of dietary adequacy. The focus should be on obtaining nutrients through consumption of a nutrient-dense, balanced diet.
    b. In certain cases, supplement usage may be warranted:

    ▶ Female athletes at risk of anemia (iron)
    ▶ Athletes with an intolerance to dairy products (calcium)
    ▶ Athletes who limit food intake to control weight
    ▶ Amenorrheic athletes

11. Discourage the use of alcohol.
    a. Alcohol adds nonnutrient calories and may alter normal energy metabolic processes.
    b. Alcohol intake negatively affects athletic performance.
    c. When they are not in training, emphasize moderate alcohol consumption in those athletes of legal drinking age who drink alcohol.

12. Discourage faddish weight-loss regimens.
    a. Over-the-counter weight-loss aids may negatively affect performance by spurring dehydration.
    b. Fast weight loss created by any modality (including fasting) typically equates with loss of lean body mass and strength.

13. Be flexible with diet planning.
    a. Any diet plan you recommend will be accepted better if it considers the athlete's schedule, which usually cannot be altered.
    b. Be prepared to follow up frequently to make adjustments to your original diet plan and fine-tune it with feedback from the athlete.

▶ GENERAL NUTRITION

Nothing makes a bigger difference to nutritional status than the way an athlete eats *most of the time*. Eating correctly most of the time sets up an athlete so that eating the right meal before a game and the right nourishment during the competition can make a difference. Without good general eating habits, no pregame meal and during-competition nourishment can do enough to make a difference. Getting this point across to athletes is critical to help ensure that nutrition will not be a limiting factor in performance.

An athlete cannot rely solely on nutrition for athletic prowess, but poor nutrition can be a limiting factor in athletic performance by limiting the benefits of training and by reducing an athlete's ability to perform to his or her conditioned ability. The dietary needs of athletes vary only slightly from those recommended for all healthy individuals. Due to an energy expenditure that is higher than those of nonathletes, the caloric needs of athletes are greater than those of sedentary people. Caloric requirement will also vary depending on body size, age, gender, sport, and conditioning. The distribution of energy nutrients in an athlete's diet should be about 15% protein, 30% (or less) fat, and 55% to 60% (or more) carbohydrate.

The athlete should have sufficient knowledge of nutrition principles to know how to select a variety of foods that will provide a balance of nutrients. Vitamin and mineral supplementation, except for specific high-risk groups, is typically unnecessary if an athlete meets basic caloric needs. The RDAs for vitamins and minerals are set higher (2 standard deviations above the mean requirement) than the requirement to include the vast majority of all people living in the United States. Virtually all nutrient requirements can be met by consuming a nutrient-dense diet of a wide variety of foods, and this is the best advice for athletes. Exceeding these requirements has not been shown to enhance performance and, in some cases, it may be detrimental to health and performance.

Carbohydrates

Carbohydrates are the ideal energy fuel for the body: they are inexpensive, readily available, easily metabolized, and metabolically efficient. Over the past 20 years, the importance of carbohydrates in athletic performance has been clearly established.

Carbohydrate is the only food component that can be metabolized anaerobically. Carbohydrate utilization occurs throughout anaerobic and aerobic metabolic processes, with a gradual increase in the metabolism of fat and protein as exercise of moderate intensity continues. To sustain energy metabolism, the body eventually turns to the storage form of carbohydrate, glycogen. Liver glycogen helps to regulate blood glucose level, while muscle glycogen is used by muscles as a source of glucose for metabolic processes. Muscle glycogen and fat supply energy during endurance activity.

Dietary manipulation can affect initial glycogen stores both in muscle and in the liver. Increased dietary carbohydrates can raise the glycogen content of the muscle by two to three times the normal level.[3] There is a high correlation between initial glycogen level and the time to exhaustion. Athletes who follow a high-carbohydrate diet (600 g per day) can maintain high-intensity exercise for a longer period than those on a lower-carbohydrate diet (350 g per day). Complex carbohydrates seem to allow for a greater glycogen storage than simple sugars.[3] However, the advantage of complex carbohydrates over simple sugars appears to be more clearly related to their ability to provide more nutrients for the same level of energy.

Both training and proper diet are important to optimize athletic performance. Diet provides the body with the needed fuels, while training helps improve the body's utilization of fuel and its muscle glycogen storage capacity. A more fit individual uses less glycogen, is better able to conserve the limited glycogen stores in the body, and utilizes more fat as a fuel source during endurance events.

Carbohydrates are often categorized as either simple or complex. Simple carbohydrates are sugars (including sucrose, fructose, and glucose). Fruits and many vegetables have a desirable mix of both simple and complex carbohydrates. Cereals and starchy vegetables are high in complex carbohydrates. Complex carbohydrates should make up the largest portion of the athlete's diet (55% or more of total calories). Athletes who train exhaustively on successive days, or who compete in more prolonged endurance events, would benefit from a diet that contains even more energy from carbohydrates (65% to 70% of total calories).[4] As a general rule, complex carbohydrates are the most valuable food sources for energy to the athlete. Complex carbohydrates increase glycogen stores more efficiently than sugars.

Different sources of carbohydrates have different rates of absorption, and therefore affect blood glucose uniquely. The differential effect of carbohydrates on blood glucose is categorized in the glycemic index (see *Table 4.3*). It has been found, for instance, that dried legumes (beans, lentils, chickpeas) produce the lowest peak in blood glucose, but sustain blood glucose longer. Certain root vegetables (potatoes and carrots) produce a blood glucose rise similar to that of sugar (sucrose).[5] Breads, cereals, grains, and fruits all produce a lower glucose peak than sugar. To be assured of providing energy when he or she needs it the most, it is important to refer to the glycemic index when planning snacks or meals for the athlete. It is equally important to remember, however, that there is a great deal of individual variation in the way people respond to different foods.

TABLE 4.3   Glycemic Index* of Foods

Milk products		Grains	
Yogurt	36	Cornflakes	80
Ice cream	36	Whole-wheat bread	72
Whole milk	34	White rice	72
Sugars		Shredded wheat	67
Maltose	95	Sweet corn	59
Glucose	100	Oatmeal	49
Honey	87	Vegetables	
Sucrose	59	Carrots	92
Fructose	20	Potatoes	70
Fruits		Potato chips	51
Bananas	62	Peas	51
Orange juice	46	Baked beans	40
Apples	39	Peanuts	13

From Jenkin DJA, et al. The glycemic index of foods: a physiological basis for carbohydrate exchange. *Am J Clin Nutr.* 1981;34:362. © American Society for Clinical Nutrition.

*The blood glucose response following the feeding of a test dose of the food relative to glucose (glucose = 100).

Fats

Utilization of fats, like that of carbohydrates, is controlled by the duration and intensity of exercise. Training causes physiologic adaptation in muscle and adipose tissue that enhances free fatty acid mobilization and delivery to muscles during exercise. The most important role of fat is to spare carbohydrates (which are in limited supply) in exercise of long duration and low intensity.[3]

Fat is a concentrated source of energy, providing 9 kcal/g. One of the adaptations the body makes to endurance exercise is increased accommodation for fat metabolism.[6] This adaptation enables the athlete to perform longer without exhaustion. During light to moderate (aerobic) exercise, stored fat supplies 50% to 60% of the energy needed, while in prolonged aerobic exercise, its contribution increases to 70%.[3] The athlete capable of using the abundant supply of fat in the body can spare limited glycogen reserves. The average 150-lb person with 10% to 20% body fat has 63 000 to 126 000 kcal as fat, but only 1800 to 2000 kcal as carbohydrate (glycogen and glucose). Even the leanest athletes have sufficient fat storage to meet the metabolic demands of strenuous exercise.

Fatty acids are supplied from triglyceride deposits within the adipose tissue. The concentration of free fatty acids in the blood that is delivered to the exercising muscles is one factor that determines the amount of fatty acids oxidized (greater supply, greater oxidation). Consuming a high-fat diet will result in a larger proportion of fats used during exercise, but this limits the amount of carbohydrate storage, which ultimately limits endurance.[7] It is also important to consider that fat requires carbohydrate for complete oxidation. Some studies have shown that caffeine ingestion of 250 to 350 mg can increase free fatty acid concentration in the blood, which may then increase oxidation of fat by 30% to 50%.[7] However, these findings are still controversial.

Protein

There is a general misunderstanding about the protein needs of athletes. Many believe that large quantities of protein foods (and supplements) are necessary to enhance muscle growth. There is no evidence, however, that protein requirements would ever exceed 2 g/kg body weight, a level that is easily and commonly achieved from food alone.

Protein contributes 1% to 2% of the total energy needed during normal exercise. In more prolonged exercise, protein can provide up to 5.5% of the total caloric needs.[7] Evidence suggests skeletal muscle has a good capacity to oxidize amino acids for energy, particularly the branched chain amino acids (commonly derived from animal protein).[7] Amino acids, therefore, have the potential to provide the working skeletal muscle with energy during sustained exercise periods, when glycogen stores are depleted or very low. However, amino acid metabolic waste products (urea and ketones) must be eliminated via the urine, increasing the chance of dehydration. Because of this waste-product production, amino acids are not good fuels for exercise. To avoid protein energy utilization, meals consumed before exercise should be high in carbohydrates and low in protein.

Protein can be supplied from animal or vegetable food sources, such as beef, chicken, eggs, milk, cheese, dried beans and peas, peanut butter, nuts, seeds, and tofu. Plant protein from vegetable sources is usually low in one or more of the nine essential amino acids. Vegetable protein sources, in combination, can complement one another to provide a high-quality protein. (See *Table 4.4.*)

TABLE 4.4   Protein Complementation

Vegetable Protein	Vegetable Protein	Animal Protein
Legumes (beans)	Cereals (corn, wheat, rice)	Milk, cheese, eggs
Beans + tortillas		Pasta + cheese
Pea soup + cornbread		Oatmeal + milk
Soybean curd + rice		Toast + eggs
Baked beans + brown bread		Rice pudding
Seeds (sesame, sunflower)	Legumes (beans, peas, lentils)	Cheese, eggs
Hummus (tahini + chickpeas)		Beans + cheese
Mixed seed + soynut snack		Beans + eggs
Seeds (sesame, sunflower)	Leafy green vegetables	Cheese, eggs
Sesame seeds + bok choy		Broccoli + cheese sauce
Sunflower seeds + broccoli		Spinach souffle

Adapted from the book: *The Eater's Guide* by: Candy Cumming and Vicky Newman © 1981. Used by permission of the publisher, Prentice Hall/A Division of Simon & Schuster, Englewood Cliffs, NJ.

Hydration

Water is a nutrient often undervalued by athletes, but it may be the most critical one for ensuring that an athlete can perform up to his or her trained and conditioned ability. Because heat production rises as a result of an increased rate of energy metabolism, it is critical that athletes have enough body water to help dissipate this heat through sweat. When sweat evaporates, heat is released from the blood circulating near the skin, cooling the body. Even an untrained, unacclimatized body has a large capacity for sweat production. Sweat losses of 1 to 2 L per hour are not uncommon during exercise in the heat. In trained athletes, sweat losses can exceed 3 L per hour. Fluid losses in excess of 6% of body weight can occur during a 1- to 2-hour training session in high heat.

Dehydration occurs when fluid loss exceeds 1% of body weight. Work capacity and temperature control can be impaired with a loss of as little as 2% of body weight.[8] When dehydration becomes sufficiently severe, sweating ceases in an attempt to conserve body water. As a result, body temperature quickly rises, increasing the chance of heat cramps, exhaustion, or stroke. Therefore, adequate fluid intake before, during, and following exercise is critical in preventing dehydration. Unfortunately, thirst is not a reliable gauge of fluid needs, and significant dehydration can occur before the thirst mechanism is triggered.

Inadequate fluid replacement during exercise can result in heat injury. Dehydration increases the concentration of electrolytes in extracellular and intracellular water, and can result in muscle cramping and impairment of temperature control. Dehydration can also result in pronounced thirst, fatigue, loss of coordination, mental confusion, irritability, dry skin, and decreased urine output that, with elevated body temperature, are common symptoms of heat exhaustion. Heat stroke, the most dangerous heat injury, has a mortality rate of 80%, and many survivors suffer from permanently impaired hypothalamic thermoregulatory control, predisposing themselves to future heat injury.[8]

Although electrolytes (sodium, potassium, chloride, and magnesium) are lost in sweat, the loss of water is considerably greater. However, conditions exist in which electrolyte loss, particularly sodium loss, can be significant. During hard physical work in hot climates, sodium loss may exceed 8 g per day. In these extreme situations, in which large volumes of fluid (>3 L) are required to replace sweat loss, a carbohydrate-electrolyte solution should be provided.

The environmental conditions, the fitness and acclimatization of the workers, and the severity of sweat losses are all factors to be considered when evaluating and recommending electrolyte replacement.

Another type of electrolyte disturbance can occur when only water is consumed during prolonged physical activity, such as marathons, triathlons, ultramarathons, or similar prolonged work. Hyponatremia (low plasma sodium concentration) can be produced by consuming plain water during prolonged work.[9] This condition can cause diarrhea, exhaustion, mental confusion, syncope, pulmonary edema, and ECG alterations. Although hyponatremia may not constitute a major health risk, the increasing popularity of long-duration athletic competitions may spark an increase in occurrence. Consumption of sports beverages appears to be an effective way of preventing this condition.

Some researchers consider potassium losses during exercise in the heat to constitute a potential health problem,[10,11] but the significance of potassium loss is controversial.[12,13]

Fluid needs can be effectively monitored by recording pre- and postexercise body weights. The following guidelines will help athletes meet fluid needs:

▶ Adequate daily hydration with water and other fluids (care should be taken to limit consumption of fluids containing caffeine or alcohol; each acts as a diuretic and can increase fluid loss).
▶ Drink at least 8 to 16 oz of fluid 2 hours before exercise.
▶ Drink at least 4 to 8 oz of fluid immediately before exercise.
▶ Drink at least 4 to 8 oz of fluid every 15 to 20 minutes during exercise to obtain a maximum of 26 oz per hour.
▶ Drink at least 8 to 16 oz of fluid after exercise.
▶ Drink at least 8 oz of fluid with each meal.
▶ Drink at least 8 oz of fluid between meals.

Gastric Emptying of Fluids

The rate at which the stomach can empty fluids is affected by the volume, temperature, and composition of the fluid consumed. Ingesting a large volume of fluid at one time during exercise can cause a feeling of fullness and sluggishness, and may lead to cramping. Since the upper limit for gastric emptying during exercise is about 800 mL per hour (26 oz per hour), a balance must be attained between fluid loss and fluid intake. Research has demonstrated that if fluid is consumed in relatively small volumes at regular intervals, severe dehydration can be prevented and bloating can be avoided. Therefore, the goal should be small, frequent drinks (see guidelines above).[14]

As the carbohydrate content of a fluid increases above 8%, the rate of gastric emptying decreases. Fluids with more than 8% sugar may produce a decrease in gastric emptying rate sufficient to produce a feeling of fullness, and may slow fluid absorption.[14]

Plain, cool water (5° to 10°C; 40° to 50°F) is an effective fluid replacement, and it is the most readily available and least costly alternative. However, in sport or training that requires more than 1 hour of continuous effort, fluids that contain both glucose and electrolytes might improve performance.

▶ THE PREEXERCISE/PRECOMPETITION MEAL

The goals of the preexercise/precompetition meal (PEPCM) follow:

▶ Prevention of hypoglycemia and associated symptoms (light-headedness, blurred vision, needless fatigue, and indecisiveness)

▶ Prevent feelings of hunger
▶ Provide energy for working muscles
▶ Provide fluids to begin exercise in a fully hydrated state

Since a single precompetition meal inadequately compensates for a poor training diet, athletes should eat a carbohydrate-rich diet every day to enhance muscle glycogen storage. The PEPCM should be an extension of this general training regimen, but with a greater focus on carbohydrates and a lower concern for nutritional balance.[15,16]

Although an athlete may want to know exactly when, what, and how much to eat, specific recommendations can be made only with a knowledge of the individual athlete and the athlete's sport. For example, some runners can eat within 1 hour before racing, while others avoid food to reduce the risk of gastrointestinal distress. Some gymnasts want a little food to settle a nervous stomach, while others are so nervous they feel sick and are unable to eat. The PEPCM food preferences also vary from sport to sport. For example, cyclists are likely to eat more than runners, who fear gastrointestinal problems related to the jostling that occurs with running. Since each athlete has unique food preferences and aversions, it is impossible to recommend a single food or meal that will ensure top performance. Therefore, individualized recommendations must be made on a case-by-case basis.

In general, the PEPCM should emphasize complex carbohydrates, because they are quickly digested and absorbed, they leave the stomach quickly, and they are the ideal fuel for muscular work. However, not all carbohydrate-containing foods are good choices for the PEPCM. Foods high in fiber (raw fruits and vegetables with seeds and tough skin; bran; nuts; and seeds) are not recommended because they may cause intestinal discomfort. Heavy use of simple sugars are also not recommended, because they may cause a sudden rise in blood glucose with an overresponse of insulin, resulting in low blood glucose and a feeling of tiredness. Some foods high in carbohydrates are gas-forming, and may cause discomfort during the game. These foods, such as dried beans, cabbage, onions, radishes, cauliflower, and turnips, although excellent choices for general nutrition, are not recommended for the PEPCM. The best high-carbohydrate foods are those high in starch: pastas, breads, potatoes, and rice are excellent. See *Table 4.5* for sample precompetition dinners of approximately 1000 kcal each.

Although many athletes have traditionally exercised and competed on an empty stomach, current research supports the benefits of the PEPCM consumed within 4 hours of the event.[17] Contrary to popular belief, food eaten within 4 hours of exercise is used to fuel working muscles. In one study, five males who consumed 400 kcal of sugar 3 hours before running for 4 hours at 45% $\dot{V}O_2$max, oxidized 68% of the glucose.[18] In another study, cyclists consuming 400 kcal of sugar 1 hour before cycling for 2 hours at 35% $\dot{V}O_2$max oxidized 41% of the consumed sugar.[19]

The PEPCM is especially important before morning exercise, because athletes who compete after an overnight fast have depleted liver glycogen stores. Consuming a meal, or at least a light snack, before morning exercise helps to replenish liver glycogen and helps to maintain normal blood sugar levels and endurance.[20]

Timing of the Meal

When planning the preexercise meal, the athlete should allow adequate time for the food to leave the stomach. Fatty foods delay gastric emptying, but add to the satiety value of foods and may be important for long-endurance exercise. Therefore, a low level of fat in the PEPCM (<25% of calories) is acceptable, but

TABLE 4.5   Sample Precompetition Dinners of Approximately 1000 kcal Each

Foods	Serving Size	kcal
Dinner 1		
Spaghetti	2 cups	395
Meatless spaghetti sauce	¾ cup	203
Parmesan cheese	2 tbsp	46
Tossed salad	¾ cup	17
Salad dressing	1 tbsp	67
Dinner rolls	2	156
Apple juice	8 oz	116
	Total kcal:	1000
	% kcal from CHO:	69
	% kcal from protein:	11
	% kcal from fat:	20
Dinner 2		
Baked chicken, no skin	4 oz	187
Stuffing	½ cup	208
Mashed potato	1 cup	162
Green beans	1 cup	44
Sherbet	½ cup	135
Blueberries	¾ cup	61
Dinner rolls	2	156
	Total kcal:	953
	% kcal from CHO:	58
	% kcal from protein:	20
	% kcal from fat:	22

the focus should be high-carbohydrate foods. Since large, high-fat meals take longer to leave the stomach than smaller, low-fat meals, the general rules are as follows.

The meal should be finished . . .

▶ Three and a half to four hours before exercise or competition if the meal contains more than 25% of calories from fat

▶ Three and a half to four hours before exercise or competition if the meal is relatively large (high in calories, multiple courses)

▶ Two to three hours before exercise or competition if the meal is low in fat (<25% of total calories), high in carbohydrates, and moderate in amount (this is the recommended intake for a PEPCM)

▶ One to two hours before exercise or competition for a blended or liquid meal

▶ Less than one hour before exercise or competition for a light carbohydrate snack, as tolerated

Preparing for morning events.   The night before morning events, athletes should eat a hearty, high-carbohydrate dinner and bedtime snack. That morning, they should eat a light, high-carbohydrate snack or breakfast to abate feelings of hunger, replenish liver glycogen, and absorb some gastric juices. Mealtimes should also provide ample amounts of fluid (see fluid consumption recommendations). For example, a runner who is going to participate in a 10 AM road race may require only a bowl of cereal with skim milk to provide around 300 kcal. However, this amount of food may not be adequate if the athlete did not consume a high-carbohydrate dinner and bedtime snack the night before.

Preparing for afternoon events.   Athletes should plan a hearty, carbohydrate-rich dinner and breakfast, to be followed by a light lunch. A runner racing at noon can enjoy a heartier breakfast (such as four or five pancakes to provide about 600 kcal), but he or she should keep the lunch before the race moderate in calories and high in carbohydrates. As recommended earlier, all meals should provide ample amounts of fluid.

Preparing for evening events.   Athletes should plan a hearty, carbohydrate-rich breakfast and lunch, followed by a moderate-calorie, high-carbohydrate snack 1 or 2 hours prior to the event. As recommended earlier, all meals should provide ample amounts of fluid.

Athletes With High Stress

Some athletes who are overly nervous, stressed, or have sensitive stomachs may prefer to abstain from food the day of competition. They should make a special effort to eat extra food the day prior to the event to be well fueled for competition. This situation may also be ideal for using quickly absorbed liquid meals or liquid carbohydrate-containing supplements. However, liquid meals should be tested and found to be acceptable before they are tried on a competition day.

Liquid Meals

Since liquid foods leave the stomach faster than solid foods, the athlete may want to experiment with blenderized, liquid meals to determine if they offer any advantage. In one report, a 450-kcal meal of steak, peas, and buttered bread remained in the stomach for 6 hours.[21] A blenderized version of the same meal emptied from the stomach in 4 hours. Before converting to blenderized or commercial liquid meals, the athlete should keep in mind anecdotal reports that too much liquid may "slosh" in the stomach and contribute to nausea. Therefore, any new meal should be experimented with during training to determine its level of acceptance.

Preexercise Sugar

Historically, athletes have been advised to avoid sugary foods prior to exercise, with the belief that the "sugar high" will trigger a rebound hypoglycemic effect that will hinder performance.[22] More recent studies suggest that preexercise sugar may actually enhance stamina and endurance or at least not affect it adversely. Gleeson and colleagues reported that subjects who consumed 280 kcal of carbohydrate as glucose 45 minutes prior to hard exercise (73% $\dot{V}O_2$max) improved their time to exhaustion by 12%.[23] Alberici and colleagues reported no adverse effects from consuming a milk-chocolate candy bar 30 minutes before bicycle ergometry (70% $\dot{V}O_2$max) to exhaustion.[24] Because of the inconclusiveness of the findings in this area, athletes who perceive themselves as *sugar sensitive* should abstain from concentrated sweets and rely more on carbohydrate from starch in the preexercise hours. Given the higher nutrient density of starchy foods as compared with simple sugars, it would be preferred if all athletes tried to obtain more energy from foods high in complex, rather than simple, carbohydrates.

High-sugar foods are often consumed as a quick-fix to make up for poorly timed meals before an event. The high-school athlete who craves a sugary quick-energy food before an afternoon workout could remedy this need by consuming a wholesome breakfast and lunch. Not only would this pattern be an investment for better performance in the short term, but the long-term investment would be improved nutrient intake.

Psychological Value of Foods

Preexercise and precompetition food have both physiologic and psychological value. If an athlete firmly believes that a specific food or meal enhances performance, then it may actually enhance performance (the placebo effect). (A cinematic example: Rocky's brew of raw eggs in the morning.) Athletes who believe that a "magic" food helps to ensure athletic performance end up requiring this food to perform at an optimal level. As long as the food consumed is not detracting from the client's nutritional status, it may be important for the sports nutritionist to find other battles to fight rather than trying to give rational arguments for why the "magic" food is not what the athlete believes it to be.

Practice Precompetition Eating

Experience has shown that all athletes must learn, often through trial and error, what foods work best for them. Food preferences may vary depending on the type of exercise, the level of intensity, and the time of day they are consumed. Hence, the guidelines for the PEPCM should be viewed as a starting point for recommendations that can be tried during training. Ideally, the best combination of foods, timing, and amounts will be established in time for competition.

▶ DURING-EXERCISE NOURISHMENT

Athletes who perform exhaustive endurance exercise that lasts for 1 hour or more will have greater stamina and enhanced performance if they consume carbohydrates during the event. Depending on the sport, the carbohydrate can be provided as a solid food or as a liquid. These carbohydrates help to maintain normal blood sugar levels as well as provide an active source of energy for exercising muscles.[25]

It has been found that cyclists can derive an 18% increase in time to exhaustion when they consume 1 g carbohydrate per kilogram body weight per hour.[26] This amounts to approximately 70 g carbohydrate (280 kcal) per hour for a 150-lb athlete and is more than many athletes voluntarily consume. It is important, therefore, that athletes practice consuming carbohydrate-containing foods and beverages during training. This is difficult, because the greater the intensity of exercise, the less likely athletes are to want to consume a food or drink. During intense exercise (>70% $\dot{V}O_2$max), the stomach may get only 20% of its normal blood flow.[21] This slows the digestive process, so any food in the stomach may feel uncomfortable. Sports drinks with sugar solutions of 5% to 8%, on the other hand, tend to be readily accepted. Athletes should plan on programmed drinking (and, where acceptable, programmed eating) to maintain energy levels and hydration status. Although many athletes fear that taking nourishment during an event may cause stomach problems, research suggests that those who do not drink enough and lose more than 4% of body weight have an increased prevalence of gastrointestinal disorders.[27]

During exercise of moderate intensity, blood flow to the stomach is 60% to 70% of normal, so the athlete can still digest food.[21] Therefore, solid-food snacks commonly consumed by skiers, cyclists, and ultramarathon runners do contribute to energy needs and are better tolerated.

▶ POSTEXERCISE REPLENISHMENT

Many of the same athletes who carefully select a high-carbohydrate diet prior to exercise and competition neglect their recovery diet. Since muscles are most receptive to replacing muscle glycogen within the first 2 hours after a hard workout, failure to consume carbohydrates at this time may hinder optimal glycogen recovery and endurance.[28] This could develop into a serious deficit in stored glycogen, especially for those athletes who train or compete daily.

A carbohydrate-deficient recovery diet is common in athletes who eat:

▶ too much protein after the event, often as a reward for eating little protein before the event,

▶ too much fat, typically for those who dine at fast-food restaurants after training,

▶ too many "treats" such as cookies and ice cream, which are actually high in fat and low in carbohydrates, and

▶ too few calories, in those who are taking steps to control weight. These athletes often consider carbohydrate foods "fattening," and they consume high-protein foods like cottage cheese or tuna.

To optimize the recovery process after a hard workout, an athlete should eat 200 to 400 kcal of carbohydrates within 2 hours immediately following exercise, repeating it 2 hours later.[28] This recommended "dose" represents approximately 0.5 g carbohydrates per pound of body weight (or 1 g/kg body weight). For a 150-lb athlete, the recommended postexercise replenishment could be 300 kcal from a juice or carbohydrate-containing fluid within the 2 hours immediately following exercise, followed by a carbohydrate-rich meal after stretching, showering, and recovering from the workout. Examples of some high-carbohydrate snacks (with their calorie content) are:

▶ 2 slices of bread (135 kcal; 81% carbohydrate)

▶ 1 bagel (165 kcal; 76% carbohydrate)

▶ 1 cup pasta (215 kcal; 81% carbohydrate)

▶ 1 medium-sized baked potato (100 kcal; 88% carbohydrate)

▶ 3 cups air-popped popcorn (70 kcal; 79% carbohydrate)

▶ 1 medium-sized apple (80 kcal; 100% carbohydrate)

▶ 1 medium-sized orange (65 kcal; 100% carbohydrate)

▶ 1 cup vegetable juice (55 kcal; 93% carbohydrate)

For those who report that exercise "kills the appetite," juices or sports drinks can provide adequate carbohydrates and also supply needed fluids. Commercial carbohydrate supplements can also be helpful after exercise when an athlete is unlikely to make appropriate selections, or when the right foods are unavailable. In general, however, a hungry athlete can easily consume the recommended amount of carbohydrates from food, and benefit from the nutritional value of these foods.

In addition to replacing carbohydrates, the athlete should be careful to replace fluids lost through sweat. Carbohydrate-containing fluids, such as juices and sports beverages, replace both muscle glycogen and water losses; they are the best choice for both good nutrition and top performance.

Beer is popular as a postexercise "recovery drink," but it is not recommended for this purpose for several reasons:

▶ Alcohol in beer has a dehydrating effect.

▶ Carbonation in beer gives a sense of fullness that limits fluid consumption, just at a time when fluid consumption should be high.

▶ Alcohol in beer may have a depressant effect, just at a time when the athlete should be experiencing an invigorating "natural high."

Although many athletes are concerned about replacing the sodium and potassium that are lost in sweat, only athletes who exercise more than 1 hour daily with heavy water losses from sweat are at risk for depleting these electrolytes. Most can easily replace these minerals with the foods and fluids they consume after the event without the need for special supplements.

To determine how much fluid they must replace, athletes should weigh themselves before and after exercise. The difference in pre- and postexercise weights is equal to the number of pints of fluid that should be replaced (1 pint of fluid for 1 lb lost). Athletes can also monitor their urine: dark-colored urine is a sign that it is concentrated with metabolic waste and the athlete needs more water; clear and voluminous urine is a sign that the athlete is adequately hydrated.

REFERENCES

1. *Report of the Ross Symposium on the Theory and Practice of Athletic Nutrition: Bridging the Gap*. Columbus, Ohio: Ross Laboratories; 1990.
2. National Research Council. *Recommended Dietary Allowances*. 10th ed. Washington, DC: National Academy Press; 1989.
3. Mattson FH. Fat. In: Hegstead DM, et al, eds. *Present Knowledge in Nutrition*. 4th ed. New York, NY: Nutrition Foundation Inc; 1976.
4. Sherman W. Carbohydrates, muscle glycogen, and muscle glycogen supercompensation. In: Williams MH. *Ergogenic Aids in Sports*. Champaign, Ill: Human Kinetic Publishers; 1983.
5. Consensus conference: lowering blood cholesterol to prevent heart disease. *JAMA*. 1985;253:2080.
6. Costill DL, Miller JM. Nutrition for endurance sport: carbohydrate and fluid balance. *Int J Sports Med*. 1980;1:2.
7. Lemon PWR, Nagle FJ. Effects of exercise on protein and amino acid metabolism. *Med Sci Sports Exerc*. 1981;13:141.
8. Knochel JP. Clinical physiology of heat exposure. In: Maxwell MH, Kleeman CR, eds. *Clinical Disorders of Fluid and Electrolyte Metabolism*. New York, NY: McGraw-Hill; 1980.
9. Noakes TD, Goodwin N, Raynor BL, et al. Water intoxication: a possible complication during endurance exercise. *Med Sci Sports Exerc*. 1985;17:370.
10. Knochel JP, Sclein EM. On the mechanism of rhabdomyolysis in potassium depletion. *J Clin Invest*. 1972;51:1750.
11. Knochel JP, Dotin LN, Hamburger RJ. Pathophysiology of intense physical conditioning in hot climate: mechanisms of potassium depletion. *J Clin Invest*. 1972;51:242.
12. Costill DL, Cote R, Miller E, et al. Water and electrolyte replacement during repeated days of work in the heat. *Aviat Space Environ Med*. 1975;46:795.
13. Costill DL. Sweating: its composition and effects on the body fluids. *Ann N Y Acad Sci*. 1977;301:160-174.
14. Costill DL, Saltin B. Factors limiting gastric emptying during rest and exercise. *J Appl Physiol*. 1974;37(5):679.
15. Sherman WM, Costill DL, Fink WJ, Miller JM. The effect of exercise and diet manipulation on muscle glycogen and its subsequent use during performance. *Int J Sports Med*. 1981;2:114-119.
16. Sherman WM. Muscle glycogen supercompensation during the week before athletic competition. *Sports Science Exchange*. June 1989;2:16.
17. Jandrain B, Krentowski G, Pirnay F, et al. Metabolic availability of glucose ingested three hours before prolonged exercise in humans. *J Appl Physiol*. 1984;56:1314-1319.
18. Ravussen L, Pahus P, Dorner A, et al. Substrate utilization during prolonged exercise preceded by ingestion of 13-C glucose in glycogen-depleted and control subjects. *Pflugers Arch*. 1979;382:197-202.

19. Neufer PD, Costill DL, Fink WJ, Wirwan JP, Fielding RA, Flynn MC. Effects of exercise and carbohydrate composition on gastric emptying. *Med Sci Sports Exerc.* 1986;18:658-662.
20. Nilsson LH, Hultman E. Liver glycogen in man: the effect of total starvation or a carbohydrate-poor diet followed by carbohydrate feedings. *Scand J Clin Lab Invest.* 1973;32:325-330.
21. Brouns F, Saris W, Rehrer NA. Abdominal complaints and gastrointestinal function during long-lasting exercise. *Int J Sports Med.* 1987;8:175-189.
22. Costill DL, Coyle E, Fink WJ, et al. Effects of elevated plasma FFA and insulin on muscle glycogen usage during exercise. *J Appl Physiol.* 1977;43:695-699.
23. Gleeson M, Maughan R, Greenhaff P. Comparison of the effects of preexercise feedings of glucose, glycerol, and placebo on endurance and fuel homeostasis in man. *Eur J Appl Physiol.* 1988;55:645-653.
24. Alberici JC, Farrell PA, Kris-Etherton PM, Shively CA. Effects of preexercise candy-bar ingestion on substrate utilization and performance in trained cyclists. *Med Sci Sports Exerc.* 1989;21:547.
25. Costill DL. Carbohydrates for exercise: dietary demands for optimal performance. *Int J Sports Med.* 1988;9:1-18.
26. Coogan AR, Coyle EF. Effect of carbohydrate feedings during high-intensity exercise. *J Appl Physiol.* 1988;65:1703-1709.
27. Rehrer N, Beckers EJ, Brouns F, Hoor FT, Saris W. Effects of dehydration on gastric emptying and gastrointestinal distress while running. *Med Sci Sports Exerc.* 1990;22:790-795.
28. Ivy J. Muscle glycogen synthesis after exercise and effect of time of carbohydrate ingestion. *J Appl Physiol.* 1988;64:1480-1485.

Exercise in Extreme Temperatures

Peggy H. Paul and Charlene Harkins

▶ EXERCISING IN COLD WEATHER

Physiological adaptations that accompany exercising in the cold allow most athletes to continue their training programs during the winter months. The following factors affect an athlete's tolerance to cold-weather exercise.

Cold Acclimatization

The process of cold-weather acclimatization is less understood and less documented than warm-weather acclimatization, but it is known that cold-weather acclimatization is more difficult. Athletes who have become acclimatized to cold-weather training typically demonstrate increased blood flow to peripheral areas,[1] increased skinfold thickness for greater insulation, and elevated metabolic rate for greater heat production.[2] This greater metabolic rate translates into a greater caloric requirement for weight maintenance, regardless of the intensity and duration of exercise.

Fitness Level

Maintaining body temperature in a cold climate requires harder work, and harder work requires a higher level of fitness.[3] Intensive exercise training seems to improve an athlete's tolerance to cold, so there is a premium in developing the highest possible level of fitness.[2]

Body Fat

Athletes with slightly higher body fat levels can usually tolerate cold-weather exercise better than leaner athletes. Because the peripheral blood temperature does not drop as dramatically in "more insulated" individuals as it does in leaner individuals, core temperature does not decrease as rapidly.

Temperature and Wind (Windchill Factor)

Air temperature alone is not an adequate measure of the true temperature felt on the exposed portions of the athlete's body (eg, hands, face, neck) (see *Table 4.6*). On a windy day, blowing air magnifies heat loss via convection because the warm layer of air surrounding the body is constantly being replaced by cooler air.[4,5] In addition to determining the wind velocity, a runner, skier, skater, or cyclist must also determine his or her own exercise velocity because it

TABLE 4.6 Windchill Factor and Safety of Exercise

Estimated Wind Speed	Actual Temperature Reading (°F)											
	50	40	30	20	10	0	-10	-20	-30	-40	-50	-60
(in mph)	Equivalent Chill Temperature (°F)											
Calm	50	40	30	20	10	0	-10	-20	-30	-40	-50	-60
5	48	37	27	16	6	-5	-15	-26	-36	-47	-57	-68
10	40	28	16	4	-9	-24	-33	-46	-58	-70	-83	-95
15	36	22	9	-5	-18	-32	-45	-58	-72	-85	-99	-112
20	32	18	4	-10	-25	-39	-53	-67	-82	-96	-110	-121
25	30	16	0	-15	-29	-44	-59	-74	-88	-104	-118	-133
30	28	13	-2	-18	-33	-48	-63	-79	-94	-109	-125	-140
35	27	11	-4	-20	-35	-51	-67	-82	-98	-113	-129	-145
40	26	10	-6	-21	-37	-53	-69	-85	-100	-116	-132	-148

(Wind speeds greater than 40 mph have little additional effect.)	LITTLE DANGER in less than 1 hour with dry skin. Maximum danger of false sense of security.	INCREASING DANGER Danger from freezing of exposed flesh within 1 minute.	GREAT DANGER Flesh may freeze within 30 seconds.

Note: 1. Trench foot and immersion foot may occur at any point on this chart.
2. °F = ⅘°C +32.

is directly related to the overall windchill factor. Thus, running at 6 mph into a 20-mph head wind has a combined wind speed of 26 mph. As a general rule, there is little exercise risk when the outside temperature is 20°F or higher, regardless of wind speed. Cooler outside temperatures pose greater dangers, especially when coupled with windy conditions.

Cold-Weather Clothing

When choosing to exercise in the cold, an athlete should prepare appropriately and use common sense. When dressing for cold-weather exercise, the goal is to insulate while allowing perspiration to be absorbed by the garments. Multiple layering of garments is an excellent practice for cold-weather exercise. A polypropylene-type garment is an ideal first layer; middle layers should be good insulators (goose down, hollow-fill synthetic fibers, or wool are excellent); and outer garments should be resistant to a variety of weather conditions (Gore-Tex* is often selected). Outdoor gear should also include proper head, ear, face, and neck coverings.

Winter Camping and Expeditions

The nutrient needs of survival in the cold differ from the nutrient needs of physical performance in winter sports. Sports require intense physical effort within a confined time, while living in the cold may require extended effort.

Menu planning for an expedition should first ensure the availability of a source of safe water or other acceptable fluids. Although it is a tedious process, water can be obtained by melting snow. Five cups of snow are needed to obtain 1 cup of water, and a filtering or chemical purification system ensures bacteria-free water. Expedition members should be encouraged to avoid both caffeinated products and alcohol-containing products because of their diuretic effect.

---

*W.L. Gore and Associates, Newark, DE 19711.

It is important to prepare to meet adequately the extremely high caloric needs of participants in cold-weather expeditions. Past Arctic expeditions have demonstrated a need for 6000 to 8000 kcal per day to maintain body weight.[6] These caloric needs are generally met through consumption of a diet that has a higher distribution of fat than typically recommended for athletes. Among the reasons for this is that (1) on an isocaloric basis, fat takes up less space than either carbohydrate or protein—this makes it easier to transport a greater amount of calories in a package of a set size; and (2) fats provide a greater level of satiety than carbohydrates.

Members of the Steger North Pole expedition consumed a monotonous diet that derived 66% of its calories from fat, half of which was saturated. Blood lipid analysis demonstrated little or no change among the seven participants of the expedition. Researchers at the University of Minnesota postulated that the high physical activity counterbalanced the potential cholesterol-raising effect of the high-fat diet.[6]

The differential needs of trace nutrients in cold-weather expeditions have not been adequately studied. However, the higher rate of energy utilization (mainly from fat) suggests a greater need for certain vitamins and minerals associated with oxidative metabolism. Fresh vegetables and fruits should be included when practical, but it is often necessary to bring dehydrated forms on expeditions to reduce the weight of provisions. When it is known that foods will be of limited variety and the trip will be long, a multivitamin-mineral supplement is advisable. (See *Table 4.7* for suggested menu items.)

▶ EXERCISING IN HOT WEATHER

It is no secret that an exercising person's ability to generate heat is often better than the ability to remove it. Competition between these two mechanisms is especially intense during hot and humid weather. The training regimen (frequency, intensity, and duration of exercise) during hot weather ultimately determines how well an athlete compensates for the added heat stress. Care should be taken to avoid or curtail exercise when the combination of heat and humidity reaches dangerous levels. The wet-bulb temperature, which takes humidity into account, is a good guide for evaluating safety of activity (*Table 4.8*).

TABLE 4.7   Suggested Menu Items for Cold-Weather Expeditions

Milk	Powdered milk, cocoa mixes, powdered breakfast drink
Grains	Instant whole grain cereals, instant rice or potatoes, pasta, crackers, soup mixes, cookies (especially fig, apple, or blueberry types), breakfast bars or pastries
Fruit	Fresh apples, oranges, grapes, etc; dried fruit–raisins, prunes, apricots, bananas, apples, fruit leathers; freeze-dried dessert products
Vegetables	Freshly cut and peeled, packaged, and ready-to-go; freeze-dried.
Protein	Peanut butter, nuts, seeds; cured meats–ham, sausage, etc; dried meat sticks and jerky; assorted cheese; dried eggs
Snacks	Chocolate, peanut-chocolate candy, cookies, gumdrops, hard candies, licorice, pudding, trail mixes
Beverages	Fruit juices and drinks, lemonade, apple cider, Russian tea, herbal teas, cocoa, fluid-replacement products, any powdered drink mixes
Others	Margarine, condiments

TABLE 4.8   Wet-Bulb Temperature Ranges and Safety of Exercise

°F	°C	Condition
60	15.5	No prevention necessary
61-65	16.2-18.4	Alert
66-70	18.8-21.1	Insist on frequent fluid consumption; watch for signs of heat stress
71-75	21.6-23.8	Insist on frequent rest periods and frequent fluid consumption; watch for signs of heat stress
76-79	24.5-26.1	Modified or curtailed training only; cancel competitive event
80	26.5	Cancel training; cancel competitive event

Adapted from Murphy RJ, Ashe WF. Prevention of heat illness in football players. *JAMA*. 1965;194:650. Copyright 1965, American Medical Association.

Heat Acclimatization

Consistent training in heat produces several physiologic adjustments that make athletes more tolerant of hot-weather exercise, yet do not make them immune to the threat of heat illness.[5] The process of heat acclimatization, or the physiologic adjustments that improve an athlete's heat tolerance, can be achieved best when the athlete trains in a warm environment.[1] Recent studies indicate that it is possible to become fully acclimatized with as little as 30 minutes per day of exercise over an 8- to 12-day period at a relatively intense level (70% $\dot{V}O_2$max).[5]

The physiologic adjustments that accompany acclimatization are critical to enhance an athlete's performance in the heat. With acclimatization, larger quantities of blood transport metabolic heat from deep tissues to the body's shell, cooling the inner core more effectively. The threshold for the onset of sweating also is lowered, allowing the cooling process to begin earlier in exercise. After 10 days of heat exposure, the sweating capacity is nearly doubled; the sweat is more evenly distributed over the entire body and becomes more dilute (which preserves the body's electrolytes in the extracellular fluid). Extracellular fluid also increases in volume by 8% to 20%.[5] Unfortunately, the benefits of the acclimatization process can quickly be attenuated if the athlete is not well hydrated or if training in the heat is postponed for 2 or 3 weeks.[4]

Performance Expectations

Although an acclimatized athlete would undoubtedly perform better in high heat than someone not acclimatized to heat, neither athlete would perform at a "personal best." Exercise in heat increases the rate of muscle glycogen use, contributing to earlier fatigue and exhaustion than in a cooler climate. Athletes who must train in the heat for repeated days without being acclimatized experience a rapid depletion of energy reserves and may feel the onset of chronic fatigue symptoms. Acclimatization can reduce the rate of glycogen usage by as much as 50%, thereby enhancing hot-weather training capacity and performance.[5]

Exercising in hot weather puts special emphasis on the importance of adequate hydration and the replacement of glucose during exercise. In hot conditions, water loss through sweat can exceed 2 L per hour,[7] and may peak around 3 L per hour in an acclimatized athlete.[1] Without adequate replacement of lost fluids, circulating blood volume decreases, stroke volume decreases, and heart rate increases, causing an overall deterioration in circulatory efficiency.

Adequate hydration is essential for meeting the metabolic and thermic needs of exercise in the heat. There is, however, some question about the optimal makeup of the rehydration fluid. Some researchers find no evidence to support the need for anything other than water to replace fluid lost during hot-weather exercise.[1]

Another found that the addition of salt to drinking water was of minimum value to men and women who were dehydrated (3% body weight) from sweating for each of 5 consecutive days.[4]

Rats supplied with sodium in their drinking water rehydrated more completely than when supplied with water alone.[8] Similar findings are also reported with humans. It was found that people who became mildly dehydrated (2.3% body weight) and were then offered water, voluntarily restored 68% of lost fluid. The same individuals, when offered water and sodium capsules with a sodium content comparable to that of sweat, voluntarily rehydrated 82% of lost fluids.[9] It appears that sodium does help to maintain the drive to drink, and also helps to maintain plasma volume and reduce urine production.

REFERENCES

1. McArdle WD, Katch FI, Katch VL. *Exercise Physiology: Energy, Nutrition, and Human Performance.* 2nd ed. Philadelphia, Pa: Lea & Febiger; 1986.
2. Pate RR. Special considerations for exercise in cold weather. *Sports Science Exchange.* 1988;1:10.
3. Horvath SM. Exercise in a cold environment. *Exerc Sport Sci Rev.* 1982;9.
4. Costill DL, et al. Water and electrolyte replacement during repeated days of work in heat. *Aviat Space Environ Med.* 1975;46:795.
5. Costill DL. Heat acclimatization: preparing for exercise in hot weather. *Sports Med Digest.* 1989;11:7.
6. Steger W, Schurke P. *North to the Pole.* New York, NY: Times Books; 1987.
7. Nadel ER. New ideas for rehydration during and after exercise in hot weather. *Sports Science Exchange.* 1988;1:3.
8. Nose H, Morita M, Yawata T, Morimoto T. Recovery of blood volume and osmolality after thermal dehydration in rats. *Am J Physiol.* 1986;251:R492-R498.
9. Nose H, Mack GW, Shi XR, Nadel ER. Role of osmolality and plasma volume during rehydration in humans. *J Appl Physiol.* 1988;65:325-331.

Exercise at High Altitude

Charlene Harkins and Jill Mielcarek

Physical performance at high altitudes is dependent on many factors, including:

▶ Actual elevation
▶ Physical training of the individual
▶ Acclimatization to the new environment
▶ The task to be performed

Competition and training for athletic events generally takes place at moderate altitudes of 1000 to 3000 m above sea level. Mountain-climbing expeditions may reach altitudes as high as 7500 m above sea level.

▶ PHYSICAL PERFORMANCE

Altitude does not appear to affect muscle strength and flexibility, but endurance is affected. Due to a lower-density atmosphere at high altitude, performance on speed events like sprinting may be improved.[1] However, performance on endurance events may suffer from a lower oxygen availability and a de facto lowering of $\dot{V}O_2$max. This means that performance in events such as Nordic (cross-country) skiing, biathlon, hockey, distance running, and distance speed skating may be related to how well the participant has adjusted to the lower oxygen environment. Because there is a training effect and adaptation to high-altitude training, some athletes have used high-altitude training as a means of improving low-altitude performance. However, data on the effectiveness of this type of training regimen are lacking.

Acute altitude exposure usually results in a somewhat easier water loss and, therefore, a greater chance of dehydration. This water loss may be compounded by anorexia, difficulty in acquiring sufficient fluids, and loss of thirst.[2,3] Acclimatization can be aided by gradually going to higher and higher altitudes, moving higher only when the athlete feels that adaptation had taken place. It is possible that altitude illness may occur if an athlete makes a radical and sudden change in altitude and begins to train as usual. This is a reversible failure of the body's ability to handle sodium and water, which may result in tissue edema. To counteract this condition, a low to moderate sodium intake coupled with a high fluid intake may be desirable.

It has been recommended that those who compete at high altitude consume a mixed diet composed of 65% carbohydrates, 20% fat, and 15% protein, distributed throughout the day in small, frequent feedings.[4]

TABLE 4.9   Altitude-Adjustment Menus for the Aggressive Sportsperson

Food	Serving Size	Calories	Carbohydrate (g)	Protein (g)	Fat (g)
Breakfast					
Applesauce	½ cup	52	13.8	0.2	0.1
Oatmeal	1 package	104	18.1	4.4	1.8
Sugar	2 tsp	31	8.0	0	0
Skim milk	1 cup	86	11.9	8.4	0.4
Cracked-wheat bread	1 slice	66	13.0	2.2	0.6
Margarine	1 tsp	34	tr*	tr	3.8
Jelly	1 tsp	13	3.3	tr	0
Fluids (ad lib)					
Milk cocoa	2 cups	227	49.4	6.8	2.7
Sweetened tea	1 cup	88	22.0	0.3	0
Water	2 cups	0	0	0	0
Lunch					
Granola bars	2	594	67.3	15.0	33.2
Banana chips	1 cup	346	88.3	3.9	1.8
Raisins	½ cup	217	57.4	2.3	0.3
Fluids (ad lib)					
Eggnog	1 cup	261	38.9	8.2	8.4
Lemonade	2 cups	223	57.5	0	0
Sweetened tea	1 cup	88	22.0	0.3	0
Water	2 cups	0	0	0	0
Dinner					
Vegetable soup	1 cup	122	19.0	3.5	3.7
Macaroni and cheese	1 cup	430	40.2	16.8	22.2
Pita bread	1	203	38.8	6.4	2.1
Fruit cocktail	½ cup	57	14.7	0.6	tr
Fluids (ad lib)					
Apple juice	1½ cups	175	43.5	0.2	0.4
Drinking gelatin	2 cups	267	41.9	24.5	1.1
Water	2 cups	0	0	0	0
Snacks					
Fig bars	8	401	84.5	4.4	6.3
Dried apricots	½ cup	155	40.1	2.4	0.3
Hard candy	1 oz	108	27.2	0	0.3
Totals		4348	820.7 (75% of calories)	110.6 (10% of calories)	89.5 (19% of calories)

*tr = trace, <0.05 g.

General hints
▶ Gradually increase calories as activity increases.
▶ Plan one-pot meals that cook in 15 min.
▶ Drink 3-5 L water per day, drink frequently.
▶ It takes 15-20 min to melt snow to water; it takes 10-15 min to boil water.
▶ Increase carbohydrate intake drastically.

Moderate climbing, 3500 kcal
▶ 4.4 kg (2 lb) dry food per person
▶ 75% kcal from carbohydrate
▶ 15% kcal from fat
▶ 10% kcal from protein
▶ 4 L fluid

Heavy climbing, 5000 kcal
▶ 5 kg (2¼ lb) dry food per person
▶ 5 L fluid

▶ ACUTE MOUNTAIN SICKNESS

Altitude sickness or acute mountain sickness (AMS) may occur when a person receives lower levels of oxygen than she or he is accustomed to.[5] Symptoms of AMS include:

- ▶ headache
- ▶ anorexia
- ▶ nausea
- ▶ fatigue
- ▶ shortness of breath

These symptoms occur most often at elevations of 8000 ft (2400 m) or higher, and are most dependent on the rapidity with which one ascends to this height. Symptoms may be caused by the inability to properly control intercellular and

TABLE 4.10   Altitude-Adjustment Menus for the Casual Sportsperson

Food	Serving Size	Calories	Carbohydrate (g)	Protein (g)	Fat (g)
Breakfast					
Orange juice	½ cup	56	13.4	0.9	0.1
Cornflakes	¾ oz	83	18.3	1.7	0.1
Sugar	2 tsp	31	8.0	0	0
Skim milk	1 cup	86	11.9	8.4	0.4
Cracked-wheat bread	1 slice	66	13.0	2.2	0.6
Margarine	1 tsp	34	tr*	tr	3.8
Jelly	1 tsp	13	3.3	tr	0
Fluids (ad lib)					
Sweetened tea	1 cup	88	22.0	0.3	0
Water	2 cups	0	0	0	0
Lunch					
Chicken noodle soup	½ cup	26	3.7	1.5	0.6
Saltine crackers	6	74	12.2	1.5	2.0
Low-fat cottage cheese	½ cup	82	3.1	14.0	1.2
Gelatin salad	½ cup	80	19.7	1.6	0.1
Canned peaches	½ cup	55	14.3	0.8	tr
Fluids (ad lib)					
Lemonade	2 cups	223	57.5	0	0
Water	1 cup	0	0	0	0
Dinner					
Broiled salmon	3 oz	184	0	23.2	9.3
Baked potato	1 small	124	28.6	2.6	0.1
Mixed vegetables	½ cup	54	11.9	2.6	0.1
Sherbet	½ cup	135	29.4	1.1	1.9
Fluids (ad lib)					
Sweetened tea	1 cup	88	22.0	0.3	0
Water	2 cups	0	0	0	0
Snacks					
Banana	½	52	13.4	0.6	0.3
Apple	1 medium	81	21.1	0.3	0.5
Totals		1714	326.8 (76% of calories)	63.4 (15% of calories)	21.1 (11% of calories)

*tr = trace, <0.05 g.

General hints

- ▶ Resume normal patterns after 36-48 h.
- ▶ Keep exercise to a minimum.
- ▶ Avoid alcohol; increase other fluids.
- ▶ Drink 2 to 3 L water per day, drink frequently.

extracellular fluid balance. Most people eventually adapt to high altitudes, with this acclimatization process dependent on four factors: speed of ascent, altitude reached, work intensity, and the amount and type of food and fluid consumed.

In general, a low-salt, high-fluid intake is recommended for the acclimatization process. (See *Tables 4.9* and *4.10* for altitude-adjustment menus for aggressive and casual sportspeople.) Ideally, dietary modifications should take place at sea level, with a transition as the individual moves to higher altitudes. Carbohydrate and fluid consumption should increase the day before departure and be maintained throughout the stay. Fat intake should be kept to a minimum, because it may contribute to feelings of nausea. There should also be a total cessation of alcohol consumption, since the alcohol may contribute to both dehydration and nausea. It should be understood that loss of appetite is normal and may decrease food intake by 40% to 60%. To counteract this, encourage the consumption of small, frequent meals. The avoidance of AMS depends on eating and drinking normally, taking time to reach higher elevations, and being sensitive to how well one's own body has adapted to the current elevation before going higher.[5]

REFERENCES

1. Daniels J. Altitude training. In: Casey MJ, Foster C, Hixson EG, eds. *Winter Sports Medicine*. Philadelphia, Pa: FA Davis Co; 1990;14-21.
2. Boyer SJ, Blume FD. Weight loss and changes in body composition at high altitude. *J Appl Physiol*. 1984;57:1580-1585.
3. Rowell A, Cove DH. Birmingham Medical Research Expeditionary Society 1977 expedition: the diuresis and related changes during a trek to high altitude. *Postgrad Med J*. 1979;55:471-491.
4. Lickteig JA. Nutrition for high altitudes and mountain sports. In: Casey MJ, Foster C, Hixson EG, eds. *Winter Sports Medicine*. Philadelphia, Pa: FA Davis Co; 1990;383-392.
5. Casey MJ, Foster C, Hixson EG, eds. *Winter Sports Medicine*. Philadelphia, Pa: FA Davis Co; 1990.

Time Zone Changes

Jill Mielcarek and Susan Kleiner

International competition is commonplace for elite athletes, yet few take steps to counteract the desynchronization of physiologic and psychological cycles that occurs as a result of long-distance travel. To make matters worse, many athletes exacerbate the problems of travel by leaving very little time to adjust before a competition.[1] Symptoms of jet lag include general malaise, appetite loss, and disturbed sleep. Two forms of travel can contribute to jet lag: (1) travel involving small but consecutive trips causing multiple shifts in normal eating and sleeping behaviors, and (2) a single trip crossing many time zones, causing a major change in eating and sleeping behaviors. The following recommendations may help to alleviate the effects of jet lag:

For small, consecutive time zone changes (phase shifts):

▶ Eat meals at regular times after arriving at the new destination.
▶ Drink plenty of liquids. The controlled environment of the plane cabin is dry, and dehydration is the cause of many complaints, including headaches and mild constipation.
▶ Alternate light meals with heavy meals before the flights. Eat a high-protein breakfast and a low-protein, high-carbohydrate dinner following phase advance.
▶ Avoid caffeine until the end of the flight.
▶ Avoid alcohol during and after the flight. If you wish to drink alcohol, limit yourself to one drink, and order a light one, such as a wine spritzer.
▶ Indulge in social activity or exercise after the flight.

For a large phase shift:

▶ Arrive at your destination at least 1 day early for each time zone crossed. For flights crossing more than six time zones, allow 1 week for resynchronization.
▶ Indulge in exercise and social activity upon arrival in the new environment.
▶ Maintain regular sleeping times (ie, anchor sleep) and eating times after arrival at the destination.
▶ Alternate light meals with heavy meals 3 days before the flight. Eat a high-protein breakfast and a low-protein, high-carbohydrate dinner following phase advance.
▶ Avoid alcohol during the period of resynchronization.
▶ Drink plenty of liquids. The controlled environment of the airplane cabin is dry, and dehydration is the cause of many complaints, including headaches and mild constipation.

To avoid problems with resynchronization, the traveler should not put off eating when hungry. It may be useful to take along some foods to snack on while traveling. *Table 4.11* presents a list of easy-to-take-along foods.

TABLE 4.11 Foods for "Eating on the Road"

Milk products	Cheese wedges, string cheese, yogurt
Meats and protein foods	Beef sticks, peanut butter sandwiches, hard-cooked eggs, nuts
Fruits and vegetables	Dried apricots, apples, banana chips, raisins, fruit-filled cookies
Grains	Low-fat granola, breadsticks, bagels, crackers, bran muffins, soft pretzels
Fluids	Sports drinks, fruit juices

REFERENCE

1. Loat ER, Rhodes EC. Jet lag and human performance. *Sports Med*. 1989;8:226-238.

Meal Plans and Recipes

Patti Tveit and Dan Benardot

Providing athletes with examples of meal plans and recipes is an effective and practical way to assist them with dietary changes that are healthful and aid performance. (See the four nutrition-counseling case studies presented later in this section.) This section contains meal plans for:

- ▶ carbohydrate loading
- ▶ vegetarians
- ▶ weight gain and weight reduction
- ▶ precompetition
- ▶ adolescents
- ▶ diabetes

In general, all diets for athletes should be high in carbohydrates (55% to 60% or more of calories), low in fat (30% or less of calories), and moderate in protein (15% of calories), and should provide plenty of fluid.

▶ CARBOHYDRATE LOADING

During prolonged exercise, the depletion of muscle glycogen and exercise-induced hypoglycemia can work together or independently to cause exhaustion. Because of this, the initial glycogen store in muscle and liver is an important predictor in determining endurance potential of the athlete. Endurance athletes have learned that endurance can be improved by maximizing glycogen stores, and many have practiced one form or another of glycogen loading for that purpose. The traditional (original) method of glycogen loading has been associated with a number of problems (weakness, irritability, lethargy, postural hypotension, and ketonemia), and it is not recommended. Currently recommended is a method that avoids these problems while achieving a similar level of glycogen storage. The two methods are compared in *Table 4.12*. There is no evidence that glycogen loading is useful for sports involving less than 1 hour of continuous exercise. An example of a high-carbohydrate diet useful for maximizing stored glycogen is presented in *Table 4.13*.

▶ VEGETARIAN DIETS

Meat is not necessary for ensuring optimal athletic performance. This point is notably demonstrated by the many elite athletes who are vegetarians. There are many different types of vegetarian diets, including diets that eliminate only red meat but include fish, poultry, eggs, and dairy products; eliminate all meats, poultry, and fish, but include eggs and dairy products; and eliminate all meats,

TABLE 4.12   Traditional Method and Current Recommended Method for Glycogen Loading

Day	Traditional Method	Current Recommended Method
1	Exercise exhaustively to deplete muscle glycogen	Exercise exhaustively to deplete muscle glycogen
2	Consume a high-protein, high-fat, low-carbohydrate diet and reduce intensity and duration of exercise	Consume a mixed diet with a moderate to high amount of carbohydrate and reduce intensity and duration of exercise
3	Same as day 2	Same as day 2
4	Same as day 2	Same as day 2
5	Consume a high-carbohydrate diet (500-800 kcal from CHO), and continue reduction of intensity and duration of exercise	Consume a high-carbohydrate diet (500-800 kcal from CHO), and continue reduction of duration and intensity of exercise
6	Consume a high-carbohydrate diet, and continue reduction of intensity and duration of exercise or complete rest	Consume a high-carbohydrate diet, and continue reduction of intensity and duration of exercise or complete rest
7	Consume a high-carbohydrate diet, with very low intensity and short-duration exercise or complete rest	Consume a high-carbohydrate diet, with very low intensity and short-duration exercise or complete rest
8	Competition day	Competition day
	Problems: Hypoglycemia, weakness, lethargy, irritability, nausea, postural hypotension, ketonemia	*Problems:* None

TABLE 4.13   Example of a High-Carbohydrate Diet Useful for Maximizing Glycogen Storage

Food	Serving Size	Calories	Carbohydrate (g)	Protein (g)	Fat (g)
Breakfast					
Orange juice	1 cup	112	26.8	1.7	0.2
Cornflakes	2 cups	221	48.9	4.6	0.2
Skim milk	1½ cup	128	17.8	12.5	0.7
Cracked-wheat bread	2 slices	131	26.0	4.4	1.1
Jelly	2 tsp	36	9.2	0.1	tr*
Banana	1	105	26.7	1.2	0.6
Snack					
Whole-wheat bread	2 slices	138	28.2	5.2	1.5
Honey	2 tsp	42	11.4	tr	0
Orange juice	1 cup	112	26.8	1.7	0.2
Lunch					
Cracked-wheat bread	4 slices	263	52.1	8.7	2.2
Turkey breast	4½ oz	140	0	28.7	2.0
American cheese	2 oz	210	0.9	12.4	17.5
Granola bars	2	594	67.3	15.0	33.2
Apple juice	1 cup	117	29.0	0.2	0.3
Snack					
Low-fat frozen yogurt	¾ cup	108	12.0	8.9	2.6
Apple juice	1 cup	117	29.0	0.2	0.3
Dinner					
Spaghetti with meatless sauce and cheese	2 cups	520	74.0	17.5	17.5
Steamed green beans	1 cup	44	9.9	2.4	0.4
Whole-wheat dinner roll	1	129	26.2	5.0	1.4
Margarine	2 tbsp	203	0.3	0.3	22.7
Apple	1 medium	81	21.1	0.3	0.5
Skim milk	1 cup	86	11.9	8.4	0.4
Snack					
Cranberry juice cocktail	1 cup	144	36.4	0	0.2
Orange	1 medium	62	15.4	1.2	0.2
Gingersnap cookies	3	97	18.4	1.3	2.1
Totals		3938	625.6 (64% of calories)	141.7 (14% of calories)	107.7 (25% of calories)

*tr = trace, <0.05 g.

poultry, fish, eggs, and dairy products. A balanced diet with a focus on carbohydrates and a de-emphasis on fat is important. While most vegetarian diets easily meet this requirement, some nutrient problems may occur with pure vegans (those who consume only foods of plant origin). These nutrient concerns include the possibility of inadequate supplies of protein, vitamin B12, iron, zinc, calcium, and (for athletes with a large muscle mass) calories. The athlete who wishes to follow a vegetarian diet should combine foods to be assured of obtaining protein of high biological values (see *Table 4.14*). The vitamin B12 requirement can typically be satisfied with small amounts of milk, cheese, eggs, fortified soy products, or brewer's yeast. Foods containing iron should be consumed with high–vitamin C foods to help ensure higher rates of absorption. Some vegetarian practices limit food choices to the degree that they may increase the risk of nutrient deficiency. Diets should be evaluated to ensure the intake of a wide variety of foods. An example of a lactovegetarian diet is included in Table 4.14. This basic, 2400-kcal diet can be increased to 3000 kcal or more by increasing the size of the portions. For example, including 4 oz of nuts and seeds or 8 oz of dried fruit adds 500 calories.

TABLE 4.14   Example of a 2400-kcal* Lactovegetarian Diet

Food	Serving Size	Calories	Carbohydrate (g)	Protein (g)	Fat (g)
Breakfast					
Grapefruit juice	1 cup	94	22.2	1.3	0.3
Whole-wheat bread	1 slice	67	13.8	2.6	0.7
Peanut butter	2 tbsp	188	6.6	7.9	16.0
Skim milk	1 cup	86	11.9	8.4	0.4
Snack					
Tangerines	2	74	18.8	1.1	0.3
Lunch					
Split-pea soup	1 cup	190	28.0	10.3	4.4
Pita bread	1	203	38.8	6.4	2.1
Low-fat cottage cheese	½ cup	82	3.1	14.0	1.2
Grated carrots	1 cup	47	11.2	1.1	0.2
Canned cherries	½ cup	39	9.4	0.8	0.2
Banana	1	105	26.7	1.2	0.6
Orange juice	½ cup	56	13.4	0.9	0.1
Snack					
Dried apricots	7 halves	58	15.1	0.9	0.1
Dried dates	2½	57	15.3	0.4	0.1
Dinner					
Cheese pizza	¼ of 10-in.	280	40.9	15.3	6.4
Tossed green salad	1 cup	36.3	7.3	2.8	0.2
Italian dressing	2 tbsp	137	3.0	0.2	14.2
Sourdough bread	2 slices	203	38.8	6.4	2.1
Margarine	2 tsp	68	0.1	0.1	7.6
Apple	1 medium	81	21.1	0.3	0.5
Snack					
Plain low-fat yogurt	1 cup	144	16.0	11.9	3.5
Strawberries	¼ cup	11	2.6	0.2	0.1
Granola	¼ cup	149	16.8	3.8	8.3
Totals		2455	380.7 (62% of calories)	98.0 (16% of calories)	69.5 (25% of calories)

*This basic 2400-kcal diet can be expanded readily to ≥3000 kcal by increasing the size of the portions; eg, add 4 oz nuts and seeds or 8 oz dried fruit (500 kcal), or add fruit juices and low-fat dairy products (no more than 3-4 egg yolks per week).

▶ HIGH FIBER INTAKE

While vegetarian diets are typically high in fiber, the effect of a high fiber intake on athletic performance has not been evaluated. Epidemiologic studies suggest that high fiber intakes have benefits (the type of fiber determines the benefit) for clients with diabetes, atherosclerosis, cancer, and disorders of the gastrointestinal tract. Those who are on a high-fiber diet must take care to consume large amounts of fluid. Moreover, the fiber content of the diet should be increased gradually. (Note the precaution on high-fiber foods described in this section in the discussion about the preexercise/precompetition meal.) An example of a high-fiber diet is included in *Table 4.15*.

▶ HIGH-CALORIE DIETS

Many athletes find it difficult to maintain or gain weight during training. In some positions of certain sports, such as linemen on football teams, weight and mass are valued, and many adolescent athletes require an extremely high level of energy to meet the dual demands of growth and exercise. Therefore, a sound diet that promotes maintenance and supports optimal growth for athletes who are still growing is important.

TABLE 4.15 Example of a 2000-kcal High-Fiber Diet

Food	Serving Size	Calories	Carbohydrate (g)	Protein (g)	Fat (g)
Breakfast					
Bran cereal	⅓ cup	72	21.1	3.9	0.7
Skim milk	1 cup	86	11.9	8.4	0.4
Strawberries	1¼ cups	56	13.1	1.1	0.7
Whole-wheat bread	2 slices	135	27.6	5.1	1.5
Margarine	1 tsp	34	tr*	tr	3.8
Snack					
Grapes	15 medium	23	6.2	0.2	0.1
Whole-wheat crackers	6	202	34.1	4.2	6.9
Lunch					
Whole-wheat bread	2 slices	135	27.6	5.1	1.5
Mashed kidney beans	⅓ cup	74	13.3	5.1	0.3
Raw carrot	1 medium	31	7.3	0.7	0.1
Raw celery	1 stalk	6	1.5	0.3	0.1
Canned cherries	1 cup	78	18.9	1.6	0.5
Skim milk	1 cup	86	11.9	8.4	0.4
Snack					
Apple	1 medium	81	21.1	0.3	0.5
Low-fat vanilla yogurt	1 cup	194	31.3	11.2	2.8
Dinner					
Stir-fry:					
Skinless chicken breast	4 oz	187	0	35.2	4.1
Assorted vegetables	1 cup	107	23.8	5.2	0.3
Brown rice	1 cup	216	44.8	5.0	1.8
Tangerines	2	74	18.8	1.1	0.3
Snack					
Air-popped popcorn	3 cups	69	13.8	2.3	0.9
Seltzer water	1 cup	0	0	0	0
Totals		1945	348.0 (72% of calories)	104.2 (21% of calories)	27.6 13% of calories)

*tr = trace, <0.05 g.

It has been estimated that the amount of energy expended by a typical teenage athlete can be as much as 5000 to 6000 kcal per day. To gain weight, the athlete may have a calorie requirement that may exceed 6500 kcal each day. This requires frequent consumption of meals and snacks throughout the day. A conflict may develop between trying to provide a healthful diet (that is low in fat and high in carbohydrate) along with a high-calorie diet to maintain or increase weight (which may require a higher fat intake). This is a common problem, because high carbohydrate intakes require the consumption of a large quantity (and volume) of foods over many meals because of their relatively low calorie density. The training or school schedules of many of these athletes may demand that large amounts of calories be consumed in a maximum of three meals, because the athletes' schedules do not permit consumption of small, frequent meals. Recommending diets higher in fat may be necessary to meet energy demands, but the dietary habits these athletes develop from this type of intake may require "detraining" once they retire from the sport. An example of a 3700-kcal meal plan is included in *Table 4.16*.

▶ LOW-CALORIE DIETS

For an average person on a weight-loss program, the goal rate of weight loss should not exceed 2 lb per week. The USDA Dietary Guidelines recommend a weekly weight-loss goal of 0.5 lb. In some athletes who are involved in two sports in which weight requirements are different (eg, football and wrestling), alteration in weight to meet the specific demands for each sport is important. Registered dietitians and other appropriately certified and licensed health professionals should help guide the diet so that weight loss is slow, and the diet still supports optimal growth velocity. This means that it is critically important to plan a sound nutrient intake and to allow a reasonable amount of time for weight loss. Athletes who achieve their weight-loss goal will need continued assistance with weight maintenance.

A weight-loss program for an athlete should be carefully monitored and should stay within the reasonable bounds of good health practice. It is important that goal weights be reasonable, and not imposed arbitrarily by a coach or athletic trainer. A 1200-kcal intake is considered a minimum intake for obtaining most nutrients, but still may be inadequate in some (most notably iron). A 1200-kcal weekly menu plan is included in *Table 4.17* as a guide on which to build a reasonable weight-loss program. As a general rule, a 3500-kcal deficit is required for 1 lb of weight loss. Therefore, a daily 500-kcal deficit would lead to approximately 1 lb of weight loss per week (generally accepted as a safe rate of loss). If an athlete consumes 3000 kcal to maintain current weight, the goal diet should be approximately 2500 kcal per day.

(Text continues on page 206.)

TABLE 4.16 Example of a 3700-kcal High-Calorie Diet

Food	Serving Size	Calories	Carbohydrate (g)	Protein (g)	Fat (g)
Breakfast					
Orange juice	1 cup	112	26.8	1.7	0.2
Oatmeal	1 cup	145	25.3	6.1	2.3
Whole-wheat bread	2 slices	110	21.6	4.8	1.4
Margarine	2 tsp	68	0.1	0.1	7.6
Skim milk	1 cup	86	11.9	8.4	0.4
Snack					
Bagels	2	400	76.0	14.0	4.0
Peanut butter	2 tsp	56	2.0	2.3	4.7
Grape juice	1 cup	128	31.9	0.5	0.2
Lunch					
Tuna salad	½ cup	192	9.7	16.4	9.5
Kaiser roll	1	156	29.8	4.9	1.6
Lettuce	1 leaf	3	0.4	0.2	tr*
Tomatoes	1 slice	6	1.4	0.3	0.1
Tossed green salad	1 cup	36	7.3	2.8	0.2
Italian dressing	1 tbsp	69	1.5	0.1	7.1
Fresh peach	1 medium	37	9.7	0.6	0.1
Granola bars	2	594	67.3	15.0	33.2
Skim milk	1 cup	86	11.9	8.4	0.4
Snack					
Low-fat frozen yogurt	1 cup	231	43.2	9.9	2.5
Apricot nectar	1 cup	141	36.1	0.9	0.2
Dinner					
Vegetable soup	1 cup	122	19.0	3.5	3.7
Skinless baked chicken breast	3 oz	140	0	25.4	3.0
White rice	1 cup	200	43.3	4.0	0.5
Steamed broccoli	1 cup	44	7.9	4.7	0.6
Tossed green salad	1 cup	36	7.3	2.8	0.2
French dressing	1 tbsp	67	2.7	0.1	6.4
Dinner roll	1	119	21.2	3.3	2.2
Margarine	1 tsp	34	tr	tr	3.8
Watermelon cubes	1¼ cups	64	14.4	1.2	0.9
Skim milk	1 cup	86	11.9	8.4	0.4
Snack					
Apple juice	1 cup	112	27.6	0.3	0.2
Totals		3678	569.0 (62% of calories)	151.8 (17% of calories)	97.6 (24% of calories)

*tr = trace, <0.05 g.

Example of a 1200-kcal Low-Calorie Weekly Menu Plan

Food	Serving Size	Calories	Carbohydrate (g)	Protein (g)	Fat (g)
DAY 1					
Breakfast					
Raisin bread	1 slice	66	13.4	1.7	0.7
Reduced-calorie margarine	1 tbsp	49	0.1	0.1	5.6
Fresh blueberries	¾ cup	61	15.4	0.7	0.4
Skim milk	1 cup	86	11.9	8.4	0.4
Lunch					
Whole-wheat bread	2 slices	122	23.9	5.3	1.5
Turkey breast	2 oz	62	0	12.8	0.9
Reduced-calorie mayonnaise	1 tbsp	22	0.8	0.2	2.0
Tomatoes	2 slices	20	4.3	0.8	0.3
Alfalfa sprouts	⅛ cup	1	0.2	0.2	tr*
Fresh peach	1 medium	37	9.7	0.6	0.1
Dinner					
Skinless baked chicken breast	4 oz	187	0	35.2	4.1
Baked potato	1 medium	220	51.0	4.7	0.2
Reduced-calorie margarine	1 tbsp	49	0.1	0.1	5.6
Tossed green salad	½ cup	18	3.7	1.4	0.1
Grated carrots	½ cup	24	5.6	0.6	0.1
Reduced-calorie French dressing	1 tbsp	22	3.5	tr	1.0
Honeydew melon	⅒ melon	45	11.8	0.6	0.1
Snack					
Plain low-fat yogurt	1 cup	144	16.0	11.9	3.5
Day 1 totals		1233	171.0 (55% of calories)	85.0 (28% of calories)	26.4 (19% of calories)
DAY 2					
Breakfast					
Low-fat lemon yogurt	1 cup	194	31.3	11.2	2.8
English muffin	1	140	27.0	5.0	1.0
Peanut butter	1 tsp	28	1.0	1.2	2.4
Lunch					
Fresh fruit plate	1 cup	74	19.3	0.9	0.2
Low-fat cottage cheese	½ cup	82	3.1	14.0	1.2
Dinner roll	1	119	21.2	3.3	2.2
Dinner					
Broiled lean beef	3 oz	179	0	25.4	7.9
Brown rice	½ cup	109	22.5	2.5	0.9
Cooked spinach	1 cup	41	6.8	5.4	0.5
Reduced-calorie margarine	1 tsp	17	tr	tr	1.9
Orange	1 medium	62	15.4	1.2	0.2
Skim milk	1 cup	86	11.9	8.4	0.4
Snack					
Air-popped popcorn	3 cups	69	13.8	2.3	0.9
Seltzer water	1 cup	0	0	0	0
Day 2 totals		1199	173.2 (58% of calories)	80.7 (27% of calories)	22.4 (17% of calories) (continued)

*tr = trace, <0.05 g.

TABLE 4.17   Example of a 1200-kcal Low-Calorie Weekly Menu Plan (continued).

Food	Serving Size	Calories	Carbohydrate (g)	Protein (g)	Fat (g)
DAY 3					
Breakfast					
Hominy grits	½ cup	58	11.4	1.2	0.7
Reduced-calorie					
margarine	1 tsp	17	tr	tr	1.9
Dried prunes	½ cup	158	41.6	1.7	0.3
Skim milk	1 cup	86	11.9	8.4	0.4
Lunch					
Extra-lean hamburger	3 oz	218	0	21.6	13.9
Whole-wheat bun	1	119	19.6	2.9	3.0
Mustard	1 tsp	4	0.3	0.2	0.2
Lettuce	1 leaf	3	0.4	0.2	tr
Tomatoes	1 slice	8	1.7	0.3	0.1
Fresh strawberries	1¼ cups	56	13.1	1.1	0.7
Dinner					
Broiled fish	3 oz	99	0	20.5	1.3
Cooked beets	½ cup	26	5.7	0.9	tr
Steamed green beans	½ cup	22	4.9	1.2	0.2
Dinner roll	1	83	14.8	2.3	1.6
Fresh pineapple chunks	¾ cup	57	14.4	0.5	0.5
Snack					
Gingersnap cookies	3	97	18.4	1.3	2.1
Skim milk	1 cup	86	11.9	8.4	0.4
Day 3 totals		1194	170.2 (57% of calories)	72.6 (24% of calories)	27.4 (21% of calories)
DAY 4					
Breakfast					
Vegetable juice cocktail	1 cup	46	11.0	1.5	0.2
Low-fat cottage cheese	½ cup	82	3.1	14.0	1.2
Rye bread	1 slice	62	13.3	2.3	0.3
Reduced-calorie					
margarine	1 tsp	17	tr	tr	1.9
Fresh nectarine	1 medium	67	16.0	1.3	0.6
Lunch					
Water-packed tuna	2 oz	77	0	15.1	1.4
Saltine crackers	5	61	10.2	1.3	1.7
Broccoli florets	½ cup	22	4.0	2.3	0.3
Fresh pear	1 medium	98	25.1	0.7	0.7
Skim milk	1 cup	86	11.9	8.4	0.4
Dinner					
Flank steak	3 oz	176	0	23.0	8.6
White rice	½ cup	132	28.5	2.7	0.3
Steamed asparagus	½ cup	22.5	4.0	2.3	0.3
Fresh cantaloupe cubes	1 cup	56	13.4	1.4	0.5
Orange juice	1 cup	112	26.8	1.7	0.2
Snack					
Puffed wheat cereal	1 cup	44	9.6	1.8	0.1
Skim milk	1 cup	86	11.9	8.4	0.4
Day 4 totals		1244	188.6 (61% of calories)	88.2 (28% of calories)	19.0 (14% of calories)
DAY 5					
Breakfast					
Fresh grapefruit	½	37	9.5	0.7	0.1
Oatmeal	1 cup	145	25.3	6.1	2.3
Skim milk	1 cup	86	11.9	8.4	0.4

TABLE 4.17   Example of a 1200-kcal Low-Calorie Weekly Menu Plan (continued).

Food	Serving Size	Calories	Carbohydrate (g)	Protein (g)	Fat (g)
DAY 5 (continued)					
Lunch					
Roast chicken breast	2 oz	94	0	17.6	2.0
Whole-wheat bread	2 slices	122	23.9	5.3	1.5
Reduced-calorie					
mayonnaise	1 tsp	6	0.2	0.1	0.6
Lettuce	1 leaf	3	0.4	0.2	tr
Tomatoes	1 slice	9	1.9	0.4	0.1
Watermelon cubes	1¼ cups	64	14.4	1.2	0.9
Dinner					
Spaghetti	1 cup	159	33.7	5.2	0.7
Tomato sauce	½ cup	37	8.8	1.6	0.2
Extra-lean ground beef	3 oz	214	0	21.0	13.8
Tossed green salad	1 cup	36	7.3	2.8	0.2
Reduced-calorie blue					
cheese dressing	1 tbsp	12	0.7	0.5	0.9
Fresh blueberries	¾ cup	61	15.4	0.7	0.4
Snack					
Graham crackers	2 squares	55	10.4	1.1	1.3
Skim milk	1 cup	86	11.9	8.4	0.4
Day 5 totals		1224	175.5 (57% of calories)	81.1 (27% of calories)	26.0 (19% of calories)
DAY 6					
Breakfast					
Orange juice	½ cup	56	13.4	0.9	0.1
Bran flakes	½ cup	64	15.3	2.5	0.4
Skim milk	1 cup	86	11.9	8.4	0.4
Lunch					
Whole-wheat bread	2 slices	135	27.6	5.1	1.5
Turkey breast	2 oz	62	0	12.8	0.9
Reduced-calorie					
mayonnaise	1 tbsp	22	0.8	0.2	2.0
Lettuce	1 leaf	3	0.4	0.2	tr
Tomatoes	1 slice	9	1.9	0.4	0.1
Low-fat frozen yogurt	½ cup	115	21.5	4.9	1.2
Dinner					
Roast pork loin	3 oz	208	0	24.0	11.7
Boiled potatoes	2 small	232	54.0	4.6	0.3
Steamed brussels					
sprouts	½ cup	30	6.8	2.0	0.4
Fresh pineapple	¾ cup	57	14.4	0.5	0.5
Snack					
Banana	½	52	13.4	0.6	0.3
Skim milk	½ cup	43	5.9	4.2	0.2
Day 6 totals		1173	187.3 (64% of calories)	71.0 (24% of calories)	20.1 (15% of calories)
DAY 7					
Breakfast					
Cream of wheat	1 cup	133	27.6	3.8	0.5
Skim milk	1 cup	86	11.9	8.4	0.4
Lunch					
Pita bread	½	102	19.4	3.2	1.1
Mashed garbanzo beans	⅓ cup	89	14.8	4.8	1.4
Lettuce	1 leaf	3	0.4	0.2	tr
Plain low-fat yogurt	½ cup	72	8.0	5.9	1.8
Fresh plum	1	36	8.6	0.5	0.4

(continued)

TABLE 4.17   Example of a 1200-kcal Low-Calorie Weekly Menu Plan (continued).

Food	Serving Size	Calories	Carbohydrate (g)	Protein (g)	Fat (g)
DAY 7 (continued)					
Dinner					
Baked salmon	3 oz	184	0	23.2	9.3
Egg noodles	1 cup	213	39.7	7.6	2.4
Cooked spinach	½ cup	27	5.1	3.0	0.2
Fresh mango cubes	1 cup	107	28.1	0.8	0.5
Snack					
Fresh apple	1 medium	81	21.1	0.3	0.5
Skim milk	½ cup	43	5.9	4.2	0.2
Day 7 totals		1174	190.5 (65% of calories)	65.8 (22% of calories)	18.6 (14% of calories)

▶ DIET FOR ADOLESCENTS

Care is needed in planning a diet for growing adolescent athletes who engage in competitive sports. The energy needs of these athletes may be great, but the combined pressures of the sport and society may easily induce many adolescent athletes to consume diets too low in calories and nutrients. Parents should be advised to keep plenty of fresh fruit, vegetables, juices, whole-grain breads, and skim-milk products available. The average caloric requirement for children aged 7 to 10 years is 2400 kcal (range: 1650 to 3300 kcal) and for adolescents aged 11 to 18 years is 2750 kcal (range: 2500 to 3000 kcal). These average calorie ranges are for the US population. Therefore, adolescents who exercise will have considerably greater caloric requirements. *Table 4.18* presents a 2400-kcal diet for adolescents that should be considered a baseline *minimum* intake for most athletes in this age group.

▶ DIET FOR ATHLETES WITH DIABETES

Exercise and good eating habits are the cornerstones of diabetes control. Because exercise causes a decrease in blood glucose, the insulin levels of exercising people who have diabetes can be decreased. Ideally, exercise should take place at about the same time each day to keep the relationship between food intake and insulin stable. If exercising before a meal, the athlete with diabetes should eat a small carbohydrate (nonsugar) snack. Before each hour of exercise, one fruit or bread-starch serving should be eaten. Before every 2 hours of activity, the meal eaten should be half a sandwich or six crackers and two slices of cheese, or one piece of toast with a half cup of skim milk. These preexercise meals are in addition to the daily meal plan. Exercise has a long-lasting effect on blood glucose level. Exercise may elevate the BMR for several hours after an event or workout, causing blood glucose to drop. Therefore, the athlete with diabetes should carry some form of carbohydrate (fruit, fruit juice, candy) to be prepared to handle a drop in blood glucose.

TABLE 4.18   Example of a 2400-kcal High-Calorie Diet

Food	Serving Size	Calories	Carbohydrate (g)	Protein (g)	Fat (g)
Breakfast					
Orange juice	½ cup	56	13.4	0.9	0.1
Cornflakes	1 cup	110	24.4	2.3	0.1
Skim milk	1 cup	86	11.9	8.4	0.4
Raisin bread	2 slices	133	27.1	3.4	1.4
Margarine	2 tsp	68	0.1	0.1	7.6
Snack					
Fresh peach	1 medium	37	9.7	0.6	0.1
Lunch					
Whole-wheat bread	2 slices	122	23.9	5.3	1.5
Water-packed tuna	2 oz	77	0	15.1	1.4
Mayonnaise-type salad dressing	2 tsp	37	2.3	0.1	3.2
Lettuce	1 leaf	3	0.4	0.2	tr*
Tomatoes	1 slice	9	1.9	0.4	0.1
Celery	1 stalk	10	2.2	0.5	0.1
Raw carrot	1 medium	31	7.3	0.7	0.1
Oatmeal cookies	2	117	19.1	1.6	4.0
Skim milk	1 cup	86	11.9	8.4	0.4
Snack					
Low-fat fruit yogurt	1 cup	231	43.2	9.9	2.5
Granola bar	1	277	31.4	7.0	15.4
Dinner					
Skinless baked chicken breast	3 oz	140	0	25.4	3.0
Baked potato	1 medium	220	51.0	4.7	0.2
Steamed green beans	½ cup	22	4.9	1.2	0.2
Dinner roll	1	119	21.2	3.3	2.2
Margarine	2 tsp	67.6	0.1	0.1	7.6
Apple	1 medium	81	21.1	0.3	0.5
Skim milk	1 cup	86	11.9	8.4	0.4
Snack					
Apple juice	1 cup	117	29.0	0.2	0.3
Air-popped popcorn	3 cups	69	13.8	2.3	0.9
Totals		2409	382.9 (64% of calories)	111.2 (18% of calories)	53.8 (20% of calories)

*tr = trace, <0.05 g.

Feeding Stations for Various Events

Dan Benardot, Mildred Cody, Ann Grediagen, and Page Love

There do not appear to be any established rules on what products to have available at feeding stations, how often (distance/frequency) to have products available, how much product to have available, and product sanitation. Often, these questions are based on the advice and desires of race sponsors. What follows are general guidelines and considerations for providing drinks and foods for races of different distances and environmental conditions.

▶ WHAT TO HAVE AVAILABLE

Most races 5 km or longer provide water or a sports beverage at periodic intervals. Marathons also occasionally include fruits (bananas are popular) and carbohydrate supplements at selected food stations and at the end of the race. Typically, the type of sports beverage available is controlled by the sponsor of the race. Ideally, there should be at least the following at all races 5 km or longer:

> ▶ *Cool, clean, unflavored water.* In some locales, the water may be heavily chlorinated or have a sulfurous taste that some people find displeasing. If this is the case, noncarbonated bottled water may be a desirable alternative to tap water.
> ▶ *A cool sports beverage.* Many athletes have become accustomed to training with a sports beverage, and many find that it aids endurance. Ideally, this beverage should contain no more than 8% glucose or sucrose, and should not derive most of its sugar from fructose.
> ▶ *High-carbohydrate food.* This is not necessary for most races, but athletes appreciate having some food available at the end of the race. A bagel, fruit, bread, or other high-carbohydrate food is desirable. For marathons or ultramarathons, high-carbohydrate foods (with fluids) should be available for the athletes at the water-food stations, especially those stations beyond the 10-km point and at the end of the race.

▶ HOW OFTEN PRODUCTS SHOULD BE AVAILABLE

The frequency with which drinks and food are made available to racers varies with the distance of the race and the sponsor of the race. The following frequency is recommended:

> ▶ *For races less than 5 km.* Water and sports beverages should be made available at the beginning and end of the race.
> ▶ *For a 5-km race.* Water and sports beverages should be made available at the beginning, midpoint, and end of the race.

▶ *For a 10-km race.* Water and sports beverages should be made available at the beginning of the race, at every 2-km marker (or more frequently on a hot and humid day), and at the end of the race. Carbohydrate foods should be available at the end of the race.

▶ *For a marathon or ultramarathon.* Water and sports beverages should be made available at the beginning of the race, at every 2-km marker (or more frequently on a hot and humid day), and at the end of the race. Carbohydrate foods should be available at all stations following the 10-km point of the race.

Stations should be close to the course, and positioned so that racers can easily consume the product. In general, this means they should not be at the top of a long hill where exhaustion might make it difficult to swallow. If possible, products should be available where there is a slight downhill grade or where the grade is level. The stations should be situated such that athletes have easy access to the product(s) without waiting for or getting in the way of other athletes. This generally means a long serving area or a serving area on both sides of the course. If the terrain makes it difficult to space the serving areas equally, signs at each area should be posted to remind the athlete of the distance to the next area.

The race information packet provided to athletes should furnish information on food, beverage, and aid-station locations on the course map. There should also be information on the specific products available, and the concentration of the products (for instance, "full-strength Gatorade,"* "half-strength Exceed"†).

▶ HOW MUCH PRODUCT TO HAVE AVAILABLE

It is difficult to predict how much fluid and food should be made available, because the amount consumed has much to do with ambient temperature and the general fitness level of the runners in a particular race. It is important to remember that fluid losses in hot and humid environments may be as high as 2 to 3 L per hour. As a general guide, the minimum fluid available should follow these formulas.

Thirty minutes before the race:

0.5 to 1 L × number of racers
Use the higher value (1 L) for hot or humid environments

During the race:

0.25 L every 10 to 15 minutes × number of racers
The total number of minutes in a race is determined by the average predicted finishing time for the race. Use the higher value (10 minutes) for hot or humid environments.

After the race:

0.25 L for every 10 to 15 minutes spent racing × number of racers
Use the higher value (10 minutes) for hot or humid environments.

▶ SANITATION CONCERNS FOR PRODUCT DISTRIBUTION

Foods selected for athletic events must be held at appropriate temperatures and kept clean. Table tops should be kept clean and garbage and food waste must

---

*Quaker Oats Co, Chicago, IL 60654.
†Ross Laboratories, Columbus, OH 43216.

be removed regularly to reduce insect problems around the food and drink to be provided. It is almost inevitable that a great deal of spillage of water and sugar-containing sports beverages will occur near drink stations. Athletes commonly take one or two sips of drink from a cup, and discard the remainder by throwing it to the side of the running area or track. To avoid attracting insects, there should be a means (water hose with drainage would be most desirable) for periodically washing these areas to keep insect problems to a minimum.

Foods available at athletic events require the same holding temperatures recommended for safe home storage. Foods such as breads, unopened canned beverages, and fruits can be safely held at ambient temperatures. Foods that require refrigeration, such as yogurt and opened milk-based beverages, can be held iced. Maintain hot foods at 160°F or above in separate insulated containers that have been sanitized.

Food handling should be kept to a minimum, and all food must be protected from dust and insects. Distributing water and sports beverages from open wide-mouth containers creates an invitation to corrupt the drink quality. Servers should take whatever means possible to maintain sanitary serving practices, including wearing protective gloves and hair coverings. This is especially important with certain serving practices that involve dipping a serving cup (and often a hand and portion of one's arm) into an open container to serve an athlete.

Presenting food in single-serving units improves safety and reduces garbage accumulation. Holding partially consumed food safely is difficult at athletic events, since most foods would be difficult to label and many foods require refrigeration (which is largely unavailable) after opening. In addition, single servings are easier to pick up, which reduces handling by athletes and servers.

Packaging should be minimal to reduce both the time required to access food and the amount of garbage that accumulates. Wide-opening garbage cans should be readily available for food and packaging refuse.

Case Studies

Joan Buchbinder and Nancy Clark

▶ CASE STUDY A. FOOD AND WEIGHT OBSESSION

"This is my career... I can't be 1 lb overweight or I can't ride. I need to know what foods cause fluid. I mean, I've even picked up a paranoia about which foods will cause me to retain water weight. Water pills are frowned upon at the stables. . .but I could use the sweatbox. I've heard that if I use the sweatbox I should probably get B_{12} shots...."

At age 23, Ellen has been training to be a horse jockey for many years. She has just passed her equestrian examinations and has been offered a position as a first-year apprentice at a popular Boston race track. To maintain this qualification during her first year, she can weigh no more than 110 lb and no less than 105 lb for her height of 5 ft 3 in.

Ellen weighed 122 lb 6 weeks ago; she reduced to 105 lb by markedly reducing her food intake, galloping horses for hours each day, and running 1 to 5 miles a few times a week, rowing, aerobic dancing, or swimming. While a freshman in high school, Ellen weighed 105 lb, but by her senior year she weighed as much as 148 lb. She has been struggling with her weight ever since, and she admits to having turned to vomiting in the past to control her weight.

She is pleased with her recent weight loss, but she is now struggling to maintain the 105 lb. She is afraid to drink fluids for fear it will cause her to weigh more through retained fluid weight. She now admits that she has taken the weight off "unhealthfully," and she wants to learn how to eat and train "normally" to maintain her weight loss. She is anxious and troubled by the fact that she has begun to experience uncontrollable food binges again at this new weight. After a few days of binge eating, her weight will increase to 113 lb. She cannot be at this weight and qualify as a professional jockey.

Ellen's Typical Reducing Diet and Training Schedule

4:00 AM	Awaken
4:05 AM	Two rice cakes, cantaloupe quarter
5-8:00 AM	Ride horses
8:00 AM	Break
10:30 AM	Ride and groom horses
12:00 PM	Cantaloupe
1:00 PM	Jogging, groom parents' horses
7:00 PM	Chicken, broccoli, spinach, carrots, rice

Assessment

Ellen has a long-standing underlying eating disorder commonly described as bulimorexia. She is so determined not to lose her position as a jockey that she has succumbed to old, unhealthful weight-loss tactics to lose weight quickly. Her loss of 17 lb in less than 2 months, with a resulting body fat percentage estimated at 11.4% of her weight, most likely explains her amenorrhea, fatigue, and mounting appetite.

Ellen suffers from severe asthma, which is often triggered by pollen, hay, dust—and horses. She claims to be affected by these elements when grooming her parents' horses on their farm, but not when working the horses at the race track.

Coincidentally, Ellen claims to only binge-eat at her parents' home. Here, she says, her asthma worsens and she must take more asthma medication; she states that the medication increases her appetite. Ellen also expresses resentments for having to travel 1.5 hours per day to her parents' farm to groom and care for their horses; this cuts into her own horse training and equestrian study time. She claims that she is worn out by all of the work and that when she is tired and fatigued she has less control with food.

Ellen's food binges at her parents' farm are more likely triggered by a long history of emotional strain between Ellen and her parents. She is currently angry with her parents for the demands they have placed on her to care for their horses; these demands disrupt her own training and eating routines. Additionally, she is most likely binge-eating in response to her very low calorie intake and the body's need to replenish her glycogen stores. She is vulnerable to the availability of tempting foods in her parents' well-stocked kitchen. She will also binge-eat in response to her sense of weight gain; the more she weighs the more she eats. Ellen views her 6- to 8-pound weight gain after a few days of binge eating as a gain in pure body fat, whereas her weight gain after binges is semireflective of stored glycogen and water weight.

Solutions

Ellen must work to unlabel her days as "good" or "bad," "out of control" or "in control," based on her food intake. Unfortunately, with respect to her food and weight history, she has chosen a career path that places daily emphasis on her food and weight.

To Create More Normalcy in Her Food Intake
1. Stop labeling "allowed" and "forbidden" foods and thinking of foods in terms of whether they are "fueling her body" or "feeding her fat cells."
2. Increase the frequency of her food intake by incorporating small, high-energy snacks between meals, thus allowing less time between meals.
3. Increase her daily calorie intake to approximately 1800 to 2300 kcal per day versus her swings from 800 kcal per day when "dieting" to more than 3000 kcal per day when "bingeing."

To Improve Nutritional Quality
4. Incorporate more nutrient-dense carbohydrate foods, including whole-grain breads, cereals, bagels, English muffins, fresh fruits, fruit juices, dried fruits, pasta, rice, potatoes, lentils, soups, and whole-grain crackers.

Target Diet: 55% to 65% Carbohydrate Calories per Day
5. Add more calcium to diet, through low-fat or nonfat yogurt, skim or low-fat milk, part-skim string cheese, and homemade thick-crust pizza.

6. Add more low-fat animal proteins each day for daily protein, iron, zinc, and other vitamin and mineral needs (eg, turkey breast, tuna packed in water, skinless chicken breast, extra-lean ground beef, lower-fat cuts of red meat, lentils, etc). Target diet: 10% to 20% protein calories per day.

7. "Allow" herself some more freedom to incorporate fats and refined sugars into diet (eg, lower-fat ice milks, frozen yogurt, fig bar cookies, graham crackers). Target diet: 20% to 30% fat calories per day; 10% simple sugar calories per day.

To Improve Energy Level

8. Improve quality and quantity of 4:00 AM breakfast meal (eg, whole-grain bagel, low-fat cottage cheese, tomato slices; frozen waffles with applesauce and skim milk; whole-grain cereal, fruit, milk).

9. Incorporate 8:00 AM snack during training break (eg, graham crackers and low-fat yogurt; fresh fruit and fig bar cookies).

10. Drink more hydrating fluids throughout the day to prevent dehydration headaches and fatigue (eg, water, seltzer waters, fruit juices, low-fat/skim milk, sports beverages). Avoid dehydrating beverages, including colas, diet colas, tea, coffee, and alcohol.

To Improve Morale and Sense of Control

11. Stop going to sweatbox to lose body water weight.

12. Concentrate only on horse training and conditioning needs; avoid overexertion with other aerobic activities.

13. Establish more efficient schedule for working at parents' farm, studying, and riding and training. Bring own food to parents' home so as not to be as tempted by foods in the refrigerator at home, until she has a handle on her food intake. She must also speak to her parents about her inability to control herself around tempting foods such as cake, brownies, and ice cream.

Changes

4:05 AM	Cereal, banana, skim milk
8:00 AM	Skim milk, graham crackers
12:00 PM	Non-fat vanilla yogurt, bagel
2:00 PM	Cantaloupe, fruit juice
6:00 PM	Skinless chicken, pasta, steamed vegetables, sorbet
9:00 PM	Fresh fruit

The Bottom Line

"I am not walking around all day hungry, irritable, or thinking about food. My energy level is much better, and I don't succumb to the food cravings when at my parents' home.

"I'm back to 105 lb and have maintained it now for a few months rather than a few days. I don't need the sweatbox or water pills to step on the scale before my competition rides.

"My parents understand my need to keep my weight down during this apprentice year, and they will support my food needs. They are trying to find a rider to come to the farm a few times a week to work the horses and relieve me from having to go there as much.

"I think my dream of being a jockey is finally coming true!"

▶ **CASE STUDY B. PREMENSTRUAL FOOD CRAVINGS AND WEIGHT GAIN**

"I just can't stand it. I'm so good for 3 weeks each month: I don't cheat, I'm a perfect eater, I run 8 to 12 miles a day and do my conditioning exercises for 30 to 60 minutes every day. . . . And then I get premenstrual and I'm double-*O-C: out of control*. I can't get enough chocolate or peanut butter, and I look as though I am 4 months pregnant. Forget wearing stretch pants—my legs blow up like tree stumps. And I know what I'm doing—I just can't get myself to stop eating. It's like there's a power stronger than me causing me to binge-eat. . . . *I am so miserable*."

Thirty-year-old Carol is a weight-conscious, sports-active female who has battled premenstrual food cravings and cyclical weight gain since the age of 20, when she developed premenstrual syndrome (PMS) as a sophomore in college. She had gained the notorious "freshman 10," so she went on her first self-imposed "diet" and exercise program. By the end of the summer she had lost 20 lb, returning as a sophomore at 98 lb and amenorrheic. Over the first semester she slowly returned to her former college eating habits, got too busy to exercise regularly, and regained most of her lost weight. With the weight gain, her menstrual cycles returned. However, when her periods returned they were associated with marked food cravings, breast tenderness, fluid retention, irritability, mood swings, and anxiety. Since that time she experiences PMS monthly. For more than 10 years she has felt controlled by PMS.

Carol's Typical Nonpremenstrual Diet

5:30 AM	Awaken; coffee; calisthenics (1 hour)
6:00 AM	Bagel with jam; coffee
8:00 AM	Coffee
10:00 AM	Seltzer water
12:00 PM	Bagel, coffee, seltzer water
2:00 PM	Pear, seltzer water
6:00 PM	Run 8-12 miles
7:45 PM	Pasta and tomato sauce, Parmesan cheese, steamed vegetables, cottage cheese, coffee
9:00 PM	Frozen yogurt, water

Carol's Typical Premenstrual Diet

5:30 AM	Awaken; coffee
5:40 AM	Bagel with jam, bakery muffin or Danish, coffee
8:00 AM	Coffee
10:00 AM	Bagel, coffee
11:00 AM	Apple, coffee
1:00 PM	Frozen yogurt and cone, trail mix, coffee
3:00 PM	Graham crackers (too many), coffee
6:00 PM	Run 5-6 miles
7:15 PM	Pasta and tomato sauce, Parmesan cheese, steamed vegetables, cottage cheese, two fudge ice milk bars, wine
9:00 PM	Ice milk
9:30 PM	Homemade chocolate-chip cookies, peanut butter
9:45 PM	Brownie, peanut butter
10:30 PM	Ice cream
2:00 AM	Blueberry muffin, peanut butter, ice milk

Assessment

At 5 ft 3 in, 110 lb, 16% body fat, Carol works hard to maintain her physique and to stay a size 2 or 4. She is caught up in a cycle of starve-stuff over a typical month. Carol eats a very low-fat, high-carbohydrate diet to keep her body fat low, yet she binges on higher-fat "forbidden" foods in response to hormonal changes in the luteal or second phase of her menstrual cycle. She takes daily megadoses of vitamins C and E.

Carol is a self-employed professional who works 7 days a week, 12 hours a day. Over the years she has placed more emphasis on running and calisthenic exercises to help control her body size—and stress level. Intellectually, she realizes what she is doing as she spreads high-fat peanut butter on a high-fat bakery muffin; however, she seems unable to stop. Many of the foods she eats premenstrually are easily consumed carbohydrates, yet higher in fat than she would allow herself when not premenstrual.

She is able to maintain her training regimen premenstrually, but she does so less intensely because she feels crampy, bloated, or lethargic. Keeping up with her exercises is essential in helping her believe she is fighting back against the inability to control her food cravings and body bloat.

Solutions

Carol needs to work on making dietary modifications over the entire menstrual cycle in an effort to alleviate her premenstrual symptomology.

Reduce

1. Caffeine and other dehydrating beverages (eg, coffee, soda, diet soda, tea, ice tea, and alcohol) to prevent fluid retention, headaches, and agitation.
2. Chocolate and other caffeinated foods or medications.
3. Excessive sodium and salt intake to reduce fluid retention.
4. Foods high in simple sugars (eg, candy, cakes, cookies, ice cream, muffins) to avoid fluctuations in blood sugar levels and resulting hypoglycemic feelings.
5. Excessive intake of high-fat foods (eg, peanut butter, cheese, ice cream) to decrease her self-induced feelings of guilt about needing to eat more frequently premenstrually.
6. Megadoses of any vitamin-mineral supplement.

Increase

7. A variety of foods high in complex carbohydrates, balanced with a low-fat, moderate protein intake.
8. Hydrating beverages (eg, water, sugar-free seltzer, caffeine-free beverages, herbal teas, sports drinks, low-fat or skim milk).
9. 500 kcal per day more than usual caloric intake due to hormonally controlled metabolic changes during the luteal phase of the menstrual cycle. Increased appetite premenstrually may be related to these changes.
10. Smaller, more frequent meals and snacks to keep blood glucose (sugar) levels normal; eat every 3 hours.
11. A multivitamin-mineral supplement meeting 100% of the RDA, for nutritional insurance.

Changes

5:30 AM	Awaken; water; calisthenics (45 minutes)
6:00 AM	High-fiber cereal, banana, strawberries, low-fat yogurt, coffee
9:00 AM	Bagel, water
12:00 PM	Turkey sandwich, vegetables, fruit, graham crackers
3:00 PM	Fruit
6:00 PM	Run 8 miles
7:30 PM	Pasta, vegetables, cottage cheese, fudge ice milk bars
10:00 PM	Ice milk

The Bottom Line

"My cravings are better. I can control my food intake much better pre-menstrually when I reduce my caffeine intake all month, and when I don't overtrain. By 'allowing' myself more food during this one week, I don't feel as guilty when my appetite naturally peaks. I 'allow' myself peanut butter (if I want it) and chocolate (in the form of fudge ice milk bars) all month long, so they don't seem so special to me premenstrually. I guess I won't rush my life away waiting for menopause."

▶ CASE STUDY C. TOO MUCH FAT

"My eating is pretty bad.... I'm so busy with work and workouts that I don't take the time to eat as well as I should. I know I could perform better if I ate better...."

After Brian, a 34-year-old construction superintendent, has worked from 7 AM to 3:30 PM, he jumps into his second job—training from 4 PM to 9 PM for stair races, such as a race up the Empire State Building. Brian runs stairs 5 days per week; on weekends, he bikes and runs trails. Needless to say, this rigorous schedule leaves little time for cooking up a creative sports diet.

Brian's Typical Diet and Exercise Schedule

6:30 AM	Large bowl of cereal; banana; whole milk
7:00 AM	Coffee with cream and sugar; doughnut
12:00 PM	Spaghetti with butter (prepared and eaten at home), 1-2 slices bread with butter, 3-4 sandwich cookies, 2 cups whole milk
4-5:30 PM	Drives into city
5:30-7:30 PM	Training session
7:30-9:00 PM	Drives home
7:30 PM	16 oz sports drink (while driving home)
10:00 PM	Macaroni and cheese (frozen dinner) or fast-food hamburger with french fries; six or more butter-flavored crackers; 2 cups milk; 3-4 sandwich cookies

Diet Composition

Actual:	4000 kcal,	50% carbohydrate,	15% protein,	35% fat
Target:	4000 kcal,	60%-70% carbohydrate,	10%-15% protein,	20%-25% fat

Assessment

Brian tries to make carbohydrate-rich food choices, but he admits that he knows little about nutrition. He struggles with "solo cooking," time constraints, and the "hungry horrors" that constantly confront him. He generally succumbs to the fastest and easiest foods around—often fast-food burgers, boxfuls of crackers, or high-fat frozen dinners. Eating fruits and vegetables is hit-or-miss. Salads are limited to the two or three days just after grocery shopping. "Foods that spoil are a real headache. I end up throwing them away most of the time."

Solutions

Although Brian tries to eat a carbohydrate-rich diet, his 50% carbohydrate intake misses the recommended target of 60% to 70% carbohydrate. He consumes far more fat than he realizes. It was suggested that Brian incorporate the following dietary improvements:

To Lower Fat, Boost Carbohydrates, and Improve Nutritional Quality

1. Switch from whole milk (3.5% fat) to 2% milk. As he learns to like the lower fat taste, progress to 1% fat milk, and eventually to skim milk (0% fat).
2. Trade in butter (fat) on spaghetti for tomato sauce (carbohydrate).
3. Spread bread with jam or honey, or eat it plain.
4. Trade in the butter-flavored crackers with 48% calories from fat to lower-fat crackers, such as stoned wheat, RyKrisp,* Ak-mak,† or pretzels (approximately 5% to 20% fat).
5. Boost fruit intake: drink more juices, and eat more bananas. (Keep bananas in the refrigerator to reduce spoilage. Their peels may turn black, but the fruit will be fine.)
6. Boost vegetable intake: top spaghetti with tomato sauce rather than butter; add chopped broccoli, green peppers or other vegetables (frozen or fresh) to the tomato sauce.

To Improve Stamina and Endurance

7. Plan an after-work snack that would digest easily in the 2 hours before the workout. These carbohydrates would help maintain a normal blood sugar level after his busy workday, and improve his stamina and endurance during his workout. Experiment to determine what snacks settle best (suggestions include juice, yogurt, bagel, crackers, pretzels, bananas, and dried fruits). These preexercise and postexercise snacks would help abate Brian's "hungry horrors," so that he would have more energy and patience to choose and cook a simple meal upon getting home, instead of stopping for fast-but-fatty foods along the way.
8. Drink juices as well as sports drinks after workouts. Fruit juices have more nutritional value; in the long run, that will prove to be useful for training and performance.
9. Change his training schedule to include more rest days (or easy days), to provide the opportunity for his muscles to recover and to replace depleted glycogen stores—and thereby be able to do better-quality workouts as well as reduce his risks of getting injured.
10. Go food shopping on the rest days; stock up for the week.

---

*Ralston Purina Co, St Louis, MO 63164.
†Ak-mak Bakeries, Sanger, CA 93657.

Changes

6:30 AM	Cereal, banana, 2% milk, juice
7:00 AM	Coffee with milk, bagel with jam
12:00 PM	Spaghetti with tomato sauce, 1 or 2 slices hearty, whole-grain bread, 2 cups 2% milk, 2 cups orange juice
3:30 PM	Four fig bar cookies
6:30 PM	Workout, alternating hard days, easier days, and days off
7:30 PM	32 oz cranberry-apple juice
10:00 PM	Canned soup (minestrone) and sandwich (turkey, lean meat), 2 cups 2% milk

Diet Composition

4000 kcal,   68% carbohydrate,   12% protein,   20% fat

The Bottom Line

"I came in second in the Empire State Building Run-up with energy to spare, and I was feeling stronger than ever. Two weeks later, I not only won a stairclimb in Indianapolis, but also set a record by 12 seconds—and still felt good at the end. By cutting back on fats, eating more carbs and training harder (but only every other day), I feel great."

▶ CASE STUDY D. INJURED AGAIN

"First I got a stress fracture. Then a cold that I couldn't shake. Then the flu. Then another stress fracture. I think I eat healthfully. I eat lots of fresh fruits and vegetables, but maybe you can find something wrong with my diet."

Janice, a 32-year-old nurse and mother of two, is frustrated by her injuries. Her goals of qualifying for the Boston Marathon were fading away. She felt lucky if she was able to get her training up to 4 miles a day, far from the longer distances she wanted to do.

Janice's Typical Diet and Exercise Schedule

9:00 AM	Large bowl of cut-up fruit (brought to work)
1:00 PM	Large salad (from a salad bar), juice
4:00 PM	Rice cakes
4:30 PM	Run 2-4 miles, if not injured or sick
6:30 PM	Large plateful of stir-fried vegetables, brown rice
9:00 PM	Piece of fruit

Diet Composition

Actual:	2000 kcal,	70% carbohydrate,	8% protein,	27% fat
Target:	2000 kcal,	60%-70% carbohydrate,	10%-15% protein,	20%-25% fat

---

Assessment

True, the foods that Janice eats are highly nutritious, but her overall diet is unbalanced (see *Table 4.19*). In her effort to eat a high-carbohydrate "all-natural" diet, Janice neglected to look at the whole picture. She was eating *too many* fruits

TABLE 4.19 *Common Problems Faced by Endurance Athletes*

Problem	Symptom	Solution
Too little fat	Undesired weight loss or binge-eating	20%-25% kcal from fat
Too much fat	Muscular fatigue during training; weight gain	20%-25% kcal from fat
Too little carbohydrate	Muscular fatigue during training	60%-70% kcal from CHO or 3-5 g/lb
Too much carbohydrate	General fatigue due to insufficient protein, iron, and zinc	60%-70% kcal from CHO or 3-5 g/lb
Too little protein	Injuries that heal slowly; lack of muscular bulk; iron and zinc deficiency	10%-15% kcal from protein or 0.5-0.75 g/lb
Too much protein	Muscular fatigue due to lack of CHO	10%-15% kcal from protein or 0.5-0.75 g/lb
Too little energy (kcal)	Binge-eating on sweets, fats	Approximately 15-20 kcal/lb
Too much energy (kcal)	Undesired weight gain	Approximately 12-15 kcal/lb
Too little iron	Fatigue associated with anemia	Consume RDA (10-15 mg); generally increase iron-rich foods
Too little zinc	Slow healing of injuries; lingering colds; early fatigue	Consume RDA (12-15 mg); generally increase zinc-rich foods
Too little calcium	Suboptimal bone development and maintenance; muscle cramping	Consume RDA (800-1200 mg); generally increase low-fat, calcium-rich foods

and vegetables, not enough protein-rich foods (for protein, iron, and zinc), and not enough low-fat dairy foods (for calcium, riboflavin, and protein). Consequently, her health was suffering. (Protein helps build and maintain strong muscles. Iron helps reduce the risk of anemia. Zinc helps build a strong immune system, enhances healing, and is in numerous enzymes involved in energy metabolism. Calcium helps reduce the risk of stress fractures. Riboflavin helps convert food into energy.)

Solutions

Janice preferred to eat very little meat, fish, or chicken, and her lack of protein was having a negative impact on her overall health. Since she doubted she would make the effort to eat a high-quality vegetarian diet with plenty of beans, lentils, tofu, and whole grains that would provide the needed nutrients, the recommendation was that she include small portions of lean animal proteins at lunch and/or dinner three or four times per week, and also boost her intake of low-fat dairy foods to three or four times per day. Preferably, she would choose small portions of darker-colored proteins, since they tend to have more iron and zinc: lean beef, the thigh meat of chicken and turkey, and darker fish (such as tuna, mackerel, and trout). These would better help her rebuild her body stores and get back on the road to good health.

Once she understood that meat has a cholesterol content similar to that of chicken and fish (70 to 80 mg per 4 oz portion) and that lean meats can appropriately fit into a low-fat diet, she agreed that the nutritional benefits of these foods were important to her, and that she would include small portions as an accompaniment to her current diet. She also saw the benefits of eating more vegetarian sources of protein, since fruits and vegetables (the foundation of her current diet) lack high-quality protein.

Recommendations

1. Eat adequate protein (0.4 to 0.6 g per pound of body weight). For Janice (at 120 lb), this came to 50 to 70 g of protein per day, and contributed 10% to 15% of her total caloric intake. She could obtain this amount by:

▶ Swapping 100 kcal of fruit for 100 kcal of plain yogurt at breakfast

▶ Trading the 350 kcal of Italian dressing in her salad for a yogurt-based dressing (100 kcal), plus some tuna, garbanzo beans, or other protein-rich food

▶ Stir-frying some tofu or lean meat into her vegetables at night

▶ Trading her evening fruit snack for a yogurt snack

2. For optimal iron and zinc, eat more extra-lean meats, enriched or fortified breakfast cereals, and iron-rich vegetables, lentils, beans, and tofu. It also helps to cook food in a cast-iron skillet.

3. Include a food rich in vitamin C with each meal to enhance iron absorption. This might be orange juice at breakfast, tomatoes at lunch (in a salad or sandwich), and broccoli, spinach, or another dark green vegetable at dinner.

4. See her physician for a blood test for anemia (to include hemoglobin, hematocrit, serum ferritin, and total iron-binding capacity). At the doctor's recommendation, take iron supplements as necessary.

Changes

9:00 AM	Cut-up fruit (small bowl), 1 cup yogurt or iron-enriched cereal, fruit, milk
1:00 PM	Salad with yogurt dressing (brought from home), plus tuna, garbanzo beans, or another protein-rich food
4:00 PM	Rice cakes
6:30 PM	Stir-fried vegetables with lean meat, chicken, or tofu; brown rice
9:00 PM	Yogurt

Diet Composition

2000 kcal,   65% carbohydrate,   15% protein,   25% fat

The Bottom Line (1 Month Later)

"I'm feeling much better—I'm eating more protein, and drinking more milk. I'm not chronically fatigued, and I haven't gotten sick at all. My stress fracture is healing better. I can't wait to start running consistently."

▶ CONCLUSION

Athletes struggling with food concerns may feel embarrassed to get nutrition advice from a registered dietitian (RD) or sports nutritionist. They may think that they should be able to do something as simple as eat properly on their own. However, this is often difficult to accomplish; many athletes struggle for years on their own, trying to figure out how to eat properly.

This barrier to seeking professional advice is more easily broken if the registered dietitian or sports nutritionist makes recommendations that fit into the athlete's life-style, much like a coach helps to fine tune a training regimen. The food coach or sports nutritionist should help athletes fine tune their diets to overcome the obstacles and stumbling blocks that hinder them from being the best they can be. With the right nutrition counseling, athletes can train harder and perform up to their conditioned ability.

Controversial Practices of Athletes

Susan M. Kleiner, Editor

The primary factors responsible for successful athletic performance include proper training and conditioning, good nutrition practices, natural talent, and a positive attitude. Because competition is intense and the margin between a winning and losing effort may be extremely small, some athletes seek shortcut solutions to gain a competitive advantage. Although no fast cures or guarantees of superior performance exist, some athletes experiment with substances and techniques that may harm their health and actually impair performance. Health professionals, athletic trainers, coaches, and the athletes themselves should become aware of the fallacies of these questionable practices, and should become better equipped to recognize false claims. Popular, yet controversial, practices believed to affect metabolism and performance, and ways to detect false claims and nutrition fraud, are discussed in this section.

Recognizing Nutrition Quackery

Susan Kleiner

The US population demonstrates its susceptibility to false nutrition claims by spending millions of dollars on useless products. Athletes often look for any product that can give them a greater competitive edge, so they, in particular, are vulnerable to the claims made for a variety of "performance-enhancing" nutritional aids. According to a study by Miller that was sponsored by the Food and Drug Administration, 435 questionable advertisements appeared in newspapers and magazines over a one-month period.[1] However, because not all of the nation's newsprint and magazines were reviewed in this study, it is likely that the magnitude of false advertising is much larger.[2]

Much of the difficulty surrounding false claims about foods and nutritional supplements is due to the fact that the Food and Drug Administration regards nutritional supplements as foods (not drugs), so health claims made about supplements do not need to be proved prior to introducing them to the market. This policy has put the US Postal Service, which requires truth in mail-order advertising, on the front line in the battle against nutrition quackery.[2]

In a summary of indications of nutrition fraud based on information from Monaco,[3] Kleiner suggests the use of the following points when evaluating potential nutrition fraud[2]:

▶ Treatment is based on an unproved theory that usually calls for painless, nontoxic therapy.
▶ The credentials of the author or purveyor are not recognized in the scientific community.
▶ No reports about the product are published in scientific, peer-reviewed journals; the mass media are used for marketing.
▶ Purveyors claim that the medical establishment is against them; they play on the public's paranoia about the phantom greed of the medical establishment.
▶ The "treatment" is known only to the author or purveyor; drugs and preparations are manufactured according to a "secret" formula.
▶ Excessive claims promise a dramatic, miraculous cure, including prolonging life and preventing disease.
▶ Emotional images, rather than facts, are used to support the claims.
▶ The "treatment" calls for special nutrition support that includes vitamins, minerals, or "health" food products.
▶ Purveyors often caution clients or readers against discussing the program, so they do not get discouraged by those who are "negative."
▶ Programs are based on drugs, treatments, or tests that have not been labeled for such uses.

REFERENCES

1. Miller RW. *Critiquing Quack Ads.* Washington, DC: Federal Drug Administration; 1985. US Dept of Health and Human Services publication FDA 8885-4196.
2. Kleiner SM. Beware of nutrition quackery. *Phys Sports Med.* 1990;18(6):46-50.
3. Monaco GP. The primary care physician: the first line of defense in the battle against health fraud. *Medical Times.* 1986;114:43-48.

Nutritional and Nonnutritional Factors That May Influence Metabolism and Performance

Julane Contursi, Susan Kleiner, Kathy Quinn, and Jill Mielcarek

▶ CAFFEINE

The use of caffeine as an ergogenic aid has been the subject of many investigations. Its effectiveness, however, remains controversial. Results of early studies showed that caffeine ingestion prior to cycling and Nordic skiing improved performance, and the subjects perceived the work as easier than without caffeine. In contrast, other studies have found caffeine to be of no ergogenic benefit during exercise.[1-3]

As a central nervous system stimulant, caffeine increases alertness, attention, and mental ability.[4] In addition, caffeine has been shown to stimulate the cardiovascular, respiratory, metabolic, gastrointestinal, and renal systems. The degree to which intake alters the psychological and physiologic states varies, depending on individual caffeine tolerance.[5]

While the mechanisms responsible for the influence of caffeine on energy metabolism have not been completely elucidated, several theories exist. Caffeine ingestion triggers hormonal production of epinephrine, elevating the release of free fatty acids in the blood by inhibiting phosphodiesterase, making more cyclic adenosine monophosphate available for lipolysis. Consequently, more fat is available as an energy source, and limited glycogen stores can be spared, thereby delaying the onset of fatigue. Additionally, caffeine may directly stimulate intramuscular triglyceride utilization and inhibit glycogenolysis. Caffeine may also facilitate neuromuscular function.[3]

Other factors may be related to caffeine's effectiveness as an ergogenic aid. For instance, a high-carbohydrate meal eaten at the time of caffeine ingestion and prior to competition has been shown to prevent the rise in free fatty acid levels, thus limiting the ergogenic potential of caffeine.[6] Athletes who habitually use moderate amounts of caffeine do not respond to either the metabolic or neuromuscular effects related to caffeine as an ergogenic aid.[3] Considering the small subject pools of the research studies investigating this area, these factors may cause enough intersubject variation to explain the differing results reported on the ergogenic properties of caffeine.[7]

It is important to note that caffeine is a drug that acts as a stimulant to the central nervous system. Caffeine ingestion causes an increased heart and metabolic rate, resulting in a feeling of alertness and, for some, nervousness. Blood levels of caffeine peak within 30 to 60 minutes of consumption. The physiologic effects of caffeine vary among individuals and are dependent on dosage, body composition, and past usage habits. Some people, especially young children, are highly sensitive to the stimulating effect of caffeine in the bloodstream.

Caffeine also has negative effects that could impair performance. Some individuals complain of stomach upset due to the stimulating effect of caffeine on gastric acid secretion. Caffeine tablets, which can irritate the gastrointestinal mucosa, should be avoided. Doses in excess of 250 mg can cause unwanted side effects, including[8]:

- ▶ increased anxiety
- ▶ nervousness
- ▶ irritability
- ▶ headaches
- ▶ diarrhea

Caffeine is a diuretic, stimulating water loss. Without a corresponding increase in water intake, particularly in hot weather, athletes are at greater risk of dehydration with caffeine consumption.

Caffeine is on the International Olympic Committee's and United States Olympic Committee's lists of banned substances. A urinary concentration of 12 µg/mL represents a positive drug test for caffeine, resulting in the athlete's elimination from competition. Levels exceeding this standard have been noted in individuals ingesting 900 to 1000 mg of caffeine.[9]

It is clear that the potential benefits of caffeine use must be weighed against the risks of its use. If an athlete wishes to use a moderate amount of caffeine, his or her response should be tested during training bouts in advance of competition.

A wide range of foods and beverages contain caffeine. Coffee, tea, cocoa, chocolate, many cola and noncola soft drinks, and over-the-counter and prescription medications (decongestants, pain relievers, and diet aids) contain various amounts of caffeine (see *Table 5.1*). The caffeine content of coffee and tea depends on the method of preparation and the brewing time. Nutrition and ingredient labels on products will often specify caffeine content. Failure to consider the caffeine content of food and drug products can result in gross underestimation of actual daily consumption.

▶ TOBACCO

One of the best available methods to assess an individual's fitness is to measure $\dot{V}O_2$max. This value estimates the efficiency of respiratory and circulatory systems to deliver oxygen to the working muscles. Anything that interferes with this oxygen-delivery process will negatively affect exercise performance. Because cigarette smoking interferes with oxygen delivery, it has a measurably negative effect on fuel utilization and exercise performance.

Cigarette smoking impairs both the circulatory and respiratory systems. Cigarettes contain numerous toxic substances—tar, nicotine, and other chemicals—which form harmful agents or act as direct irritants to the lungs. The tars of cigarette smoke can progressively destroy the protective surface lining of the lungs. This protective lining is a vital medium for the transfer of gases to the cells, and its destruction leaves the smoker with varying degrees of pulmonary emphysema. Smoking can, therefore, diminish the oxygen-intake efficiency of the lungs and decrease the supply of oxygen to respiratory, cardiac, and skeletal muscles. The effect of limited oxygen supply is even more critical during intense exercise, when oxygen demands are greater.

TABLE 5.1   Caffeine Content of Common Beverages, Foods, and Drug Products*

Substance	Caffeine, mg	Substance	Caffeine, mg
Coffee (5-oz cup)		Diet Pepsi	36
Drip method	110-150	Pepsi Light	36
Percolated	64-124	**Stimulants**	
Instant	40-108	NoDoz tablets	100
Decaffeinated	2-5	Vivarin tablets	200
Tea (5-oz cup)		**Pain Relievers**	
1-min brew	9-33	Anacin	32
3-min brew	20-46	Excedrin	65
5-min brew	20-50	Midol	32
Instant tea	12-28	Plain aspirin	0
Iced tea (12 oz)	22-36	Vanquish	33
Cocoa		**Diuretics**	
Made from mix	6	Aqua Ban	100
Milk chocolate (1 oz)	6	**Cold Remedies**	
Baking chocolate	35	Coryban-D	30
		Dristan	0
Soft Drinks (12-oz)		Triaminicin	30
Mountain Dew	54	**Weight-Control Aids**	
Mello Yello	52	Dexatrim	200
Tab	46	Prolamine	140
Coca-Cola	46	**Prescription Pain Relievers**	
Diet Coke	46	Cafergot	100
Shasta Cola	44	Darvon Compound	32
Mr. Pibb	40	Fiorinal	40
Dr. Pepper	40	Migralam	100
Sugar-free Dr. Pepper	40		
Pepsi-Cola	38		

*Caffeine data obtained from Consumers Union, Food and Drug Administration, National Coffee Association, National Soft Drink Association, and *Physicians' Desk Reference for Nonprescription Drugs.*
Mountain Dew, Pepsi-Cola, Diet Pepsi, Pepsi Light, Pepsi-Cola USA, Purchase, NY 10577. Mello Yello, Tab, Coca-Cola, Diet Coke, Mr Pibb, Coca-Cola Co, Atlanta, GA 30301. Shasta Cola, Shasta Beverages Inc, Hayward, CA 94545. Dr Pepper, Sugar-free Dr Pepper, Dr Pepper Co, Dallas, TX 75265.
NoDoz, Excedrin, Bristol-Myers Products, New York, NY 10154. Vivarin, SmithKline Beecham, Pittsburgh, PA 15230. Anacin, Dristan, Whitehall Laboratories Inc, New York, NY 10017. Midol, Vanquish, Glenbrook Laboratories, New York, NY 10016. Aqua-Ban, Dexatrim, Prolamine, Thompson Medical Co Inc, West Palm Beach, FL 33407. Triaminicin, Cafergot, Fiorinal, Sandoz Pharmaceuticals, East Hanover, NJ 17936. Darvon, Eli Lilly and Co, Indianapolis, IN 46285.
Adapted from Slavin JL, Joensen D. Caffeine and sports performance. *Phys Sports Med.* 1985;13:191-193.

During breathing, respiratory muscles work against an airway resistance. Smoking a single cigarette increases this resistance. Consequently, the respiratory muscles of a smoker must work harder and consume more oxygen during normal breathing. The higher cost for the ventilation leaves less oxygen to supply other skeletal muscles. During periods of heavy exercise, the oxygen cost of ventilation for smokers is nearly twice that of nonsmokers.[10] The effect of this is premature fatigue, which is usually the cause of impaired performance. A 24-hour abstinence from smoking can help offset this increased oxygen cost; thus, to reduce the detrimental effects on performance, smoking athletes should refrain from smoking cigarettes at least 1 day prior to competition. Of course, total cessation of smoking would have the greatest positive effect.

Smoking also taxes the heart and circulatory system. Carbon monoxide is a by-product of cigarette smoke. Hemoglobin in the red blood cells will preferentially bind carbon monoxide instead of oxygen. This reduces the oxygen-carrying capacity of blood, limiting the oxygen supply to working muscles, including the heart, during exercise. The blood of a one-pack-a-day smoker has approximately a 10% reduction in oxygen-carrying capacity.[11] To compensate for this, the heart has to pump more blood more often to deliver the needed oxygen, increasing its resting and exercise rate. Exacerbating this condition, the nicotine in cigarette smoke stimulates the release of epinephrine, causing blood vessels to constrict, blood pressure to rise, and heart rate to increase. Nicotine also causes an increased release of free fatty acids into the blood.

Smoking appears to negate many of the beneficial effects that regular exercise has on the heart. While exercise leads to increases in the concentration of circulating high-density lipoprotein cholesterol (HDL-C), which is a protective factor against coronary heart disease, smoking has been shown to reduce this blood constituent. Clearly, smoking compromises both athletic performance and health.

▶ ALCOHOL

Alcohol is one of the most abused drugs in the United States. Although it is a concentrated source of kilocalories, it has limited food value. While alcohol has a relatively high caloric yield of about 7 kcal/g, it is not available to the muscles, so is not a significant energy supplier during exercise (see Table 1.5). Once metabolized, most of the alcohol's energy yield is released as heat; hence alcohol is not converted to glycogen for future use as body fuel.

Although the effect of alcohol differs widely between individuals, it is generally agreed that if it is consumed in moderate amounts (less than two drinks) and on nonexercise days, it does not negatively affect exercise performance. However, consumption of alcohol on an exercise day or on the day of a competition is known to affect performance negatively. If one drink (12 oz of beer, 4 oz of wine, or 1 oz of 80-proof liquor) is consumed before a workout or event, the alcohol will have a direct effect on the nervous system. Alcohol acts on the brain by depressing its ability to reason and make judgments. Information-related processes are slowed; fine motor skills are decreased; reaction time is reduced; coordination, balance, and visual perception are altered; and muscular reflexes are impaired. Sports that demand the athlete's rapid reflex response, such as tennis and racquetball, are most affected.

Alcohol affects carbohydrate metabolism mainly through inhibition of gluconeogenesis.[12] The oxidation of alcohol results in an elevation in the reduced form of nicotinamide adenine dinucleotide (NADH) in the cytosol, resulting in a decreased amount of NAD^+ available for gluconeogenesis. This reduces pyruvate, which subsequently decreases pyruvate carboxylase activity. Pyruvate carboxylase is necessary for gluconeogenesis. This condition may also predispose a person to hypoglycemia, especially if glycogen stores are depleted.

One of the most harmful effects of alcohol in an athletic event is evident in prolonged endurance contests. The liver is the primary organ for the detoxification of alcohol. Once alcohol is present in the blood, its metabolism takes priority over other liver functions. During prolonged exercise, when the body needs the extra glucose that can be formed by the liver, an elevated level of blood alcohol may block this biochemical pathway. A drop in blood glucose during an endurance event could lead to early fatigue. This effect may be attributable to the fact that alcohol reduces total body fat oxidation by as much as 79%.[13] Alcohol also has the effect of reducing protein oxidation by as much as 39%, and may also reduce protein synthesis.[13] Because protein metabolism only accounts for a small amount of total energy consumption (<5%) during exercise, it is not likely that this would have a major effect on performance. However, the lower rate of protein synthesis may, in the long run, reduce athletic performance.[14]

Alcohol is absorbed into the bloodstream via the stomach and small intestine. Peak concentration in the blood occurs within 1 hour of consumption, depending on whether food is in the stomach. The absorbed alcohol is distributed within the water compartments of cells. This can disturb the water balance in muscle cells and consequently alter the cellular enzymatic activity that produces adenosine triphosphate (ATP), the substrate that provides fuel for muscle contraction, active transport, and biosynthesis within the body.

Body size and composition will alter dose/response rates to alcohol. A small, lean athlete whose body has a high percentage of body water would experience fatigue from the effects of alcohol sooner than would a larger person with more body fat.

Research indicates that moderate levels of alcohol are associated with elevated levels of HDL-C. Levels of HDL-C are also increased as a result of exercise, and are associated with a reduced risk of heart disease. However, two distinct subfractions of HDL have been identified. The HDL_3-C component is increased with moderate alcohol consumption; the HDL_2-C fraction is increased as a result of exercise. It is the HDL_2-C fraction that is believed to be protective against coronary heart disease.[15]

Drinking alcohol provides relaxation and can calm precompetition nervousness, and its vasodilation effect enhances blood flow to the muscles. However, drinking before training or before a competition may not improve work capacity and may lead to decreased performance levels.

Alcohol abuse is a major cause of automobile and other serious accidents, and prolonged overconsumption can damage the liver, heart, muscles, and brain. Alcohol use should be discouraged.

▶ ANABOLIC-ANDROGENIC STEROIDS

The use of anabolic steroids is epidemic in the world of elite athletics.[16] The only sports in which steroid use has not been documented are women's field hockey and figure skating.[17] Surveys report their pervasive use by recreational and adolescent athletes.[18,19] Although most steroid users state that improvement of athletic performance is their main reason for drug use, a distinct percentage of users admit that appearance is the main reason that they use steroids.[19,20]

Anabolic-androgenic steroids are synthetic androgens that have greater anabolic activity relative to the androgenic activity of testosterone. They have been available for legitimate medical use for almost 40 years.[21] Conditions such as certain anemias, hereditary angioedema, certain cases of breast cancer and osteoporosis, and male hypogonadism may all be treated with physiologic doses of anabolic-androgenic steroid preparations.[22] When used in superphysiologic doses, as in the case of steroid abuse by athletes, these drugs have strong androgenic effects. The mechanism by which anabolic steroids exert their effect is unclear. It is claimed that steroids diffuse into cellular cytosol, combining with an androgenic virilizing receptor. The receptor-steroid complex migrates into the nucleus of the cell, interacting with DNA, to initiate transcription. Next, RNA production increases, resulting in a higher rate of protein synthesis. Steroids also induce a positive effect on nitrogen balance, necessary for development of muscle tissue.

The results of studies investigating the effectiveness of anabolic steroid use on muscle and weight gain and on increases in strength in athletes have been equivocal. However, in 1984, Haupt and Rovere concluded that the differences in the effects of anabolic steroids on human strength, size, and weight are the result of differences in the study protocols.[23] After distilling all the variables and statistically analyzing for those factors consistently associated with either the presence or absence of increases in strength, the authors determined that consistent improvements in strength, body size, and body weight will result from anabolic steroid administration in certain individuals, if the use of steroids is coupled with a continuing program of intensive strength-training exercise and a high-protein, high-calorie diet. In contrast, the use of anabolic steroids will not enhance aerobic capacity. The conclusions reached by Haupt and Rovere have been supported and restated by the American College of Sports Medicine position paper on anabolic steroids.[24]

In addition to superphysiologic dosing of 10 to 100 times the physiologic replacement dose of testosterone, patterns of steroid abuse by athletes often include the simultaneous use of different steroid preparations, called stacking. Stacking generally follows a pyramid scheme, in which a low dose of one preparation is begun, and then dosages are increased along with the number of compounds, usually a mix of oral and parenteral agents, until a peak intake is reached. After peaking, dosages and compounds are tapered off. The entire cycle usually lasts 6 to 12 weeks, and may be repeated many times throughout a training career.[25]

Adverse side effects from the misuse of anabolic steroids occur in virtually all systems of the human body.[25] Many of the minor side effects in men occur often and are usually reversible. The virilizing effects in women are profound, and often irreversible. Documentation of psychological disorders as a result of anabolic steroid abuse have indicated an increased frequency of affective and psychotic symptoms in steroid abusers.[26]

Agents that are 17-α alkylated compounds are more highly associated with liver abnormalities, including abnormal liver function test results, cholestasis, and rarely, peliosis hepatis, hepatic adenomas, and hepatocellular carcinoma, than are the 17-ß hydroxyl esterified group.[22] The alkylated agents are water-soluble (vs the fat-soluble esterified agents), allowing their metabolites to be quickly cleared from the body only 14 days after discontinuing use. They are, therefore, less detectable during drug tests after only a brief period of discontinued use. This property has recently increased the popularity of the apparently more dangerous alkylated compounds.[27]

The mechanisms of action of anabolic steroid use include the improvement of nitrogen utilization, and the promotion of positive nitrogen balance by the reversal of catabolic processes. With heavy training, an individual can maintain a relative state of chronic catabolism. Therefore, requirements for protein and energy would appear to be increased from the non-steroid-using training state. However, the actual protein and energy requirements of these athletes are unknown.[25]

▶ HUMAN GROWTH HORMONE

Human growth hormone (hGH) is a primary anabolic hormone in the body, produced by the anterior pituitary gland. Its release is stimulated by physical exercise of high intensity or long duration, physical or psychological stress, hypoglycemia, dietary protein, specific amino acids, deep sleep, and stimulatory hormones and drugs. Human growth hormone secretion is inhibited by chronic exercise or overtraining, hyperglycemia, obesity, disturbed sleep, and inhibitory hormones and drugs.[28]

Human growth hormone enhances amino acid uptake and the synthesis of protein, RNA and DNA, stimulates lipolysis, and inhibits glucose utilization in tissues (increasing blood glucose levels). It has been used effectively to treat dwarfism due to lack of hGH, and in the treatment of atrophied muscle.[22]

Due to recent advances in biomedical engineering, hGH can now be synthesized in the laboratory, and it is more readily available. Previously, pituitary-extracted hGH was available in very limited quantities. As the methods for detecting the use of anabolic steroids in competitive athletes have been perfected, anecdotal reports indicate a rise in hGH doping by athletes, since it currently cannot be detected through drug testing.[20,22,28] It is, however, included on the list of banned substances by the International Olympic Committee.

Adverse effects of hGH doping by athletes have not been documented but can be predicted on the basis of known effects of endogenous hypersecretion. These include acromegaly, which is associated with glucose intolerance, hyperlipidemia, heart disease, impotence, and bony overgrowth (eg, protruding forehead and jaw or enlarged hands and feet).[22]

An athlete can optimize the natural secretion of growth hormone by periodization of training, control of stress, adequate nutritional support, and adequate sleep and relaxation.[28] Since overtraining and overstrain will inhibit hGH release, these situations should be avoided.

The use of amino acid supplements by athletes to stimulate growth hormone secretion has led to recent scientific investigations. Arginine, histidine, lysine, methionine, phenylalanine, leucine, valine, and ornithine have been studied as potentiators of hGH secretion.[29] The majority of studies have investigated the effects of amino acid infusions on hGH secretion. Since athletes take these supplements orally, present studies are investigating the effects of oral dosing of amino acids on hGH secretion, and preliminary results from two studies indicate that there is a positive relationship between the two. However, in one study the subjects became ill on the ornithine dosage level required to stimulate hGH release, and muscle strength or growth was not measured.[30] In another study using a combined arginine-ornithine supplement where the authors concluded significant strength and lean body mass increases, hGH was not measured and diets were not controlled.[31]

▶ MARIJUANA

Although it is not an ergogenic aid, marijuana is the most widely abused illicit drug in sports.[32] Acute effects of marijuana use have been reported to last only 4 hours, but further research has demonstrated impairment for as long as 24 hours after use. According to reports, marijuana is said to decrease muscle strength. Although specific data relative to athletic performance are lacking, it would appear that the use of marijuana would have deleterious effects on athletic performance. Marijuana impairs psychomotor function. While under the influence of this drug, coordination, short-term memory, judgment, and time perception are altered.

Cardiovascular effects include tachycardia and postural fluctuations in blood pressure. Sweating is also inhibited with a resultant increase in body temperature. Performance in hot weather would be significantly hampered, with an increased risk of heat stroke. Similar to tobacco, smoking of any kind reduces the blood's oxygen-carrying capacity. Long-term use of marijuana may result in personality changes such as apathy, concentration difficulties, confusion, and memory deficits.

▶ AMPHETAMINES

Athletes use amphetamines to enhance performance and delay the point of fatigue. These drugs are psychostimulants that mimic the body's natural hormonal compound, epinephrine, causing an increased metabolic rate, elevated heart rate and breathing, increased blood pressure, release of free fatty acids, and increased blood glucose. These physiologic responses result in a feeling of increased alertness. The stimulatory effect is of short duration, and only masks (does not reduce) fatigue.[33]

Several studies have investigated the influence of amphetamines on athletic performance. These studies have looked at the use of amphetamines as performance enhancers in nonfatigued athletes. Although some of the studies have shortcomings in design, a review of available evidence[32] suggests that amphetamine use can enhance skills that play a key role in athletic performance, including speed, power, endurance, concentration, and fine motor coordination.

Laboratory-measured improvements that have been noted are not always applicable to competitive situations. An athlete who achieves a particular level of performance with the use of stimulants might be able, with proper motivation and training, to reproduce similar efforts naturally. A drug-induced mood elevation might also contribute to an athlete's perception that his or her performance was improved, when in reality it was not.

Dose response to amphetamines is highly variable among individuals. Certain doses of amphetamine may be more useful for certain athletic endeavors, that is, sport-specific or position-specific dosing.[32] However, firm data regarding amphetamine use and doses in various sports are unavailable.

Amphetamines are included on the lists of substances banned by the International and US Olympic Committees, and are part of a standard drug testing regimen. Use of amphetamines is contraindicated for all individuals, especially those with high blood pressure or nervous conditions. Side effects of amphetamines may range from mild to severe, and acute to chronic. Some of these may include restlessness, dizziness, tremor, irritability, confusion, assaultiveness, delirium, paranoia, hallucinations, convulsions, angina, myocardial infarction, addiction, psychosis, vasculitis, neuropathy. Addiction and dependency to amphetamines may further potentiate any of the above-mentioned adverse effects.

▶ BLOOD DOPING

Blood doping first became evident as an athletic practice during the 1976 Montreal Olympic Games. It was alleged to have been used as a procedure that helped an endurance athlete attain his gold medal.[34]

Doping is defined as "the use of physiological substances in abnormal amounts and with abnormal methods with the exclusive aim of attaining an artificial and unfair increase in performance."[35] Blood doping describes a medical intervention of removing, storing, and subsequent transfusion or reinfusion of a volume of blood (to a donor) whose primary effect is to increase hemoglobin concentration.[36] Blood doping is also referred to as blood boosting, blood packing, induced erythrocythemia, or polycythemia.

Blood doping involves removing a volume of blood, separating the red blood cells (RBCs) from the plasma, storing the RBCs, and then reinfusing the RBCs back into the individual at the time that normocythemia has been attained. Transfusion or reinfusion will usually be performed 5 to 6 weeks after the initial removal and 1 to 7 days prior to competition.[37]

Sustained muscle activity requires continuous oxygen transport to the muscle. Since oxygen is carried by hemoglobin in RBCs, it seems sensible that increasing this component, either by whole blood transfusions or packed RBC transfusion, will enhance performance.[38] The theory underlying blood doping, then, is contingent on the possible increases in oxygen-carrying capacity of blood, believed to be limited by physiologic rather than biochemical processes.[37]

The supposition of increased athletic performance from increased oxygen delivery is based on three assumptions[36]:

1. Maximum cardiac output is unaffected by the increase in blood viscosity.
2. Blood distribution to the working muscle is unaltered.
3. Muscle has an oxidative capacity sufficient to utilize additional oxygen.

An early review of this process did not support the suppositions of beneficial effects, due to research incontinuity and conflicting results.[36] However, two well-designed studies have shown improvements in hemoglobin, hematocrit, $\dot{V}O_2$max, and treadmill running times after blood reinfusion.[39,40] In one study the authors concluded that the increased performance could be due to the buffering capacity of blood from the additional hemoglobin concentration.[39]

Induced erythrocythemia could increase blood viscosity to the point that greater peripheral resistance is seen if the hematocrit exceeds 49%.[38] A reduced cardiac output would result, which defeats the purpose of the blood doping process. Buick and colleagues have suggested that an optimal hematocrit for oxygen delivery is in excess of 45%, but they are uncertain of the limits of the upper range before blood viscosity would begin to offset benefits.[39]

Although blood doping may appear to be a more viable, nonpharmaceutical means for enhancing performance, it is not without risks.[38] Immune side effects complicate about 3% of all transfusions. Most are mild allergic reactions, such as fever and urticaria. Hemolytic transfusion reactions occur in approximately 1 in 6000 transfusions; these could be fatal. Anaphylactic reactions and bacterial contamination may also result in transfusion-related deaths. Acquired immunodeficiency syndrome associated with transfusions is another risk. Transfusion also stimulates immune sensitization in normal, young recipients; therefore, future medical management relating to blood transfusion, pregnancy, or bone marrow transplantation may be more difficult, or even impossible.

Although doping control regulations prohibit its use, control methods to differentiate increased hemoglobin from altitude acclimatization, genetic endowment, or blood doping have yet to be devised.[36]

► SODIUM BICARBONATE DOPING

Bicarbonate doping refers to the practice of ingesting sodium bicarbonate (baking soda) before an athletic event. This is done with the hope of eliminating the anaerobic exercise-induced disturbance in muscular acid-base balance that causes fatigue and exhaustion. The accumulation of hydrogen ions in the sarcoplasm of the muscle cell contributes to the decreased ability to do work, by inhibiting contractile proteins or resynthesis of ATP. An elevation of extracellular bicarbonate has been proposed to facilitate the efflux of hydrogen ions from the muscle, thereby reducing and offsetting fatigue.[41]

Research investigating the effects of bicarbonate doping on exercise performance report conflicting results.[41-43] According to Wadler and Hainline, most studies indicate that bicarbonate doping has no significant effect on aerobic activities or on upper-body anaerobic activities.[32] They point out that one researcher suggests that bicarbonate doping may be useful in anaerobic situations because these events are more susceptible to hydrogen ion buildup.

Important points to remember before partaking in bicarbonate doping are that it is definitely ineffective for events lasting longer than 4 minutes, since the contribution of energy from anaerobic glycolysis becomes progressively smaller. Soda doping is also useless for sprint events (<30 seconds) because fatigue in those events would be unrelated to lactic acid buildup.[43] No serious side effects have been reported associated with bicarbonate loading, but it may cause gastrointestinal distress and diarrhea. Chronic doping may lead to disturbances in sodium and water balance, and it is contraindicated for individuals with high blood pressure. Massive bicarbonate ingestion may cause profound metabolic alkalosis, leading to apathy, confusion, stupor, and tetany.[32]

▶ STRESS

There are two types of stress: distress, which produces negative effects (anxiety leading to tension, pressure, pain, and poor performance), and eustress, which produces positive effects (anxiety leading to motivation and accomplishment). Either type may occur in an acute or chronic state. Exercise is classified as eustress. It helps the body relax, and works physiologically and biochemically to combat emotional distress. Distress triggers chemical changes in the brain, stimulating the release of neurotransmitters, such as serotonin, epinephrine, norepinephrine, and acetylcholine. These chemicals act as messengers to the body to prepare a response to stress. In response to those neurotransmitters, the heart rate, blood glucose production, and blood pressure may increase. The stress of exercise boosts the production of the body's natural pain relievers and mood modulators known as endorphins. These are endogenous peptides, which act chemically like morphine, and counter the effects of distress. Endorphins are thought to cause the euphoric feeling known as the "runner's high."

Acute stress may be positive or negative during periods of intensive training or prior to competition, depending on the athlete's state of preparation and response to the situation. Acute distress may cause an athlete to become so overwrought with anxiety that performance is inhibited. However, acute eustress may increase the athlete's ability to become energized and focus on the goal: enhancing performance.[32]

Too much training (a chronic stress) may exceed an individual's functional limits and become a negative stress. Consistently overexceeding this boundary may result in negative physiologic and psychological consequences, and cancel out some of the beneficial elements of exercise. Overtraining, therefore, results in impaired performance. Athletes who overtrain become intolerant to training, sleep patterns may be disturbed, they may become depressed, and lose their sense of appetite and thirst. Exercise that is within an individual's trained capabilities and is done regularly is the least expensive and most effective method of stress management available.

▶ FASTING

Many athletes fast or drastically reduce their caloric intakes to maintain an unnaturally low body mass for performance, or to achieve an acute state of reduced body weight for competition. Dancers, gymnasts, figure skaters, and divers (especially females) are notorious for their drive to attain a sylphlike physique through short-term fasting or chronic reduced-calorie dieting. Wrestlers, weight lifters, bodybuilders, boxers, and oarsmen want to compete at a body weight that is below their natural level so they can be the largest competitor in a lower weight class. In addition to fasting, these athletes may also restrict fluids, abuse laxatives and diuretics, and promote fluid loss via sweating (eg, saunas, rubber suits) and expectorating.

Fasting is never recommended for athletes. It results in fatigue, reduced glycogen stores, and impaired performance. Dehydration regimens and polydrug abuse may have severe physiologic consequences. When water loss is equal to or greater than 2% of body weight, cardiovascular capacity and thermoregulatory functions are diminished due to reduced fluid volume and perspiration capabilities. Heart rate and body temperature progressively increase in parallel with hypohydration. Whether the athlete is exercising at maximum or submaximum intensities, hypohydration has a profound detrimental effect on performance.[44] Severe water restriction (4% to 5% or more of total body weight) and polydrug abuse may result in life-threatening heat stroke, kidney damage, and electrolyte imbalances.

Fasting-induced weight loss, a common practice among wrestlers, rowers, jockeys, skaters, and other athletes who must "make weight," is a potentially dangerous practice. Frequent fasting or crash-dieting should be of particular concern for those whose nutrient intake is compromised during critical periods of fast physical development. Because of the potential health problems, the American College of Sports Medicine and the American Medical Association long ago issued position statements on weight loss and wrestling.[45,46] The rapid weight loss generally involves dehydration that, in the short term, may reduce strength, endurance, and temperature regulating ability.[45] In the long term, this practice may sufficiently reduce nutrient reserves to compromise nutritional status and health.[47,48]

Others abstain from food to cleanse and purify the body. They feel lighter, but often become light-headed. Fasting progressively weakens the body by draining it of its energy resources, especially glycogen reserves. During fasting, glycogen reserves are essentially exhausted within 24 hours. Aerobic and anaerobic capacity is decreased, and losses cannot be replaced until the fast is broken. Low blood sugar results from poor glucose availability, causing an apathy toward physical work. A large quantity of water is also lost when glycogen stores are depleted. Dehydration and electrolyte shifts may add to fatigue. Obligatory glucose needs for brain and blood cell function must still be met, despite the lack of available carbohydrates. After glycogen stores are depleted, amino acids from body protein and glycerol from stored body fat become suppliers of necessary glucose.

Protein tissue breakdown is an expensive fuel with significant implications to the athlete who desires to spare protein to maintain the integrity of skeletal muscle. Prior to gluconeogenesis, nitrogen is wasted from glycogenic amino acids to capture their energy capacity, making them useless for their primary functions of protein production and tissue maintenance and repair.

As the body adapts to fasting via starvation metabolism, a greater amount of fat is mobilized and used as energy, to spare protein. In the absence of carbohydrates, the complete oxidation of fats is impossible, and ketone bodies, the intermediary products of fat metabolism, accumulate in the blood. During fasting, minimal amounts of glucose supplied from gluconeogenesis allow for the complete oxidation of small numbers of fatty acids for energy. Some of this glucose, along with some ketones, can be used as energy by the brain. But the general accumulation of ketones in the blood can disrupt the body's acid-base balance in a condition called ketosis. If prolonged, this condition can be threatening to the athlete's health.

Although no immediate harm or permanent metabolic damage is seen in healthy individuals on a 1- or 2-day fast, fasting is apparently of no benefit, and may be detrimental, to athletic performance. Individuals who are fasting must ingest water and a vitamin-mineral supplement. In place of water, 600 kcal of carbohydrate (1.5 quarts orange juice or 1.25 quarts apple juice) will supply energy to minimize muscle breakdown and reduce chronic fatigue. Efforts to lose weight by fasting should be discouraged in all athletes, particularly young athletes. Weight lost by short-term fasting is typically water, which is regained quickly with refeeding, and the resulting hypoglycemia and fatigue are a detriment to the fasting athlete.

▶ FRUCTOSE

The monosaccharide fructose is an isomer of glucose. It occurs naturally in many fruits and makes up 40% of honey. Fructose is absorbed more quickly than glucose, and unlike glucose, fructose does not require insulin for cellular absorption.[49] Hence, fructose consumption prior to exercise does not promote hypoglycemia.[50] Because fructose does not promote insulin secretion, it does not inhibit the circulation of free fatty acids, and its ingestion *may* enhance free fatty acid utilization. Furthermore, fructose has been shown to promote a muscle glycogen-sparing effect during the early stages of exercise.[51]

A significant negative effect of fructose ingestion is its tendency to cause gastrointestinal distress and osmotic diarrhea. Fructose may also increase blood lactate levels.[49] These effects can clearly impair athletic performance, and are contraindications for the use of fructose prior to competition, or as a sole carbohydrate source in sports drinks.

REFERENCES

1. Casal DC, Leon AS. Failure of caffeine to affect substrate utilization during prolonged running. *Med Sci Sports Exerc.* 1985;17:174-179.
2. Costill D, Dalsky G, Fink W. Effects of caffeine ingestion on metabolism and exercise performance. *Med Sci Sports Exerc.* 1978;10:155-158.
3. Tarnopolsky M, Atkinson S, MacDougall JD, Sale D, Sutton J. Physiological responses to caffeine during endurance running in habitual caffeine users. *Med Sci Sports Exerc.* 1989;21:418-424.
4. Stephenson P. Physiologic and psychotropic effects of caffeine in man. *J Am Diet Assoc.* 1977;71:240-247.
5. Partin N. Effects of caffeine on athletes. *Athletic Training.* 1988;23:286.
6. Weir J, Noakes TD, Myburgh K, Adams B. A high-carbohydrate diet negates the metabolic effects of caffeine during exercise. *Med Sci Sports Exerc.* 1987;19:100-105.
7. Costill D. Sport nutrition—past, present, and future. Opening address at the Exceed Sport Nutrition Conference; March 7, 1991; Columbus, Ohio.
8. Slavin J, Joensen D. Caffeine and sports performance. *Phys Sports Med.* 1985;13:193.
9. Price K, Weil E. How much caffeine is too much in athletes? *Am J Hosp Pharm.* 1990;47:303. Letter.
10. Rode A, Shephard R. The influence of cigarette smoking upon the oxygen cost of breathing in near-maximal exercise. *Med Sci Sports Exerc.* 1971;3:51.
11. Weltman A, Stamford B. Exercise and the cigarette smoker. *Phys Sports Med.* 1982;10:153.
12. Wright J, Marks V. The effects of alcohol on carbohydrate metabolism. *Contemp Issues Clin Biochem.* 1984;1:135-148.
13. Shelmet JJ, Reichard GA, Skutches CL, et al. Ethanol causes acute inhibition of carbohydrate, fat, and protein oxidation and insulin resistance. *J Clin Invest.* 1988;81:1137-1145.
14. Preedy VR, Peters TJ. Acute effects of ethanol on protein synthesis in different muscles and muscle protein fractions of the rat. *Clin Sci.* 1988;74:461-466.

15. Lieber C. To drink (moderately) or not to drink? *N Engl J Med.* 1984;310:846.
16. Johnson WD. Steroids: a problem of huge dimensions. *Sports Illustrated.* 1985;62:38.
17. Cowart V. Issues of drugs and sports gain attention as Olympic Games open in South Korea. *JAMA.* 1988;260:1513-1518.
18. Pope HG, Katz DL, Champoux R. Anabolic-androgenic steroid use among 1,010 college men. *Phys Sports Med.* 1988;16:75-81.
19. Buckley WE, Yesalis CE, Friedl KE, Anderson WA, Streit AL, Wright JE. Estimated prevalence of anabolic steroid use among male high school seniors. *JAMA.* 1988;260:3441-3445.
20. Salva PS, Bacon GE. Anabolic steroids and growth hormone in the Texas Panhandle. *Tex Med.* 1989;85:43-44.
21. Hershberger JG, Shipley EG, Meyer RK. Myotrophic activity of 19-nortestosterone and other steroids determined by modified levator ani muscle method. *Proc Soc Exp Biol Med.* 1953;83:175-180.
22. Council on Scientific Affairs. Drug abuse in athletes: anabolic steroids and growth hormone. *JAMA.* 1988;259:1703-1705.
23. Haupt HA, Rovere GD. Anabolic steroids: a review of the literature. *Am J Sports Med.* 1984;12:469-484.
24. American College of Sports Medicine. Position stand on the use of anabolic-androgenic steroids in sports. *Med Sci Sports Exerc.* 1987;19:534-539.
25. Kleiner SM. Performance-enhancing aids in sport: health consequences and nutritional alternatives. *J Am Coll Nutr.* 1991;10:163-176.
26. Pope GH, Katz DL. Affective and psychotic symptoms associated with anabolic steroid use. *Am J Psychiatry.* 1988;145:487-491.
27. Cowart V. Some predict increased steroid use in sports despite drug testing, crackdown on suppliers. *JAMA.* 1987;257:3025-3026.
28. Saartok T, Haggmark T. Human growth hormone: friend or foe in sports medicine? *Bull Hosp Jt Dis Orthop Inst.* 1988;48:159-163.
29. Jacobson BH. Effect of amino acids on growth hormone release. *Phys Sports Med.* 1991;18:63-70.
30. Bucci L, Hickson JF, Pivarnik JM, Wolinsky I, McMahon JC, Turner SD. Ornithine ingestion and growth hormone release in bodybuilders. *Nutr Res.* 1990;10:239-245.
31. Elam RP, Hardin DH, Sutton RAL, Hagen L. Effects of arginine and ornithine on strength, lean body mass, and urinary hydroxyproline in adult males. *J Sports Med Phys Fitness.* 1989;29:52-56.
32. Wadler GI, Hainline G. *Drugs and the Athlete.* Philadelphia, Pa: FA Davis Co; 1989.
33. Williams MG. *Ergogenic Aids in Sport.* Champaign, Ill: Human Kinetics Publishers; 1983.
34. McArdle WD, Katch FI, Katch VL. *Exercise Physiology: Energy, Nutrition, and Human Performance.* 2nd ed. Philadelphia, Pa: Lea & Febiger; 1986.
35. Williams MH, Wesseldine S, Sonna T, Schuster R. The effect of induced erythrocythemia upon five-mile treadmill run time. *Med Sci Sports Exerc.* 1981;13:169.
36. Gledhill N. Blood doping and related issues: a brief review. *Med Sci Sports Exerc.* 1982;14:183.
37. Williams MH. Blood doping in sports. *J Drug Issues.* 1980;3:331.
38. Klein HG. Sound board: blood transfusion and athletes. *New Engl J Med.* 1985;312:854.
39. Buick FJ, Gledhill N, Froese AB, Spriet L, Meyers EC. Effect of induced erythrocythemia on aerobic work capacity. *J Appl Physiol.* 1980;48:636.
40. Spriet L, Gledhill N, Froese AB, Wilkes DL, Meyers EC. The effect of induced erythrocythemia on central circulation and oxygen transport during maximal exercise. *Med Sci Sports Exerc.* 1980;12:122.
41. Horswill C, Costill D, Fink W, et al. Influence of sodium bicarbonate on sprint performance: relationship to dosage. *Med Sci Sports Exerc.* 1988;20:566.
42. Gao J, Costill D, Horswill C, Park S. Sodium bicarbonate ingestion improves performance in interval swimming. *Eur J Appl Physiol.* 1988;58:171-174.
43. Nash H. Soda loading: athletic aid or impediment? *Phys Sports Med.* 1985;13:28.
44. Wright D. Nutrition and exercise. In: Paige DM, ed. *Manual of Clinical Nutrition.* St. Louis, Mo: CV Mosby Co; 1988:713.

45. American College of Sports Medicine. *Position Stand : Weight Loss in Wrestlers.* Indianapolis, Ind: American College of Sports Medicine; 1976.

46. American Medical Association committee on the medical aspects of sports wrestling and weight control. *JAMA.* 1967;201:541.

47. Steen SN, Brownell KD. Patterns of weight loss and regain in wrestlers: has the tradition changed? *Med Sci Sports Exerc.* 1990;22:762-768.

48. Brownell KD, Steen SN, Wilmore JH. Weight regulation practices in athletes: analysis of metabolic and health effects. *Med Sci Sports Exerc.* 1987;19:546-556.

49. Allman FL, Ryan AJ, eds. *Sports Medicine.* 2nd ed. San Diego, Calif: Academic Press; 1989.

50. Costill D, Saltin B. Factors limiting gastric emptying during rest and exercise. *J Appl Physiol.* 1974;37:679.

51. Barnes WS, Hasson SM. Carbohydrate ingestion and exercise. *Sports Med.* 1989;8:327-334.

Nutrient and Quasi-nutrient Supplement Consumption

Julane Contursi, Susan Kleiner, and Jill Mielcarek

▶ PROTEINS AND AMINO ACIDS

In 1842 John Von Liebig stated that the primary fuel for muscular contraction was protein. Although this was disproved in the late 1800s, many of today's bodybuilders, weight lifters, football players, coaches, and endurance athletes tenaciously hold to this belief.

A survey of 171 college athletes revealed that 98% felt that performance is improved with a high-protein diet, and 80% indicated that large amounts of protein are necessary to increase muscle mass.[1] These percentages are probably representative of what many other athletes believe. A survey of 39 weight lifters and bodybuilders revealed that 59% consumed protein supplements; however, little information exists on the effect of additional protein on strength and muscle mass.[2]

What is the attraction of these amino acids, and why are these false beliefs so pervasive? The attraction is the relentless effort by the athlete to find that magical, mystical product that either adds muscle mass or improves endurance. The belief is pervasive among athletes, coaches, and teachers because of the convincing advertisements and quasiscientific articles presented in popular muscle and fitness magazines. Much of the information conveyed is based on scientific studies, but the results are frequently misinterpreted and overgeneralized. Incorrect extrapolations from animal studies to humans are also made.[3] All this creates the basis from which a number of supplements may be recommended.

The personal testimonials by champion athletes have a significant effect on the exercising public. The endorsements relay a message attributing the champion's physique or performance to a nutritional supplement.

Research Design Differences

Determining protein needs in athletes has been attempted by many researchers, but there still is no one definitive answer. Research designs differ in many ways as listed below; therefore, comparisons among studies may not be valid.

1. Collection of urinary or sweat urea nitrogen may be done at different training periods. A few days of sample collection after an activity may show greater nitrogen losses (and, hence, greater protein losses) than those studies where collections were done for a longer period.[4]

2. Some studies may have underestimated actual nitrogen losses due to the inability to measure or difficulty in measuring sweat urea nitrogen.
3. Because exercise decreases kidney function and the glomerular filtration rate (GFR), the greater levels of blood urea nitrogen measured may be due to the decreased clearance by the kidney.[5]
4. The exercise type, duration, and intensity affect fuel type and utilization.[6] A person exercising at a higher intensity or for a longer duration will have greater nitrogen losses than a person exercising less or for a shorter duration.
5. Diet affects protein use.[6] More protein will be used as a fuel by a person on a high-protein diet because of protein's greater availability.
6. Current fuel stores affect utilization. If glycogen storage is less than what is needed for the activity, then protein (from either diet or muscle) will be used, depending on what is available.
7. The fitness level of the individual determines the proportion of fuel utilization. A more fit individual is better able to use fat as an energy source and will, therefore, use less protein for energy than a less trained athlete.
8. The energy content is extremely important when determining protein needs, because nitrogen retention depends on adequate caloric intake. Some studies resulted in a negative nitrogen balance, but caloric intake was not a consideration.[7]

More research is necessary to determine conclusively whether chronic physical activity significantly alters daily requirements for protein.

Protein Needs of Athletes

Because physiologic and training factors affect protein needs, a range is given for both bodybuilders and endurance athletes. An important question regarding protein needs must be carefully phrased. If the question reads, "Does exercise increase protein needs above what we currently consume?" then the response will be different from the answer to this question: "Does exercise increase protein needs above the RDA of 0.8 g/kg body weight?" The answer to the second question is yes. Physical activity does seem to increase protein needs above the RDA for both endurance and strength-training activities. The current consensus of research yields a recommended range of 1 to 2 g protein per kilogram of body weight. Weight lifters may need 1.2 to 1.5 g protein per kilogram of body weight, while endurance athletes may need slightly more. These levels of protein are adequate when caloric intake is sufficient; however, if insufficient, then a higher proportion of protein to calories must be consumed to maintain a positive nitrogen balance.

Athletes in early stages of training may require up to 2 g (but rarely more than 1.5 g with a high-carbohydrate diet) protein per kilogram body weight to meet the increased synthesis of enzymes, myoglobin (oxygen-carrying protein specific to muscle only), hemoglobin, and the increased number of mitochondria that develop during the early training periods.[7] This amount equates to 140 g protein per day for a 70-kg athlete. This quantity is obtainable in 9 oz meat, chicken, fish, or cheese; 3 cups low-fat or skim milk; 2 cups vegetables; and 15 servings of bread or starchy foods (including pasta, rice, cereals, and bread). The average American consumes about 100 g protein per day, and athletes are usually greater consumers of protein than the average American. This is probably the one nutrient athletes need to worry the least about.

A study looking at the effects of diet on muscle and strength gains during resistance training[8] indicated that a hypercaloric 65% carbohydrate diet increased more lean body mass than a hypercaloric 40% carbohydrate diet. Thus, although protein may be a focus for many athletes, consuming adequate carbohydrate may be a more important issue for these reasons:

1. Carbohydrate is the primary fuel used in anaerobic activity and, up until a certain point, in aerobic activity.
2. A hypercaloric high-carbohydrate diet (60% to 65+%) appears to result in a smaller gain in body fat than a hypercaloric, low-carbohydrate diet (40%).[8]
3. Carbohydrate consumption elicits an insulin response, the hormone that facilitates the transport of glucose and amino acid into the working muscle cell, thereby increasing protein synthesis and decreasing protein degradation.[8]

The ingestion of a high-carbohydrate diet, along with increased muscle contractile activity (which increases amino acid uptake by the muscle in itself), exerts a synergistic anabolic effect on lean body mass development.[8]

Although muscle contains protein, approximately 20% of it is protein, 70% of it is water, and 8% of it is lipid. This translates into an additional 100 g protein per week in the diet to add 1 lb muscle per week.[7] This is only 14 g protein per day, which is obtainable in 2 oz meat, chicken, fish, or cheese or 2 cups low-fat or skim milk. *Extra protein is not preferentially laid down as muscle mass.* Instead, extra protein will be:

▶ used as an energy source if calories or carbohydrates are inadequate,
▶ stored as fat if protein is in excess of caloric needs, or
▶ used for its primary and structural roles (formation of tissues, hormone and antibody formation, maintenance of water and acid-base balance, and control of blood-clotting processes).[7]

Amino Acid Supplements

A number of free-form amino acids are on the market promising very specific results. Two on the market, arginine and ornithine, are popular because of their relationship to growth hormones. The claims are that, if these are taken alone or in combination with other amino acids, muscle development, increased fat loss, and decreased glycogen use will occur. Amino acids are related to growth hormone release, but the amounts necessary to stimulate growth hormone release above normal levels is extremely high and potentially dangerous. In fact, a physician may inject arginine into a patient and then measure growth hormone levels in the body to determine if production is normal or not. However, the amount injected is much greater than that contained in the supplement, and it is injected, not swallowed.[3]

Studies that have been performed on children suggest that ornithine produces a greater secretion of human growth hormone (hGH). Once past adolescence, the response of hGH to ornithine and other stimuli is much less.[9]

Branched chain amino acids (BCAA)—leucine, valine, and isoleucine—are popular based on the fact that they are oxidized to a higher degree than other amino acids. They are able to give up their amino group readily through transamination to form alanine, which is converted to glucose in the liver, where it is used as an energy source (Cori cycle).[7] Leucine oxidation, especially, is increased in aerobic activity, and the magnitude of this increased oxidation is contingent on exercise intensity and duration, fitness level, and training level. It is not known, though, whether this increased oxidation is due to an increased protein degradation (muscle breakdown), decreased protein synthesis, or both.[4]

▶ VITAMINS AND MINERALS

For a vitamin to be classified as such, a lack of it for a prolonged period must cause a specific deficiency disease that is cured when the compound is reintroduced.[10-13] Because of the intricate role that vitamins and minerals play in energy metabolism, the promises made by the manufacturers are embraced by those who use them in hopes of improved energy levels. A number of special metabolic functions require vitamins, such as the oxidation of metabolic fuels (carbohydrates, fat, and protein) to produce energy. Vitamins are essential for optimal functioning of many physiologic processes; therefore, many athletes have concluded that levels greater than the standard are a necessity for optimal performance. Approximately 23% of the US population regularly uses vitamin and mineral supplements, even though the actual benefit of taking them for persons on balanced diets is doubtful.[14] It is likely that an even higher proportion of athletes regularly consumes supplements, also with dubious outcomes.

B-complex Vitamins

B-complex vitamins include those involved in energy production from carbohydrates and fats (thiamin, riboflavin, niacin, pantothenic acid, and biotin), and those involved in erythrocyte formation (pyridoxine, folacin, and B_{12}).[15] The rationale behind the use of B vitamins is related to their physiologic role, and the fact that a prolonged deficiency of some of the B vitamins may result in a deterioration of endurance. Supplementing a diet lacking several B vitamins generally does result in improved performance; however, an athlete who obtains adequate amounts of the B vitamins will not improve endurance or increase energy levels when supplementing the B-complex vitamins. An exception to this may be riboflavin (B_2).

Riboflavin may be required in greater amounts than the RDAs for active people.[16] Riboflavin is involved in forming an enzyme (glutathione reductase) that protects hemoglobin. If hemoglobin is destroyed, as happens with insufficient riboflavin, oxygen-carrying capacity is reduced with a resultant drop in endurance. The results of one study indicate that individuals' need for riboflavin may be nearly double the RDA (ie, a level of 1 to 1.2 mg/1000 kcal may be required vs the RDA of 0.6 mg/1000 kcal).[7] No toxicity has been reported with high dosages of this vitamin.

Niacin

The popularity of this vitamin stems from its vasodilator effect,[15] which allows more oxygen to be delivered to the working muscles and tissues. However, large doses given prior to exercise have not shown any benefit. Niacin participates in many metabolic processes, including glycolysis, fat synthesis, hormone synthesis, and tissue respiration.

The two forms of niacin are nicotinic acid and nicotinamide. Nicotinamide functions in the body as a component of two important coenzymes, nicotinamide adenine dinucleotide (NAD) and nicotinamide adenine dinucleotide phosphate (NADP). Both enzymes are involved in oxidation-reduction reactions. Ingestion of large doses of nicotinic acid could increase glycogen utilization, decrease serum lipids, and decrease fatty acid mobilization from adipose tissue during exercise,[15] all of which adversely affect endurance performance. A greater glycogen utilization is undesirable because of its limited storage and high utilization rate in most sports. Additionally, a greater rate of glycogen utilization yields higher levels of lactic acid, which is an inhibitor of lipolysis, to further contribute to a diminution in performance.

The minimum toxic dose is 1000 mg (about 50 times the RDA).[17] Evidence shows that nicotinic acid greater than 500 mg may be harmful but that niacinamide (the biologically active form) may be reasonably safe (but unnecessary) up to 400 mg.[10-13] Potential toxic reactions and side effects include flushing, nausea, vomiting, diarrhea, skin rash, duodenal ulcers, pruritus, tachycardia, hypotension, hyperglycemia, hyperuricemia, and liver damage.[10-13,18]

Pyridoxine (B$_6$)

The claim that vitamin B$_6$ increases an athlete's energy level probably relates to the vitamin's physiologic role: glycogen utilization, amino acid metabolism, and formation of porphyrin.[7] Theoretically, a pyridoxine deficiency could decrease glycogen utilization as an energy source and decrease hemoglobin formation, both decreasing endurance by delivering less oxygen to the muscles and tissues. It may also be argued that a high-protein diet increases vitamin need, because of its relationship to amino acid metabolism. However, a deficiency with a high protein intake is unlikely because foods high in protein (not generally inadequate in the US diet) are also high in this vitamin. Good food sources of vitamin B$_6$ include meats, whole-grain cereals, bananas, potatoes, and lima beans. The minimum toxic dose is 2000 mg, which is about 900 times the RDA.[17] Potential side effects are nerve and liver damage and a dependency on high dosages.[10-13]

Vitamin E

The perceived benefit of vitamin E supplementation is derived from the effects that a supplement has on a person deficient in vitamin E. In a vitamin E–deficiency state, less ATP is produced for each molecule of oxygen consumed, and oxidation of cell membranes and red blood cells may occur. One of the theoretical benefits of vitamin E supplementation is the reduction of the amount of oxygen used during activity. In human adults, however, deficiency is rare because of the vitamin's presence in seeds, green leafy vegetables, margarines, shortenings, vegetable oils, and whole-grain breads and cereals.

The minimum toxic dose of vitamin E is 1200 IU, a level that is 40 times the RDA.[17] The tolerance level of vitamin E by humans varies widely. The vitamin is mostly harmless in large doses, but flulike symptoms may develop in individuals taking more than 400 IU daily for prolonged periods. Nausea, diarrhea, vomiting, pruritus, headache, fatigue, muscle weakness, prolonged clotting time, increased triglycerides, increased cholesterol, and reduced thyroid hormone are other possible side effects with dosages of 400 to 1600 IU/day.[10-13] Vitamin E can also interfere with vitamin K metabolism and blood coagulation, and with vitamin A metabolism.[19]

Iron

The claim for this micronutrient, improved performance, is associated with its actual role: iron is a component of hemoglobin, the red-pigmented protein responsible for carrying oxygen and carbon dioxide to and from the body's tissues. Iron deficiency does impair performance by decreasing aerobic capacity, and an iron-deficient athlete will benefit from supplementation. However, extra iron when hemoglobin levels are normal (13.5 to 18 g/dL for men; 12 to 16 g/dL for women) appears to have little or no effect on performance levels.[15]

Iron absorption in normal, healthy humans is regulated precisely so the possibility of toxicity from food intake is unlikely. A disorder called hemochromatosis may occur, in which iron deposits in the liver, pancreas, and heart because the normal controls that prevent excess absorption do not work properly. However, this disorder is rare.[10-13] The minimum toxic dose is 100 mg, or 5.5 times the RDA.[17]

▶ WHEAT GERM, WHEAT GERM OIL, AND OCTACOSANOL

Wheat germ and wheat germ oil are rich sources of vitamin E. These purported ergogenic aids also contain calcium, copper, manganese, magnesium, and substantial amounts of B vitamins.[20] The active incredient is believed to be octacosanol.[21]

Claims for wheat germ oil include increased physical stamina and performance. Even though some investigations have shown improvement in conditioned reflexes with wheat germ oil or octacosanol supplementation, a consensus of research results indicates that wheat germ oil probably does not improve endurance capacity.[21] There are no known adverse reactions or side effects from wheat germ or wheat germ oil ingestion.

▶ BREWER'S YEAST

Brewer's yeast (also called nutritional yeast) is a rich source of the B vitamins (except for vitamin B_{12}). Brewer's yeast may also contain protein and some trace minerals.[22] Brewer's yeast supplementation has been claimed to decrease constipation, treat diabetes mellitus, lower cholesterol, and enhance athletic performance. There is no scientific evidence to support these claims. Possible side effects from ingestion of brewer's yeast include nausea and diarrhea.

▶ BEE POLLEN

Bee pollen has been reported to cure a multitude of diseases, as well as enhance athletic performance. The reports and observations proclaiming the ergogenic properties of bee pollen have been anecdotal. The product sold as bee pollen is actually a mixture of bee saliva, plant nectar, and pollen, and is generally a loose powder compressed into tablets or capsules of 400 to 500 mg with or without other nutritional supplements. The protein content averages 20%, but ranges from 10% to 36%, with a measurable essential amino acid content. Ten percent to 15% of the content is simple sugars, and it contains small quantities of fats and significant amounts of minerals.[22]

According to a review by Hickson and Wolinsky,[21] the effects of bee pollen on human athletic performance are unclear. European studies tend to find benefits from bee pollen supplementation, but American studies find no benefit. Study protocols are inconsistent, and most studies use pure sources of pollen extract from a single manufacturer, unlike that available to the average consumer.

Adverse side effects from bee pollen supplementation have been reported. Allergic reactions are the most commonly reported, with anaphylactic reactions a documented possibility. Due to its content of nucleic acids, bee pollen should be avoided by those predisposed to gout or with signs of renal disease.[21,22]

▶ PANGAMIC ACID

Pangamic acid, also known as "pangamate" and "vitamin B_{15}" (although it should not appropriately be considered a vitamin), has been extolled as an ergogenic aid for athletes. Originally, pangamic acid was composed of a mixture of calcium gluconate and N,N-dimethylglycine in a 60-40 ratio.[23] However, it appears that products that sell under the name "pangamic acid" are made of an inconsistent array of compounds.[24]

In theory, pangamic acid functions as an aid to aerobic endurance by enhancing oxidative metabolism. This action is said to occur by an increase in oxygen utilization through an increase in the muscular content of creatine phosphate and glycogen.[7] However, the proposed action has not been supported by studies investigating the effects of pangamic acid supplementation on $\dot{V}O_2$max and athletic endurance.[7,25,26] The lack of effectiveness of this substance, plus the finding that several compounds marketed under the label of "pangamic acid" are potentially hazardous,[7] should be sufficient to discourage its use by athletes seeking a substance with ergogenic potential.

▶ CARNITINE

The ergogenic claims for carnitine supplementation include:

- ▶ Increased aerobic power
- ▶ Increased energy levels
- ▶ More intense workouts
- ▶ Reduction in body fat

These claims are closely tied to carnitine's actual function. It is part of the shuttle mechanism that transports long-chain fatty acids across the mitochondrial membrane where beta-oxidation of fats occurs.[27] The claim makes sense based on the substance's physiologic role, but humans synthesize adequate carnitine with two essential amino acids—lysine and methionine.[27] Carnitine is also prevalent in animal foods, so a deficiency is highly unlikely. Infants, especially preterm infants, may lack sufficient carnitine synthesis, but they do not seem to run the risk of a deficiency because carnitine is plentiful in human milk and cow's milk and it is fortified in soy-based formulas.

▶ CHROMIUM PICOLINATE

Chromium picolinate is advertised to increase glucose tolerance and stabilize blood sugar levels in athletes. Chromium is an essential element for the normal functioning of human carbohydrate, lipid, and nucleic acid metabolism. Many sources of dietary chromium are biologically unavailable. Picolinic acid, a metabolite of tryptophan, forms a stable complex with chromium, possibly improving its bioavailability.[28]

Chromium's role in carbohydrate and lipid metabolism is related to insulin. Chromium potentiates the action of insulin, and less insulin is required if sufficient chromium, in a usable form, is present. Chromium deficiency results in impaired glucose tolerance, decreased insulin receptor number, increased serum triglyceride and cholesterol levels, decreased HDL cholesterol levels, and increased incidence of atherosclerotic disease.[29,30]

Strenuous exercise stimulates urinary chromium losses, and research studies indicate that chromium status of exercising individuals may be compromised, particularly if their dietary chromium intakes are marginal.[30] Poor chromium status could result in diminished athletic performance due to the impairment of carbohydrate and fat metabolism. In such cases, adding good sources of chromium to the diet, and using a biologically available supplement, could return physical performance parameters to predeficiency levels. However, if chromium status is normal, there are no scientific data that indicate chromium supplementation will improve physical performance. Good sources of dietary chromium include mushrooms, oysters, and apples with skins. Poor sources of chromium include highly processed or refined foods, such as sugar and white flour. Carbohydrate loading with refined carbohydrates not only results in a chromium-poor diet, but highly refined carbohydrates also stimulate chromium losses. Carbohydrate loading should be done with unrefined carbohydrates, such as whole grains and cereals, legumes, and starchy vegetables.[30]

► LECITHIN

Lecithin is a phospholipid similar in structure to a triglyceride, except the third fatty acid is replaced with choline and includes phosphorous and nitrogen. The advertising claim for lecithin is that it dissolves cholesterol deposits in arteries and prevents or cures arthritis, gallstones, nervous disorders, and skin problems. Taking supplemental lecithin seems to be of no nutritional significance because humans are capable of synthesizing it, and synthetic lecithin is not well absorbed.[31]

Some have confirmed the benefits of lecithin in decreasing triglyceride and cholesterol levels while others have not. Because supplemental lecithin or choline may increase levels of a neurotransmitter (acetylcholine), it may be of some benefit to patients with tardine dyskinesia and Alzheimer's disease.

► HERBS

Hundreds of herbal preparations are available to consumers, all with manufacturers' claims that are, for the most part, scientifically unsubstantiated. Many of the claims are based on historical anecdote or cultural myths, where herbs have been used for centuries as medicines and remedies. Many herbs are potent medications and many of our modern-day medicines were originally derived from herbal extracts. However, the common notion that because herbs are natural, they are also safe, is a dangerous misconception. Manufacturers of herbal teas do not submit their products to the Food and Drug Administration for product safety or quality control regulation. Animal studies are not required for a determination of their safety. If allergic reactions can occur from medicines tested under strict safeguards, it is likely that herbal substances that have not been tested, and which are consumed in large amounts, may also produce allergic reactions. This concern is a reality, sometimes occurring with fatal results.

This section lists some of the most popular herbs used by athletes. Unless otherwise noted, the information was drawn from *The New Honest Herbal* by V. E. Tyler.[32]

Buchu. Dried leaves of three species of the genus *Barosma*, usually sold in tea form; possesses mild diuretic and antiseptic properties. Safe for human use.

Burdock. Dried first-year root of *Arctium Lappa L.* or *Arctium minus (Hill) Bern.* Usually sold in dried tea form. Recommended primarily as blood purifier; used in treatment of psoriasis and acne; also said to have diuretic and diaphoretic properties. None of these effects has been verified by clinical trials, and no solid evidence exists that burdock exhibits any useful therapeutic activity. Burdock appears to be safe, but there have been reports of teas contaminated with belladonna root that have caused poisonings.

Canaigre. The root of *Rumex hymenosepalus Torr.* has been recently marketed as wild red American ginseng, and wild red desert ginseng. This plant, native to the southwestern United States and to Mexico, is absolutely unrelated to ginseng, either botanically or in its active properties. It is deceptively promoted as a less-expensive American alternative to bona fide ginseng, and is recommended for maladies ranging from lack of vitality to leprosy. Conaigre does not contain any of the active constituents found in ginseng, and is more useful for tanning leather and dyeing wool than therapeutics. Due to its high tannin content, it may be carcinogenic, and should be avoided.

Damiana. From the leaves of the Mexican shrub *Turnera diffusa Willd. var. aphrodisiaca Urb.* Touted as a powerful aphrodisiac, any physiologic activity in various preparations marketed in the late 1800s and early 1900s was actually due to the presence of other drugs. On the basis of scientific investigations, the herb contains no aphrodisiac activity or any beneficial physiologic activity.

Fo-ti. The dried tuberous root of *Polygonaceae.* The Chinese believe that the root exhibits different properties depending on the size and age of the plant. A 200-year-old root is believed to preserve youth and energy. The only real action of fo-ti is as an effective cathartic and laxative, and it is probably safe for human use.

Garlic and other alliums. Garlic, onion, leek, and shallot all belong to the genus *Allium.* Bulbs and occasionally leaves are used as food and medicines. There is both animal and preliminary human research supporting the efficacy of their use in the treatment of atherosclerosis, high blood pressure, and gastrointestinal ailments. The herbs are safe for human use, although preparation and amount may alter their potency and therapeutic effects.

Ginseng and related drugs. Following American authorities, the designation *Panax pseudoginseng Wallich* designates the Oriental species. The native American species is *Panax quinquefolius L.* Ginseng is claimed to be a cure-all or panacea; also an aphrodisiac, and an adaptogen (producer of a state of increased resistance to body stress). Some favorable effects by ginseng on stress have been recorded. Studies with human subjects have failed to find ergogenic effects from ginseng root preparations.[21] There is no evidence supporting claims of enhanced sexual experience or potency. Obtaining authentic ginseng may be difficult. High-quality root is expensive; the best grades cost more than $20 per ounce. This high cost yields a lack of quality control, and many so-called ginseng products (teas, powders, capsules, extracts, tablets) are of variable quality and content. The safety of ginseng consumption is questionable. High intakes and long-term consumption can cause harmful side effects, including high blood pressure, nervousness, sleeplessness, low blood pressure, tranquilizing effects, corticosteroid poisoning–like effects, painful breasts, breast nodules, and vaginal bleeding. Due to safety concerns and difficulty in obtaining pure products, few clinical studies on the effects of ginseng have been conducted. Its reported actions and efficacy remain unsubstantiated.

Gotu kola.   Leaves from *Centella asiatic (L.) Urb.* Purported to promote longevity and act as an aphrodisiac. No current evidence exists to support these claims. The safety of this herb for human consumption is inconclusive.

Guarana.   A dried paste made chiefly from the crushed seed of *Paullinia cupana H.B.K.* Marketed as an ergogenic aid, it contains a high caffeine content, ranging from 2.5% to 5%, and averaging about 3.5%.

Maté.   The dried leaves of *Ilex paraguariensis St. Hill.* Promoted as an ergogenic aid, it contains up to 2% caffeine, and is often found as maté tea or Paraguay tea.

Pau d'arco.   Bark of various species of *Tabebuia*, usually found as a tea. Marketed as a cancer cure, a "powerful tonic and bodybuilder" effective against a multitude of diseases. The bark contains 2% to 7% of a napthopuinone derivative known as lapachol, which, if given in effective doses, produces intolerable side effects. The therapeutic effectiveness of pau d'arco is unproved, and the drug is potentially toxic.

Sassafras.   Root bark from the *Sassafras albidum* tree; usually found as a tea. Promoted as a stimulant, antispasmodic, sweat producer, purifier, and as a treatment for several diseases and conditions. No claims have been supported or documented in modern medical literature. More important, sassafras contains a highly carcinogenic constituent, safrole, as well as other unidentified cancer-causing agents. Both sassafras oil and safrole were prohibited by the FDA from use as flavors or food additives in the early 1960s. Because of the drug's harmful properties, sassafras should be avoided.

Saw palmetto.   Ripe or dried berries of *Serenoa repens*, a fan palm; usually found as a tea. Once used medically as a mild diuretic, it is presently marketed as a substance that increases the size of underdeveloped female breasts, builds sexual vigor, increases sperm production, reverses atrophy of testes and mammary glands, and relieves catarrhal soreness of the genitourinary system. When administered by injection into immature female mice, some small estrogenic activity was exhibited. However, when taken orally, it is poorly dissolved in water and poorly absorbed intestinally. It exhibits no influence on mammary glands or any therapeutic characteristics.

▶ Conclusion

Top performance cannot be achieved through pills, powders, drinks, or injections but only through a rigorous training schedule, sufficient energy needs provided from a variety of foods composed mainly of complex carbohydrates, and adequate fluid. The micronutrient requirements will then be met without all the complicated and expensive combining of quasifoods and supplements.

REFERENCES

1. Grandjean AC. Current nutrition beliefs and practices in athletics for weight/strength gains. In: *Report of the Ross Symposium on Muscle Development: Nutritional Alternatives to Anabolic Steroids.* Columbus, Ohio: Ross Laboratories; 1988.

2. Meredith CN. Protein needs and protein supplements in strength-trained men. In: *Report of the Ross Symposium on Muscle Development: Nutritional Alternatives to Anabolic Steroids.* Columbus, Ohio: Ross Laboratories; 1988.

3. Meister KA. Growth hormone releasers: amino acid magic? *News and Views Newsletter.* March/April 1985:6(2):12-13.

4. Dohm GL. Protein as a fuel for endurance exercise. *Exerc Sport Sci Rev.* 1986;14.

5. Goodman MN. Amino acid and protein metabolism. In: *Exercise, Nutrition and Energy Metabolism.* New York, NY: Macmillan Publishing Co; 1988.

6. Evans WJ, Fisher EC, Hoerr RA, Young VR. Protein metabolism and endurance exercise. *Phys Sports Med.* July 1983;11:7.

7. Williams MH. The role of protein in physical activity. In: *Nutritional Aspects of Human Physical and Athletic Performance.* Springfield, Ill: Charles Thomas Publishers; 1985.

8. Rinehfardt KF. Effects of diet on muscle and strength gains during resistive training. In: *Report of the Ross Symposium on Muscle Development: Nutritional Alternatives to Anabolic Steroids.* Columbus, Ohio: Ross Laboratories; 1988.

9. Lemon PWR, Chaney MM. Physiologic effects of amino acid supplementation. In: *Report of the Ross Symposium on Muscle Development: Nutritional Alternatives to Anabolic Steroids.* Columbus, Ohio: Ross Laboratories; 1988.

10. Marshall CW. B vitamins can help or harm. In: *Vitamins and Minerals. . .Help or Harm?* Philadelphia, Pa: George F Stickley Co; 1986.

11. Marshall CW. Iron, iodine, fluorine, and other microminerals. In: *Vitamins and Minerals. . .Help or Harm?* Philadelphia, Pa: George F Stickley Co; 1986.

12. Marshall CW. Vitamin E can help or harm. In: *Vitamins and Minerals. . .Help or Harm?* Philadelphia, Pa: George F Stickley Co; 1986.

13. Marshall CW. What is a vitamin? In: *Vitamins and Minerals. . .Help or Harm?* Philadelphia, Pa: George F Stickley Co; 1986.

14. Combs GF. *The Vitamins: Fundamental Aspects in Nutrition and Health.* San Diego, Calif: Academic Press; 1992.

15. Haymes EM. Proteins, vitamins, and iron. In: *Ergogenic Aids in Sport.* Champaign, Ill: Human Kinetics Publishers; 1983.

16. Belko A. Vitamins and exercise—an update. *Med Sci Sports Exerc.* 1987;19:S191-S196.

17. Hathcock JN. Quantitative evaluation of vitamin safety. *Pharm Times.* May 1985.

18. Dubick M. Dietary supplements and health aids: a critical evaluation. III. Natural and miscellaneous products. *J Nutr Ed.* 1983;15:4.

19. Dubick M, Rucker RB. Dietary supplements and health aids: a critical evaluation. I. Vitamins and minerals. *J Nutr Ed.* 1983;15:2.

20. Williams MH. *Ergogenic Aids in Sports.* Champaign, Ill: Human Kinetics Publishers; 1983.

21. Hickson JF, Wolinsky I. *Nutrition in Exercise and Sport.* Boca Raton, Fla: CRC Press, Inc; 1989:147-148.

22. Peterson M, Peterson K. *Eat to Compete: A Guide to Sports Nutrition.* Chicago, Ill: Year Book Medical Publishers, Inc; 1988:84-86.

23. McArdle WD, Katch FI, Katch VL. *Exercise Physiology: Energy, Nutrition, and Human Performance.* 2nd ed. Philadelphia, Pa: Lea & Febiger; 1986.

24. Berning JR, Steen SN. *Sports Nutrition for the 90s: The Health Professional's Handbook.* Gaithersburg, Md: Aspen Publishers Inc; 1991.

25. Check W. Vitamin B_{15}—whatever it is, it won't help. *JAMA.* 1980;243:2473-2480.

26. Gray M, Titlow L. B_{15}: myth or miracle? *Phys Sports Med.* 1982;10:107-112.

27. Ensminger ME, et al, eds. *Foods and Nutrition Encyclopedia.* Clovis, Calif: Pegus Press; 1983.

28. Press RI, Geller J, Evans GW. The effect of chromium picolinate in serum cholesterol and apolipoprotein fractions in human subjects. *West J Med.* 1990;152:41-45.

29. Offenbacher EG, Pi-Sunyer FX. Chromium in human nutrition. *Annu Rev Nutr.* 1988;8:543-563.
30. Anderson RA, Guttman HN. Trace minerals and exercise. In: Horton ES, Terjung RL, eds: *Exercise, Nutrition, and Metabolism.* New York, NY: Macmillan Publishing Co; 1988:188-190.
31. News America Syndicate. *The Health Letter.* Irvine, Calif; July 1986.
32. Tyler VE. *The New Honest Herbal: A Sensible Guide to the Use of Herbs and Related Remedies.* Philadelphia, Pa: George F Stickley Co; 1987.

SECTION

VI

Appendix

251

Appendix 1
Energy Distribution in Foods*

Description	Serving Size	kcal	CHO % kcal†	Pro % kcal†	Fat % kcal†
Apple juice, canned	1 cup	116	100	0	0
Apples, raw, peeled, sliced	1 cup	64	100	0	0
Apples, raw, unpeeled, 3/lb	1	84	100	0	0
Applesauce, canned, sweetened	1 cup	204	100	0	0
Applesauce, canned, unsweetened	1 cup	112	100	0	0
Apricots, canned, heavy syrup	3 halves	72	100	0	0
Barbecue sauce	1 tbsp	8	100	0	0
Catsup	1 tbsp	16	100	0	0
Celery, raw, stalk	1 stalk	4	100	0	0
Coffee, instant, prepared	6 fl oz	4	100	0	0
Cola, regular	12 fl oz	164	100	0	0
Cranberry juice cocktail	1 cup	152	100	0	0
Cucumber, with peel	6 slices	4	100	0	0
Fondant, uncoated	1 oz	108	100	0	0
Fruit punch drink, canned	6 fl oz	88	100	0	0
Ginger ale	12 fl oz	128	100	0	0
Grape drink, canned	6 fl oz	104	100	0	0
Grape soda	12 fl oz	184	100	0	0
Grape juice, frozen, diluted	1 cup	128	100	0	0
Grapes, raw, Thompson	10	36	100	0	0
Gumdrops	1 oz	100	100	0	0
Hard candy	1 oz	112	100	0	0
Honey	1 tbsp	68	100	0	0
Imitation whipped topping, from powder	1 tbsp	4	100	0	0
Italian salad dressing, diet	1 tbsp	8	100	0	0
Jams, jellies, and preserves	1 tbsp	56	100	0	0
Jelly beans	1 oz	104	100	0	0
Lemon juice, canned	1 tbsp	4	100	0	0
Lemon-lime soda	12 fl oz	156	100	0	0
Lemonade, frozen, diluted	6 fl oz	84	100	0	0
Limeade, frozen, diluted	6 fl oz	80	100	0	0
Molasses, cane, blackstrap	2 tbsp	88	100	0	0
Orange soda	12 fl oz	184	100	0	0
Parsley, raw	10 sprigs	4	100	0	0
Peaches, canned, heavy syrup	½	64	100	0	0
Peaches, canned, juice pack	½	36	100	0	0
Pears, canned, heavy syrup	½	60	100	0	0
Pears, canned, juice pack	½	40	100	0	0
Pepper-type soda	12 fl oz	164	100	0	0
Peppers, sweet, cooked	1	12	100	0	0
Pickles, cucumber, dill	1	4	100	0	0
Pickles, cucumber, sweet gherkin	1	20	100	0	0
Pineapple, canned, heavy syrup	1 slice	48	100	0	0
Pineapple, canned, juice pack	1 slice	36	100	0	0
Pineapple-grapefruit juice drink	6 fl oz	92	100	0	0
Plums, canned, heavy syrup	3	124	100	0	0
Plums, canned, juice pack	3	56	100	0	0
Plums, raw, 1½-in diameter	1	16	100	0	0

* Organized from highest to lowest in carbohydrate as a percentage of total calories.

† Percentages may not add up to exactly 100 due to rounding.

Description	Serving Size	kcal	CHO % kcal†	Pro % kcal†	Fat % kcal†
Popsicle	1	72	100	0	0
Pretzels, stick	10	108	100	0	0
Radishes, raw	4	4	100	0	0
Raisins	0.5 oz	44	100	0	0
Relish, sweet	1 tbsp	20	100	0	0
Root beer	12 fl oz	168	100	0	0
Seaweed, kelp, raw	1 oz	12	100	0	0
Sugar, white, granulated	1 tbsp	48	100	0	0
Table syrup (corn and maple)	2 tbsp	128	100	0	0
Tea, from instant, unsweetened	8 fl oz	4	100	0	0
Tea, from instant, sweetened	8 fl oz	88	100	0	0
Vinegar, cider	1 tbsp	4	100	0	0
Rhubarb, cooked, with sugar	1 cup	304	99	1	0
Strawberries, frozen, sweetened	1 cup	268	99	1	0
Blueberries, frozen, sweetened	1 cup	204	98	2	0
Fruit cocktail, canned, heavy syrup	1 cup	196	98	2	0
Plantains, cooked	1 cup	196	98	2	0
Apples, dried, sulfured	10 rings	172	98	2	0
Tangerines, canned, light syrup	1 cup	168	98	2	0
Grapefruit, canned, syrup pack	1 cup	160	98	2	0
Grape juice, canned	1 cup	156	97	3	0
Apricot nectar	1 cup	148	97	3	0
Pineapple juice, canned	1 cup	140	97	3	0
Raspberries, frozen, sweetened	1 cup	268	97	3	0
Prunes, dried	5 large	128	97	3	0
Dates	10	252	97	3	0
Peaches, frozen, sweetened	1 cup	248	97	3	0
Prunes, dried, cooked, unsweetened	1 cup	248	97	3	0
Fruit cocktail, canned, juice pack	1 cup	120	97	3	0
Grapefruit juice, canned, sweetened	1 cup	116	97	3	0
Sugar Frosted Flakes	1 oz	108	96	4	0
Orange and grapefruit juice, canned	1 cup	104	96	4	0
Orange juice, canned	1 cup	104	96	4	0
Grapefruit juice, frozen, diluted	1 cup	100	96	4	0
Marshmallows	1 oz	96	96	4	0
Prune juice, canned	1 cup	188	96	4	0
Grapefruit juice, canned, unsweetened	1 cup	92	96	4	0
Lime juice, raw	1 cup	92	96	4	0
Syrup, chocolate flavored, thin	2 tbsp	92	96	4	0
Peaches, raw, sliced	1 cup	80	95	5	0
Papayas, raw	1 cup	72	94	6	0
Water chestnuts, canned	1 cup	72	94	6	0
Oranges, raw	1	64	94	6	0
Parsnips, cooked	1 cup	128	94	6	0
Sweet potatoes, baked, peeled	1 small	120	93	7	0
Orange juice, frozen, diluted	1 cup	116	93	7	0
Potatoes, boiled, peeled	1 small	116	93	7	0
Plantains, raw	1	245	93	3	4
Orange juice, raw	1 cup	112	93	7	0
Super Sugar Crisp cereal	1 oz	112	93	7	0
Rice Krispies cereal	1 oz	108	93	7	0
Rice, white, cooked	1 cup	216	93	7	0
Trix cereal	1 oz	108	93	7	0
Apricots, raw	3	52	92	8	0
Cornflakes	1 oz	104	92	8	0
Honeydew melon, raw	1/10	52	92	8	0
Peaches, dried	1 cup	425	92	6	2
Figs, dried	10	530	92	5	3
Potatoes, baked, flesh only	1 medium	148	92	8	0
Apricots, dried, uncooked	1 cup	349	92	6	2

Description	Serving Size	kcal	CHO % kcal†	Pro % kcal†	Fat % kcal†
Cherries, sour, red, canned in water	1 cup	96	92	8	0
Kiwifruit, raw	1	48	92	8	0
Mangos, raw	1	153	91	3	6
Oranges, raw, sections	1 cup	92	91	9	0
Corn grits, cooked	1 cup	136	91	9	0
Potatoes, baked with skin	1 large	224	91	9	0
Apricots, canned, juice pack	3 halves	44	91	9	0
Grapefruit, raw, white	½	44	91	9	0
Peaches, raw	1	44	91	9	0
Rice, white, instant, cooked	1 cup	176	91	9	0
Angelfood cake, from mix	1 piece	128	91	9	0
Pears, raw, d'Anjou	1	113	90	3	7
Corn grits, cooked, instant	1 pkt	80	90	10	0
Plums, raw, 2⅛-in diameter	1	40	90	10	0
Tangerines, raw	1	40	90	10	0
Jerusalem artichoke, raw	1 cup	116	90	10	0
Gelatin dessert, prepared	0.5 cup	76	89	11	0
Bananas	1	105	89	3	7
Sweet potatoes, canned, mashed	1 cup	265	89	8	3
Carrots, canned	1 cup	36	89	11	0
Carrots, cooked from raw	1 cup	72	89	11	0
Onions, raw, sliced	1 cup	36	89	11	0
Product 19 cereal	1 oz	108	89	11	0
Sweet potatoes, canned	1 piece	36	89	11	0
Turnips, cooked, diced	1 cup	36	89	11	0
Pears, raw, Bartlett	1	113	88	4	8
Grape-Nuts cereal	1 oz	104	88	12	0
Wheaties cereal	1 oz	104	88	12	0
Corn, canned, cream style	1 cup	209	88	8	4
40% Bran Flakes	1 oz	100	88	12	0
Cream of Wheat, cooked	1 cup	132	88	12	0
Popcorn, sugar syrup coated	1 cup	137	88	6	6
Beets, cooked, drained, whole	2	32	88	12	0
Cabbage, cooked	1 cup	32	88	12	0
Carrots, raw, whole	1 medium	32	88	12	0
Corn, cooked from frozen	1 ear	64	88	12	0
Cream of Wheat, cooked, Mix n' Eat	1 pkt	96	88	12	0
Rice, brown, cooked	1 cup	229	87	9	4
Corn, cooked from frozen	1 cup	156	87	13	0
Malt-O-Meal, cooked	1 cup	120	87	13	0
Onions, cooked from raw	1 cup	60	87	13	0
Chestnuts, European, roasted	1 cup	351	87	6	8
Pears, raw, Bosc	1	97	87	4	9
Tomato puree, canned	1 cup	116	86	14	0
Blueberries, raw	1 cup	93	86	4	10
Beets, canned	1 cup	56	86	14	0
Carrots, cooked from frozen	1 cup	56	86	14	0
Eggplant, cooked, steamed	1 cup	28	86	14	0
Popcorn, air-popped	1 cup	28	86	14	0
Pumpkin, cooked from raw	1 cup	56	86	14	0
Tomato sauce, canned	1 cup	84	86	14	0
Potatoes, mashed with milk	1 cup	173	86	9	5
Froot Loops cereal	1 oz	117	85	7	8
Sugar Smacks cereal	1 oz	117	85	7	8
Cocoa powder, plain	0.75 oz	89	85	4	10
Italian bread	1 slice	80	85	15	0
Corn, canned, whole kernel	1 cup	193	85	10	5
Golden Grahams cereal	1 oz	113	85	7	8
Blackberries, raw	1 cup	85	85	5	11
Malted milk, chocolate, powder	0.75 oz	85	85	5	11
Vegetable juice cocktail, canned	1 cup	52	85	15	0

Description	Serving Size	kcal	CHO % kcal†	Pro % kcal†	Fat % kcal†
Sherbet, 2% fat	1 cup	280	85	3	13
Cantaloupe, raw	½	105	84	8	9
Lemons, raw	1	24	83	17	0
Sauerkraut, canned	1 cup	48	83	17	0
Snap beans, raw, cooked	1 cup	48	83	17	0
Tomato juice, canned	1 cup	48	83	17	0
Tomatoes, raw	1	25	83	17	0
Boston brown bread	1 slice	101	83	8	9
Nectarines, raw	1	77	83	5	12
Vegetables, mixed, cooked from frozen	1 cup	116	83	17	0
Watermelon, raw	1 piece	150	82	7	11
Pretzels, twisted, thin	10	240	82	11	8
Macaroni or spaghetti, cooked, tender	1 cup	157	82	13	6
Honey Nut Cheerios cereal	1 oz	113	81	11	8
Lucky Charms cereal	1 oz	113	81	11	8
Shredded Wheat cereal	1 oz	113	81	11	8
Raspberries, raw	1 cup	69	81	6	13
Squash, winter, baked	1 cup	89	81	9	10
Macaroni or spaghetti, cooked, firm	1 cup	193	81	15	5
Cocoa powder with nonfat dry milk	1 oz	109	81	11	8
Total cereal	1 oz	109	81	11	8
Artichokes, globe, cooked	1	60	80	20	0
Cabbage, raw	1 cup	20	80	20	0
Melba toast, plain	1 piece	20	80	20	0
Onion soup, dehydrated	1 pkt	20	80	20	0
Peppers, hot or sweet, raw	1	20	80	20	0
Pita bread	1	165	80	15	5
Raisin bran	1 oz	105	80	11	9
Snap beans, cooked from frozen	1 cup	40	80	20	0
Fig bars	4	212	79	4	17
Pumpkin, canned	1 cup	101	79	12	9
Vegetables, mixed, canned	1 cup	76	79	21	0
Sweet potatoes, candied	1 piece	147	79	3	18
English muffins, plain	1	137	79	15	7
Spaghetti, tomato and cheese sauce, canned	1 cup	198	79	12	9
Kohlrabi, cooked	1 cup	56	79	21	0
Bran flakes	1 oz	113	78	14	8
Special K cereal	1 oz	108	78	22	0
French bread	1 slice	93	77	13	10
Cherries, sweet, raw	10	50	77	7	16
Graham crackers, plain	2 squares	60	77	7	16
Tomato paste, canned	1 cup	254	77	16	7
All-Bran cereal	1 oz	109	77	15	8
Bagels	1	198	77	14	9
Oatmeal, cooked, instant, flavored	1 pkt	162	77	12	11
Noodles, egg, cooked	1 cup	194	76	14	9
Rolls, hard	1	155	76	13	11
Rye wafers, whole-grain	2	53	75	76	17
Strawberries, raw	1 cup	53	75	76	17
Raisin bread	1 slice	69	75	12	13
Tortillas, corn	1	69	75	12	13
Vienna bread	1 slice	69	75	12	13
Pumpernickel bread	1 slice	85	75	14	11
Bread crumbs, dry, grated	1 cup	389	75	13	12
Cauliflower, cooked from raw	1 cup	32	75	25	0
Mushrooms, raw	1 cup	16	75	25	0
Okra pods, cooked	8 pods	32	75	25	0
Snap beans, canned	1 cup	32	75	25	0
Turnip greens, cooked from raw	1 cup	32	75	25	0

Description	Serving Size	kcal	CHO % kcal†	Pro % kcal†	Fat % kcal†
Cap'n Crunch cereal	1 oz	123	75	3	22
Yogurt, low-fat, fruit flavored	8 oz	230	75	17	8
Gingerbread cake, from mix	1 piece	172	74	5	21
Peas, green, cooked from frozen	1 cup	124	74	26	0
Pinto beans, dry, cooked	1 cup	265	74	23	3
Caramels, plain or chocolate	1 oz	119	74	3	23
Cracked-wheat bread	1 slice	65	74	12	14
Mixed-grain bread	1 slice	65	74	12	14
Oatmeal bread	1 slice	65	74	12	14
Rye bread, light	1 slice	65	74	12	14
Wheat bread	1 slice	65	74	12	14
White bread	1 slice	65	74	12	14
Saltines	4	49	73	8	18
Fudge, chocolate or plain	1 oz	115	73	3	23
Lima beans, dry, cooked	1 cup	269	73	24	3
Mushrooms, canned	1 cup	44	73	27	0
Rolls, frankfurter and hamburger	1 roll	110	73	11	16
Tomato soup, canned, diluted with water	1 cup	94	72	9	19
Chicken chow mein, canned	1 cup	200	72	28	0
Cauliflower, raw	1 cup	28	71	29	0
Collards, cooked from raw	1 cup	28	71	29	0
Rolls, hoagie or submarine	1 roll	404	71	11	18
Whole-wheat bread	1 slice	73	71	16	12
Tomato vegetable soup, dehydrated, prepared	1 pkt	45	71	9	20
Toaster pastries	1	214	71	4	25
Red kidney beans, dry, canned	1 cup	237	71	25	4
Oatmeal, cooked, regular, quick, instant	1 cup	142	70	17	13
Black beans, dry, cooked	1 cup	233	70	26	4
Cheerios cereal	1 oz	114	70	14	16
Tomatoes, canned	1 cup	57	70	14	16
Great northern beans, dry, cooked	1 cup	217	70	26	4
Cauliflower, cooked from frozen	1 cup	40	70	30	0
Pea beans, dry, cooked	1 cup	229	70	26	4
Peas, split, dry, cooked	1 cup	241	70	27	4
Black-eyed peas, dry, cooked	1 cup	201	70	26	4
Shakes, thick, chocolate	10 fl oz	348	69	10	21
Snack cakes, sponge, creme filling	1 small	157	69	3	29
Peas, edible pod, cooked	1 cup	64	69	31	0
Sheet cake, with white frosting, home recipe	1 piece	450	68	4	28
Rolls, dinner, commercial	1	82	68	10	22
Oatmeal, cooked, instant, plain	1 pkt	106	68	16	17
Lentils, dry, cooked	1 cup	225	68	28	4
Brussels sprouts, raw, cooked	1 cup	77	68	21	12
Pudding, instant, from mix	0.5 cup	160	68	10	22
Pudding, rice, from mix	0.5 cup	160	68	10	22
Refried beans, canned	1 cup	303	67	24	9
Rolls, dinner, home recipe	1	119	67	10	23
Peas, green, canned	1 cup	125	67	26	7
Asparagus, canned	4 spears	12	67	33	0
Bean sprouts, mung, raw	1 cup	36	67	33	0
Beet greens, cooked	1 cup	48	67	33	0
Bran muffins, from commercial mix	1	144	67	8	25
Broccoli, frozen, cooked	1 piece	12	67	33	0
Cabbage, Chinese, pe-tsai, raw	1 cup	12	67	33	0
Endive, curly, raw	1 cup	12	67	33	0
Lettuce, loose leaf	1 cup	12	67	33	0
Malted milk, natural, powder	0.75 oz	90	67	13	20

Description	Serving Size	kcal	CHO % kcal†	Pro % kcal†	Fat % kcal†
Onions, spring, raw	6	12	67	33	0
Ice milk, vanilla, soft serve 3% fat	1 cup	229	66	14	20
Pudding, tapioca, canned	5 oz	169	66	7	27
Sweetened condensed milk, canned	1 cup	1003	66	10	24
Pudding, tapioca, from mix	0.5 cup	152	66	11	24
Pudding, cooked from mix	0.5 cup	152	66	11	24
Devils food cake, chocolate frosting, from mix	1 piece	244	66	5	30
Yellow cake with chocolate frosting, from mix	1 piece	244	66	5	30
Squash, summer, cooked	1 cup	49	65	16	18
Chickpeas, cooked	1 cup	276	65	22	13
Brown gravy from dry mix	1 cup	86	65	14	21
Chicken gravy from dry mix	1 cup	86	65	14	21
Vegetarian soup, canned	1 cup	74	65	11	24
Coffee cake, crumb, from mix	1 piece	235	65	8	27
Baking powder biscuits, refrigerated dough	1	62	65	6	29
White cake with white frosting, commercial	1 piece	261	64	5	31
Broccoli, cooked from raw	1 cup	56	64	36	0
Chocolate milk, low-fat, 1% fat	1 cup	163	64	20	16
Pea soup, canned	1 cup	171	63	21	16
Snack cakes, devils food, creme filling	1 small	108	63	4	33
Bean sprouts, mung, cooked	1 cup	32	63	37	0
Broccoli, cooked from frozen	1 cup	64	63	37	0
Spinach, cooked from frozen	1 cup	64	63	37	0
Collards, cooked from frozen	1 cup	77	62	26	12
Dandelion greens, cooked from frozen	1 cup	45	62	18	20
Kale, cooked from raw	1 cup	45	62	18	20
Vanilla wafers	10	187	62	4	34
Baking powder biscuits, from mix	1	91	62	9	30
Brownies with nuts and frosting, commercial	1	104	62	4	35
Shakes, thick, vanilla	10 fl oz	325	62	14	25
Syrup, chocolate flavored, fudge	2 tbsp	137	61	6	33
Brussels sprouts, cooked from frozen	1 cup	85	61	28	11
Ice milk, vanilla, 4% fat	1 cup	190	61	11	28
Sheet cake, plain, home recipe	1 piece	316	61	56	34
Potatoes, frozen, oven fries	10	112	61	7	32
Blueberry muffins, from mix	1	145	61	8	31
Wheat Thin crackers	4	33	61	12	27
Mushrooms, cooked	1 cup	53	60	23	17
Asparagus, cooked from raw	4 spears	20	60	40	0
Milk, skim, no added milk solids	1 cup	80	60	40	0
Corn muffins, home recipe	1	141	60	9	32
Nonfat dry milk, instantized	1 cup	236	59	41	0
Yellow cake with chocolate frosting, commercial	1 piece	263	59	34	38
Lemon meringue pie	1 piece	358	59	6	35
Sandwich-type cookies	4	196	59	48	37
Potatoes, mashed, with milk and margarine	1 cup	237	59	7	34
Peach pie	1 piece	409	59	4	37
Chicken noodle soup, dehydrated, prepared	1 pkt	41	59	20	22
Clam chowder, Manhattan, canned	1 cup	82	59	20	22
Oatmeal raisin cookies	4	246	59	5	37
Fruitcake, dark, from home recipe	1 piece	171	58	5	37

Description	Serving Size	kcal	CHO % kcal†	Pro % kcal†	Fat % kcal†
Blueberry muffins, home recipe	1	137	58	9	33
Spinach, cooked from raw	1 cup	48	58	42	0
Pancakes, plain, home recipe	1	62	58	13	29
Apple pie	1 piece	414	58	3	39
Cherry pie	1 piece	422	58	4	38
Evaporated milk, skim, canned	1 cup	201	58	38	4
Chocolate milk, low-fat 2% fat	1 cup	181	57	18	25
Pudding, vanilla, canned	5 oz	230	57	4	39
Corn muffins, from commercial mix	1	154	57	8	36
Granola cereal	1 oz	133	57	92	34
Yogurt, nonfat, plain	8 oz	120	57	43	0
Blueberry pie	1 piece	389	57	4	39
Broccoli, raw	1 spear	57	56	29	16
Chocolate chip cookies, commercial	4	201	56	4	40
Beans, canned, pork and sweet sauce	1 cup	388	56	16	28
Pancakes, plain, from mix	1	58	55	14	31
Chocolate chip cookies, refrigerated dough	4	235	54	3	42
Bran muffins, home recipe	1	142	54	8	38
Pound cake	1 slice	113	53	78	40
Tomato soup, canned, diluted with milk	1 cup	166	53	14	33
Kale, cooked from frozen	1 cup	53	53	30	17
Miso	1 cup	493	53	24	24
Pizza, cheese	1 slice	297	53	20	27
Asparagus, cooked	1 cup	61	52	33	15
Turnip greens, cooked from frozen	1 cup	61	52	33	15
100% Natural cereal	1 oz	138	52	9	399
Potatoes, au gratin, from mix	1 cup	238	52	11	38
Pudding, chocolate, canned	5 oz	231	52	5	43
Waffles, from mix	1	208	52	13	35
Creme pie	1 piece	455	52	3	45
Bean and bacon soup, canned	1 cup	178	52	18	30
Sugar cookies, from refrigerated dough	4	240	52	3	45
Milk, skim, added milk solids	1 cup	93	52	39	10
Chicken noodle soup, canned	1 cup	70	51	23	26
Potatoes, scalloped, from mix	1 cup	243	51	8	41
Buttermilk, dried	1 cup	463	51	35	14
Potatoes, mashed, from dehydrated	1 cup	252	51	6	43
Minestrone soup, canned	1 cup	87	51	18	31
Milk chocolate candy with rice cereal	1 oz	143	50	6	45
Alfalfa seeds, sprouted, raw	1 cup	8	50	50	0
Cabbage, Chinese, pak-choi, cooked	1 cup	24	50	50	0
Chocolate milk, regular	1 cup	208	50	15	35
Lettuce, crisphead, raw	1 cup	8	50	50	0
Mustard greens, cooked	1 cup	24	50	50	0
Potatoes, french-fried, from frozen	10	160	50	5	45
Shortbread cookies, commercial	4	160	50	5	45
Soy sauce	1 tbsp	16	50	50	0
Spinach, raw	1 cup	16	50	50	0
Yeast, bakers, dry, active	1 pkg	24	50	50	0
Yeast, brewers, dry	1 tbsp	24	50	50	0
Malted milk, chocolate, prepared from powder	1 svg	233	50	15	35
Baking powder biscuits, home recipe	1	105	50	8	43
Chocolate chip cookies, home recipe	4	211	49	4	47
Potatoes, hash brown, from frozen	1 cup	358	49	6	45
Buttermilk, fluid	1 cup	98	49	33	18

Description	Serving Size	kcal	CHO % kcal†	Pro % kcal†	Fat % kcal†
Fried pie, cherry	1	262	49	12	39
Potatoes, scalloped, home recipe	1 cup	213	49	13	38
Vegetable beef soup, canned	1 cup	82	49	29	22
Bamboo shoots, canned	1 cup	33	48	24	27
Carrot cake, with cream cheese frosting, home recipe	1 piece	397	48	43	48
Fried pie, apple	1	258	48	3	49
Pancakes, buckwheat, from mix	1	50	48	16	36
Cheese crackers, sandwich, peanut	1	42	48	10	43
Whole-wheat wafers, crackers	2	42	48	10	43
Pecan pie	1 piece	600	47	5	48
Imitation creamer, liquid frozen	1 tbsp	17	47	0	53
Milk, low-fat, 1% fat, added solids	1 cup	102	47	35	18
Snack-type crackers	1	17	47	0	53
Ice cream, vanilla, regular 11% fat	1 cup	274	47	7	46
Shortbread cookies, home recipe	2	148	46	5	49
Spinach, canned	1 cup	61	46	39	15
Spaghetti with meatballs and tomato sauce, home recipe	1 cup	340	46	22	32
Noodles, chow mein, canned	1 cup	227	46	11	44
Croissants	1	236	46	8	46
Danish pastry, fruit	1	245	46	7	48
Spaghetti with meatballs and tomato sauce, canned	1 cup	254	46	19	35
Danish pastry, plain, no nuts	1	228	46	7	47
Pumpkin pie	1 piece	325	46	7	47
Macaroni and cheese, canned	1 cup	230	45	16	39
Chicken rice soup, canned	1 cup	62	45	26	29
Malted milk, natural, prepared from powder	1 svg	242	45	18	37
Doughnuts, cake-type, plain	1	216	44	6	50
Peanut butter cookies, home recipe	4	254	44	6	50
Mushroom gravy, canned	1 cup	118	44	10	46
Doughnuts, yeast-leavened, glazed	1	237	44	7	49
French toast, home recipe	1 slice	155	44	15	41
Cheese crackers, plain	10	55	44	7	50
Popcorn, popped in vegetable oil	1 cup	55	44	7	50
Beef noodle soup, canned	1 cup	83	43	24	33
Custard pie	1 piece	333	43	11	46
Hamburger, regular, on bun	1	259	43	19	38
Yogurt, with low-fat milk, plain	8 oz	148	43	32	24
Brownies with nuts, home recipe	1	102	43	4	53
Cottage cheese, creamed, with fruit	1 cup	280	43	31	26
Corn chips	1 oz	153	42	5	53
Milk chocolate candy, plain	1 oz	153	42	5	53
Waffles, home recipe	1	249	42	11	47
Clam chowder, New England, diluted with milk	1 cup	167	41	22	38
Sweet (dark) chocolate	1 oz	158	41	3	57
Roast beef sandwich	1	341	40	26	34
Onion rings, breaded, frozen	2	81	40	5	56
Ice cream, vanilla, soft-serve	1 cup	387	39	7	53
Eggnog	1 cup	347	39	12	49
Bread stuffing, from mix, dry-type	1 cup	515	39	7	54
Custard, baked	1 cup	307	38	18	44
Macaroni and cheese, home recipe	1 cup	426	38	16	46
Potato chips	10	107	37	4	59
Bread stuffing, from mix, moist	1 cup	430	37	8	54
Milk, low-fat, 2% fat, added solids	1 cup	129	37	28	35
Milk chocolate with almonds	1 oz	162	37	7	56

Description	Serving Size	kcal	CHO % kcal†	Pro % kcal†	Fat % kcal†
Fish sandwich, regular, with cheese	1	427	37	15	48
Cheeseburger, regular	1	307	36	20	44
Cheesecake	1 piece	286	36	7	57
Coconut, dried, sweetened, shredded	1 cup	485	36	2	61
Chili con carne with beans, canned	1 cup	344	36	23	42
Ice cream, vanilla, rich 16% fat	1 cup	360	36	4	60
Beef gravy, canned	1 cup	125	35	29	36
Pie crust, from home recipe	1 shell	900	35	5	60
Beans, canned, with frankfurters	1 cup	366	35	21	44
White sauce with milk from mix	1 cup	241	35	17	49
English muffin, egg, cheese, bacon	1	358	35	20	45
Hamburger, 4-oz patty on bun	1	441	34	23	43
Fish sandwich, large, no cheese	1	479	34	15	51
Potato salad with mayonnaise	1 cup	329	34	9	57
Potatoes, au gratin, home recipe	1 cup	331	34	14	52
Cream of chicken soup, canned, diluted with water	1 cup	111	32	11	57
Cream of chicken soup, canned, diluted with milk	1 cup	187	32	15	53
Yogurt, whole milk, plain	8 oz	139	32	23	45
Chicken pot pie, home recipe	1 piece	539	31	18	52
Milk chocolate with peanuts	1 oz	167	31	10	59
Soybeans, dry, cooked	1 cup	246	31	33	37
1000 Island salad dressing, diet	1 tbsp	26	31	0	69
French salad dressing, diet	1 tbsp	26	31	0	69
Imitation creamer, powdered	1 tsp	13	31	0	69
Imitation whipped topping	1 tbsp	13	31	0	69
Taco	1	195	31	18	51
Beef pot pie, home recipe	1 piece	510	31	16	53
Enchilada	1	320	30	25	45
Cheese sauce with milk, from mix	1 cup	309	30	21	50
Milk, whole, 3.3% fat	1 cup	148	30	22	49
Evaporated milk, whole, canned	1 cup	339	30	21	50
Chicken and noodles, home recipe	1 cup	354	29	25	46
Gravy and turkey, frozen	5 oz	96	29	33	37
Avocados, Florida	1	371	29	5	66
Cream of mushroom soup, canned, diluted with water	1 cup	125	29	6	65
Cheeseburger, 4-oz patty	1	559	29	21	50
Cream of mushroom soup, canned, diluted with milk	1 cup	210	29	11	60
Beef and vegetable stew, home recipe	1 cup	223	27	29	44
Cooked salad dressing, home recipe	1 tbsp	30	27	13	60
Chicken gravy, canned	1 cup	198	26	10	64
Mayonnaise-type salad dressing	1 tbsp	61	26	0	74
Seaweed, spirulina, dried	1 oz	110	25	58	16
Fish sticks, frozen	1	67	24	36	40
White sauce, home recipe	1 cup	406	24	10	66
Bouillon, dehydrated	1 pkt	17	24	24	53
Oysters, breaded, fried	1	85	24	24	53
Mayonnaise, imitation	1 tbsp	35	23	0	77
Shrimp, french fried	3 oz	198	22	32	45
Hollandaise sauce, made from mix with water	1 cup	256	22	8	70
Turkey patties, breaded, battered, fried	1	184	22	20	59
Oysters, raw	1 cup	148	22	54	24
Cashew nuts, dry-roasted	1 oz	169	21	9	69
Scallops, breaded, frozen	6	190	21	32	47
Sandwich spread, pork, beef	1 tbsp	39	21	10	69

Description	Serving Size	kcal	CHO % kcal†	Pro % kcal†	Fat % kcal†
Tuna salad	1 cup	379	20	35	45
Quiche Lorraine	1 slice	600	19	9	72
Half and half cream	1 tbsp	22	18	0	82
Imitation sour cream	1 tbsp	22	18	0	82
Cashew nuts, oil-roasted	1 oz	178	18	11	71
Chocolate, bitter or baking	1 oz	179	18	7	75
Chop suey with beef and pork, home recipe	1 cup	309	17	34	50
Coconut, raw	1 piece	167	17	2	81
Cottage cheese, low-fat, 2% fat	1 cup	192	17	65	19
Coconut, raw, shredded	1 cup	303	16	4	80
Haddock, breaded, fried	3 oz	177	16	38	46
Chicken chow mein, home recipe	1 cup	254	16	49	35
Pistachio nuts	1 oz	178	16	13	71
Ricotta cheese, part skim milk	1 cup	335	16	33	51
Beef liver, fried	3 oz	183	15	50	34
Mixed nuts with peanuts, dry-roasted	1 oz	183	15	11	74
Chicken, fried, battered, breast	4.9 oz	354	15	40	46
Ocean perch, breaded, fried	1 fillet	191	15	34	52
Avocados, California	1	334	14	5	81
Almonds	1 oz	183	13	13	74
Clams, raw	3 oz	61	13	72	15
1000 Island, salad dressing, regular	1 tbsp	62	13	0	87
Light coffee or table cream	1 tbsp	31	13	0	87
Sour cream	1 tbsp	31	13	0	87
Tofu	1 piece	93	13	39	48
Chicken, fried, battered, drumstick	2.5 oz	187	13	34	53
Mixed nuts with peanuts, oil-roasted	1 oz	188	13	11	77
Tahini	1 tbsp	96	13	12	75
Pumpkin and squash kernels	1 oz	165	12	17	71
Sunflower seeds	1 oz	170	12	14	74
Peanut butter	1 tbsp	10	12	19	69
Cottage cheese, creamed, small curd	1 cup	209	11	50	39
Peanuts, oil-roasted	1 oz	165	11	18	71
Pine nuts	1 oz	185	11	6	83
Cottage cheese, creamed, large curd	1 cup	226	11	50	40
Chicken a la king, home recipe	1 cup	462	10	23	66
Chicken frankfurter	1	117	10	21	69
Clams, canned	3 oz	78	10	67	24
Walnuts, English	1 oz	198	10	88	82
Pecans	1 oz	199	10	42	86
Cottage cheese, uncreamed	1 cup	121	10	83	7
Pasteurized process cheese spread	1 oz	82	10	24	66
Turkey roast, light and dark meat	3 oz	129	9	56	35
Pasteurized process cheese food	1 oz	95	8	25	66
Sesame seeds	1 tbsp	48	8	17	75
Filberts (hazelnuts)	1 oz	194	8	8	84
Brazil nuts	1 oz	203	8	8	84
Pork, luncheon meat, regular	2 slices	102	8	39	53
Eggs, scrambled or omelet	1 egg	108	7	26	67
Macadamia nuts, oil-roasted	1 oz	222	7	4	89
Ricotta cheese, whole milk	1 cup	428	7	26	67
Walnuts, black	1 oz	184	7	15	78
Spinach souffle	1 cup	218	6	20	74
Feta cheese	1 oz	74	5	22	73
Pork luncheon meat, lean	2 slices	75	5	59	36
Tartar sauce	1 tbsp	76	5	0	95
Blue cheese salad dressing	1 tbsp	80	5	5	90
Mozzarella cheese, part-skim	1 oz	81	5	40	56
Eggs, whole	1	82	5	29	66
Mozzarella cheese, whole milk	1 oz	82	5	29	66

Description	Serving Size	kcal	CHO % kcal†	Pro % kcal†	Fat % kcal†
Chicken roll, light	2 slices	84	5	52	43
Pork, cured, bacon, Canadian	2 slices	84	5	52	43
French or Italian salad dressing	1 tbsp	85	5	0	95
Salami, dry-type	2 slices	84	5	23	72
Bologna	2 slices	180	4	16	80
Eggs, fried	1	91	4	26	69
Pasteurized process cheese, Swiss	1 oz	95	4	29	66
Shrimp, canned	3 oz	97	4	87	9
Blue cheese	1 oz	100	4	24	72
Braunschweiger	2 slices	202	4	16	80
Cream cheese	1 oz	102	4	8	88
Provolone cheese	1 oz	104	4	27	69
Chicken, fried, floured, breast	3.5 oz	218	4	58	38
Swiss cheese	1 oz	108	4	30	67
Chicken, fried, floured, drumstick	1.7 oz	120	3	44	53
Crabmeat, canned	1 cup	123	3	75	22
Salami, cooked-type	2 slices	135	3	24	73
Frankfurter, cooked	1	141	3	14	83
Pork, luncheon meat, canned	2 slices	140	3	14	83
Cheddar cheese, shredded	1 cup	449	1	25	74
Beef broth, bouillon, consomme, canned	1 cup	21	0	57	43
Beef heart, braised	3 oz	141	0	69	32
Beef roast, eye of round, lean	2.6 oz	133	0	66	34
Beef roast, eye of round, lean and fat	3 oz	200	0	46	54
Beef roast, rib, lean and fat	3 oz	310	0	25	75
Beef roast, rib, lean	2.2 oz	149	0	46	54
Beef steak, sirloin, broiled, lean	2.5 oz	142	0	62	38
Beef steak, sirloin, broiled, lean and fat	3 oz	227	0	41	59
Beef, canned, corned	3 oz	178	0	49	51
Beef, cooked, bottom round, lean	2.8 oz	172	0	58	42
Beef, cooked, bottom round, lean and fat	3 oz	217	0	47	54
Beef, cooked, chuck blade, lean and fat	3 oz	322	0	27	73
Beef, cooked, chuck blade, lean	2.2 oz	157	0	48	52
Beef, dried, chipped	2.5 oz	132	0	73	27
Brown 'N Serve sausage, browned	1 link	53	0	16	85
Butter	1 tbsp	99	0	0	100
Camembert cheese	1 wedge	113	0	28	72
Cheddar cheese	1 oz	109	0	26	74
Chicken liver, cooked	1	29	0	69	31
Chicken, canned, boneless	5 oz	223	0	56	44
Chicken, roasted, breast	3 oz	135	0	80	20
Chicken, roasted, drumstick	1.6 oz	66	0	73	27
Chicken, stewed, light and dark meat	1 cup	233	0	65	35
Corn oil	1 tbsp	126	0	0	100
Duck, roasted, flesh only	½ duck	433	0	48	52
Eggs, raw, white	1	12	0	100	0
Eggs, raw, yolk	1	66	0	18	82
Vegetable shortening	1 tbsp	117	0	0	100
Flounder or sole, baked in margarine	3 oz	118	0	54	46
Flounder or sole, baked, no fat	3 oz	77	0	88	12
Gelatin, dry	1 envelope	24	0	100	0
Ground beef, broiled, lean	3 oz	228	0	37	63
Ground beef, broiled, regular	3 oz	242	0	33	67
Halibut, broiled, with butter	3 oz	134	0	60	40
Herring, pickled	3 oz	185	0	37	63
Lamb, rib, roasted, lean and fat	3 oz	306	0	24	76
Lamb, rib, roasted, lean	2 oz	123	0	49	51
Lamb, chops, arm, braised, lean	1.7 oz	131	0	52	48
Lamb, chops, arm, braised, lean and fat	2.2 oz	215	0	37	63
Lamb, chops, loin, broiled, lean	2.3 oz	130	0	58	42
Lamb, chops, loin, broiled, lean and fat	2.8 oz	232	0	38	62

Description	Serving Size	kcal	CHO % kcal†	Pro % kcal†	Fat % kcal†
Lamb, leg, roasted, lean	2.6 oz	134	0	60	40
Lamb, leg, roasted, lean and fat	3 oz	205	0	43	57
Lard	1 tbsp	117	0	0	100
Margarine, imitation 40% fat	1 tbsp	45	0	0	100
Margarine, regular, hard, 80% fat	1 tbsp	99	0	0	100
Margarine, regular, soft, 80% fat	1 tbsp	99	0	0	100
Margarine, spread, hard, 60% fat	1 tbsp	81	0	0	100
Margarine, spread, soft, 60% fat	1 tbsp	81	0	0	100
Mayonnaise, regular	1 tbsp	99	0	0	100
Muenster cheese	1 oz	109	0	26	74
Olive oil	1 tbsp	126	0	0	100
Olives, canned	4 medium	18	0	0	100
Parmesan cheese, grated	1 tbsp	26	0	31	69
Pasteurized process cheese, American	1 oz	105	0	23	77
Peanut oil	1 tbsp	126	0	0	100
Pork chop, loin, broiled, lean	2.5 oz	164	0	56	44
Pork chop, loin, broiled, lean and fat	3.1 oz	267	0	36	64
Pork chop, loin, pan-fried, lean	2.4 oz	175	0	43	57
Pork chop, loin, pan-fried, lean and fat	3.1 oz	327	0	26	74
Fresh ham, roasted, lean	2.5 oz	152	0	53	47
Fresh ham, roasted, lean and fat	3 oz	246	0	34	66
Pork rib, roasted, lean	2.5 oz	170	0	47	53
Pork rib, roasted, lean and fat	3 oz	264	0	32	68
Pork shoulder, braised, lean	2.4 oz	160	0	55	45
Pork shoulder, braised, lean and fat	3 oz	290	0	32	68
Bacon, regular, cooked	3 slices	105	0	23	77
Ham, canned, roast	3 oz	135	0	53	47
Ham, roasted, lean	2.4 oz	104	0	65	35
Ham, roasted, lean and fat	3 oz	198	0	36	64
Pork link, cooked	1	48	0	25	75
Pork luncheon meat, chopped ham	2 slices	91	0	31	69
Safflower oil	1 tbsp	126	0	0	100
Salmon, baked, red	3 oz	129	0	65	35
Salmon, canned, pink, with bones	3 oz	113	0	60	40
Salmon, smoked	3 oz	144	0	50	50
Sardines, Atlantic, canned in oil, drained	3 oz	161	0	50	50
Soybean oil, hydrogenated	1 tbsp	126	0	0	100
Sunflower oil	1 tbsp	126	0	0	100
Trout, broiled, with butter	3 oz	165	0	51	50
Tuna, canned in oil, drained	3 oz	159	0	60	40
Tuna, canned in water, drained	3 oz	129	0	93	7
Turkey ham, cured turkey thigh	2 slices	71	0	62	38
Turkey loaf, breast meat	2 slices	49	0	82	18
Turkey, roasted, dark meat	4 pieces	150	0	64	36
Turkey, roasted, light and dark meat	1 cup	227	0	72	28
Turkey, roasted, light meat	2 pieces	127	0	79	21
Veal cutlet, medium fat	3 oz	173	0	53	47
Veal rib, medium fat, roasted	3 oz	218	0	42	58
Vienna sausage	1	44	0	18	82
Vinegar and oil salad dressing	1 tbsp	72	0	0	100
Whipped topping, pressurized	1 tbsp	9	0	0	100
Whipping cream, unwhipped, heavy	1 tbsp	54	0	0	100
Whipping cream, unwhipped, light	1 tbsp	45	0	0	100

Popsicle, Popsicle Industries, Inc, Englewood, NJ 07631. Sugar Frosted Flakes, Rice Krispies, Product 19, Froot Loops, Sugar Smacks, Special K, All Bran, Kellogg Co, Battle Creek, MI 49016. Super Sugar Crisp, Grape-Nuts, 40% Bran Flakes, General Foods Corp, White Plains, NY 10625. Trix, Wheaties, Golden Grahams, Honey Nut Cheerios, Lucky Charms, Total, Cheerios, General Mills, Inc, Minneapolis, MN 55440. Cream of Wheat, Cream of Wheat Mix N' Eat, Shredded Wheat, Wheat Thins, Nabisco Brands, Inc, East Hanover, NJ 07936. Malt-O-Meal, Malt-O-Meal Co, Minneapolis, MN 55402. Cap'n Crunch, 100% Natural Cereal, Quaker Oats Co, Chicago, IL 60654. Brown 'N Serve Sausage, Swift/Ekrich, Oak Brook, IL 60522.

Appendix 2

Calcium Content of Selected Commonly Consumed Foods

Food	Amount	Calcium (mg)
Cereals		
Oatmeal, cooked without salt	1 cup	19
Shredded Wheat	1 oz	11
Cream of Wheat	1 pkt	20
Cornflakes	1 oz	1
Rice, white, cooked	1 cup	21
Spaghetti, cooked, tender	1 cup	11
Dairy		
Whole milk	1 cup	291
Skim milk	1 cup	302
Yogurt, plain, low-fat	1 cup	415
Swiss cheese	1 oz	272
Cheddar cheese	1 oz	204
Processed American cheese	1 oz	174
Cottage cheese, low-fat	1 cup	155
Meats		
Sirloin steak, broiled, lean	2.5 oz	8
Flounder or sole, baked with butter	3 oz	13
Chicken breast, roasted	3 oz	13
Fresh ham, roasted, lean	2.5 oz	5
Salami, cooked	2 slices	7
Frankfurter	1	5
Hamburger (with roll)	1	56
Vegetables/fruits		
Broccoli, cooked	1 cup	177
Lettuce	1 cup	38
Bean sprouts	1 cup	14
Green beans, cooked from raw	1 cup	58

Food	Amount	Calcium (mg))
Green beans, canned	1 cup	35
Squash, baked	1 cup	29
Canned green olives	4 medium	8
Pickles, cucumber, dill	1 medium	17
Chicken soup, canned	1 cup	17
Orange, raw	1 medium	52
Orange juice	1 cup	27
Tomato, raw	1 medium	9
Apple, raw	1 medium	15
Honeydew melon	1/10 medium	8
Legumes		
Peanuts, oil roasted, salted	1 cup	125
Peanuts, oil roasted, unsalted	1 cup	125
Great northern beans, cooked	1 cup	90
Condiments		
Salt	1 tsp	14
Soy sauce	1 tbsp	3
Mustard	1 tsp	4
Catsup	1 tbsp	3
Relish, sweet	1 tbsp	3
Fats/oils		
Margarine, imitation, 40% fat	1 tbsp	2
Margarine, regular, hard	1 tbsp	4
Margarine, regular, soft	1 tbsp	4
Butter, salted	1 tbsp	3
Butter, unsalted	1 tbsp	0
Corn oil	1 tbsp	0
Olive oil	1 tbsp	0

Data from Gebhardt SE, Matthews RH. *Nutritive Value of Foods.* Washington, DC: US Dept of Agriculture, Human Nutrition Information Service; 1990. Home and Garden bulletin 72.

Shredded Wheat, Cream of Wheat, Nabisco Brands, Inc.

Appendix 3

Iron Content of Selected Commonly Consumed Foods

Food	Amount	Iron (mg)
Cereals		
Oatmeal, cooked without salt	1 cup	1.6
Shredded Wheat	1 oz	1.2
Cream of Wheat	1 pkt	8.1
Cornflakes	1 oz	1.8
Rice, white, cooked	1 cup	1.8
Spaghetti, cooked, tender	1 cup	1.7
Dairy		
Whole milk	1 cup	0.1
Skim milk	1 cup	0.1
Yogurt, plain, low-fat	1 cup	0.2
Swiss cheese	1 oz	0.0
Cheddar cheese	1 oz	0.2
Processed American cheese	1 oz	0.1
Cottage cheese, low-fat	1 cup	0.4
Meats		
Sirloin steak, broiled, lean	2.5 oz	2.4
Flounder or sole, baked with butter	3 oz	0.3
Chicken breast, roasted	3 oz	0.9
Fresh ham, roasted, lean	2.5 oz	0.8
Salami, cooked	2 slices	1.5
Frankfurter	1	0.5
Hamburger (with roll)	1	2.2
Vegetables/fruits		
Broccoli, cooked	1 cup	1.8
Lettuce	1 cup	0.8
Bean sprouts	1 cup	0.9
Green beans, cooked from raw	1 cup	1.6

Food	Amount	Iron (mg)
Green beans, canned	1 cup	1.2
Squash, baked	1 cup	0.7
Canned green olives	4 medium	0.2
Pickles, cucumber, dill	1 medium	0.7
Chicken soup, canned	1 cup	0.8
Orange, raw	1 medium	0.1
Orange juice	1 cup	0.5
Tomato, raw	1 medium	0.6
Apple, raw	1 medium	0.4
Honeydew melon	1/10 medium	0.1
Legumes		
Peanuts, oil roasted, salted	1 cup	2.8
Peanuts, oil roasted, unsalted	1 cup	2.8
Great northern beans, cooked	1 cup	4.9
Condiments		
Salt	1 tsp	0.0
Soy sauce	1 tbsp	0.5
Mustard	1 tsp	0.1
Catsup	1 tbsp	0.1
Relish, sweet	1 tbsp	0.1
Fats/oils		
Margarine, imitation, 40% fat	1 tbsp	0.0
Margarine, regular, hard	1 tbsp	0.0
Margarine, regular, soft	1 tbsp	0.0
Butter, salted	1 tbsp	0.0
Butter, unsalted	1 tbsp	0.0
Corn oil	1 tbsp	0.0
Olive oil	1 tbsp	0.0

Data from Gebhardt SE, Matthews RH. *Nutritive Value of Foods.* Washington, DC: US Dept of Agriculture, Human Nutrition Information Service; 1990. Home and Garden bulletin 72.

Shredded Wheat, Cream of Wheat, Nabisco Brands, Inc.

Appendix 4
Medical History Questionnaire

Date _____

Patient's Name _____

Nutrition Counselor _____

1. Has patient had any of the following?

   (If answer is "Yes," give month and year of occurrence.)

   Hyperlipidemia ☐ Yes ☐ No _____

   Describe (type, if known) _____

   Lipid-lowering Medications _____

   Angina ☐ Yes ☐ No _____

   Heart attack ☐ Yes ☐ No _____

   Coronary bypass surgery ☐ Yes ☐ No _____

   Stroke ☐ Yes ☐ No _____

   Cardiac rehabilitation program ☐ Yes ☐ No _____

   Medications _____

2. Does patient have high blood pressure? ☐ Yes ☐ No What is his blood pressure? _____

   If "Yes," is the treatment: weight control? ☐ Yes ☐ No

   sodium control? ☐ Yes ☐ No

   medications? (specify) _____

3. Is the patient on potassium supplementation? ☐ Yes ☐ No

   Diet supplementation? ☐ Yes ☐ No

   Medications (specify) _____

4. Does the patient have elevated uric acid levels or gout? ☐ Yes ☐ No

   Medications (specify) _____

5. Does the patient have diabetes? ☐ Yes ☐ No If "Yes," age diagnosed _____

   ☐ Insulin-dependent ☐ Not insulin-dependent

   Medications (specify) _____

6. Other diseases related to hyperlipidemia:

   a. Hypothyroidism ☐ Yes ☐ No

   Medications (specify) _____

Adapted from *Heart to Heart, A Manual on Nutrition Counseling for the Reduction of Cardiovascular Disease Risk Factors.* Raab C, ed. Washington, DC; US Dept of Health and Human Services; 1983. Publication 83-1528.

266

b. Nephrosis ☐ Yes ☐ No

Medications (specify) _____

c. Liver disease ☐ Yes ☐ No

Medications (specify) _____

d. Alcohol abuse ☐ Yes ☐ No (See dietary information)

7. Oral contraceptives: Currently taking? ☐ Yes ☐ No Kind _____

Has patient ever taken? ☐ Yes ☐ No If "Yes," how long? _____

Currently taking estrogens? ☐ Yes ☐ No Kind _____

8. Nonprescription drugs (aspirin, antacids, etc)

Kind   Frequency of Use

_____   _____

_____   _____

_____   _____

_____   _____

9. Other medical problems _____

_____

Family Medical History

1. Is patient's father living? ☐ Yes ☐ No ☐ Unsure

If no, at what age did he die? _____ Cause _____

2. Is patient's mother living? ☐ Yes ☐ No ☐ Unsure

If no, at what age did she die? _____ Cause _____

3. How many brothers and sisters does patient have? _____

How many are living? _____

4. Do or did any of the brothers or sisters, mother or father, have any of the following medical problems?

(Use "b" for brother, "s" for sister, "m" for mother, "f" for father)

	1	2	3	4	5	6	7	8	9	10
Hypertension _____										
Diabetes _____										
Overweight _____										
Stroke _____										
Hyperlipidemia _____										

Type _____

Diet prescription _____

5. Does the spouse have a weight problem? ☐ Yes ☐ No

Describe _____

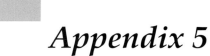

Appendix 5

Nutrition and Diet History Questionnaires for Athletes

The following questions should be answered as thoroughly as possible to gain information about your eating habits. Place a check (✔) in the appropriate column titled Yes or No; when marking "yes," fill in the further information requested.

Nutrition History		*Yes*	*No*

1. Are you pleased with your present eating habits?   ___   ___
2. Are you following a special diet or have you changed your diet in any way?   ___   ___
   If yes, what kind of diet? Check the appropriate modification(s).
   ___ Low-calorie   ___ Vegetarian
   ___ High-calorie   ___ High-protein
   ___ Diabetic   ___ Low-sodium
   ___ Low-fat   ___ High-fiber
   ___ Low cholesterol   ___ Hypoglycemic
   ___ High-carbohydrate   ___ Other
3. Were the dietary modification(s) recommended by a health professional?   ___   ___
   If yes, by whom? _____
4. Do you feel that your diet is nutritionally balanced?   ___   ___
   If you answered no, what do you feel is lacking in your diet?
   _____
5. Do you take vitamin supplements?   ___   ___
   If yes, name the vitamin, brand, and dosage if known.
   _____
6. Do you take mineral supplements?   ___   ___
   If yes, name the mineral, brand, and dosage, if known.
   _____
7. Do you take supplemental protein?   ___   ___
   If yes, name the product and dosage, if known.
   _____
8. Do you take any other food supplements?   ___   ___
   If yes, name the product and amount, if known.
   _____
9. What foods do you eat most frequently during the course of a week?
   _____
10. Do you have any food allergies?   ___   ___
    If yes, name the food(s) _____
11. Check any problems that may be indicators of increased nutritional risk:
    ___ Diarrhea   ___ Dental problems
    ___ Constipation   ___ Chewing/swallowing difficulties
    ___ Nausea/vomiting   ___ Other
12. How is your appetite? ___ Good   ___ Fair   ___ Poor
13. Who usually prepares the food at home? _____
14. Who usually does the grocery shopping for the household? _____
15. Is it difficult to obtain the kinds of foods you prefer eating?   ___   ___
    If yes, why? _____

                                                     Yes   *No*

16. How are most of your foods prepared? (Circle one or more.)
    Scratch/ready-to-eat/prepackaged mix/snack foods/other _____
17. How many meals per week do you eat at a restaurant? _____
    How many at fast-food restaurants? _____
18. What types of foods are your least favorites?
    _____
19. What is your favorite meal? _____
    What is your favorite snack? _____
    Do you have access to a training table?   ___   ___
20. Are your eating habits consistent _____, or do they change
    frequently _____?
21. What time of day are you most hungry? _____
22. Do you eat more on weekends?   ___   ___
23. What eating habits would you like to eliminate, modify, or
    incorporate into your diet?_____
24. Do you have any specific questions you would like answered about
    diet and nutrition?_____
    _____
25. Do you usually follow a special meal plan one week or less
    prior to an event?   ___   ___
26. What do you usually eat the night before an event?
    _____
27. What do you usually eat/drink the day of the event?
    _____
28. What do you usually eat/drink in the hours just prior
    to an event? _____
29. Do you consume fluids prior to exercising?   ___   ___
    If yes, specify type and amount _____
30. Do you consume fluids during exercise?   ___   ___
    If yes, specify type and amount _____
31. Do you consume fluids after exercise?   ___   ___
    If yes, please specify _____
32. How soon after an event do you consume fluids? _____
    What and how much do you consume? _____
33. Do you consume a fluid-replacement beverage containing
    carbohydrates?   ___   ___
    If yes, please specify _____
34. How soon after an event do you consume solid food?_____
    What foods do you eat? _____
35. Are you willing to change your present eating habits if a recommendation is
    made as a result of your nutrition assessment?   ___   ___

Weight History

1. Height _____ Weight _____
2. What is the most you have ever weighed? _____ pounds.
   At what age? _____ years.
3. What is the least you have weighed in your adult life? _____ pounds.
4. I presently think of myself as being:
   _____ Underweight
   _____ At a healthy weight
   _____ Mildly overweight/overfat
   _____ Moderately overweight/overfat
   _____ Very overweight/overfat

Yes   No

5. I would like to:

_____ Maintain my present weight

_____ Gain weight

_____ Lose weight

_____ Lower my percentage of body fat

_____ Increase my lean body mass

6. If you would like to gain or lose weight, what would you like to weigh? _____

In what amount of time would you like to accomplish your goal? _____

_____ weeks   _____ months   _____ years

7. Have you gained/lost (circle one) weight in the last six months?   ___   ___

If yes, how much? _____

8. Weight during: <u>Underweight</u>   <u>Normal</u>   <u>Overweight</u>

Childhood   _____   _____   _____

Teen   _____   _____   _____

Young adult   _____   _____   _____

Older adult   _____   _____   _____

9. What methods have helped you obtain/maintain a desirable weight in the past?

_____

_____

_____

_____

10. Are you or have you ever been anorexic? _____   ___   ___

If yes, at what age(s) _____?

What is the lowest you weighed? _____

How long did you remain at that weight? _____

What induced you to gain weight? _____

11. Are you or have you ever been bulimic? _____   ___   ___

If yes, at what age(s)? _____

How frequently did this occur? _____

Sports Nutrition Questionnaire (Basic)

Date:_____   Male _____   Female _____

Weight: _____ lb   Height: _____ ft_____ in   Age: _____ y

What is your desired weight? _____ lb

What sport are you in? _____What position do you play?_____

How many hours do you spend each day in sports activity?_____

*Please respond to the following questions based on **current** intake:*

	Item	Amount per day
What three foods do you eat most frequently?	_____	_____
	_____	_____
	_____	_____
What three beverages do you drink most frequently?	_____	_____
	_____	_____
	_____	_____

Place a check in the box that most describes your current intake:

	Never	Less than 1 time per day	1-3 times per day	4-6 times per day	7-9 times per day	10 or more times per day
Meat, fish, poultry						
Dairy products (Milk, yogurt, cheese)						
Bread, cereal, pasta, rice, potatoes, etc						
Vegetables or vegetable juice						
Fruits or fruit juice						
Desserts						
Water						
Sports beverages						
Alcoholic beverages						

At the present time, how much control do you have over selection of your foods? No control _____ Some control _____ Full control _____

If you could, would you change your food selections?   Yes _____   No _____

Latha Balachandran, Angela Cacciatore, Julie Field, Ann Grediagin, Susan Hagood, Linda McMurray, Stephanie Perkins, Dept of Nutrition and Dietetics, Georgia State University, Atlanta.

Sports Nutrition Questionnaire (Intermediate)

Name: _____   Age:_____y   Today's date:_____

Current weight: _____ lb   Desired weight: _____lb   Height: _____ft _____in

Sport:_____   Position:_____

Typical number of hours spent each day in sports activity:_____hr

Are you following any kind of a special diet at this time?   Yes _____   No _____

If you are following a special diet, please check all that apply below. Diet prescribed by:

Diet	Physician	Dietitian	Coach or trainer	Other health care professional	Other nonlicensed person	Self
High calorie						
Low calorie						
Diabetic						
Low fat/low cholesterol						
Vegetarian						
High carbohydrate						
Low fiber						
High fiber						
Low sodium						
Diet for low blood sugar						
Liquid diet						
Diet for allergy						
Other						

Are you taking vitamin/mineral supplements?   Yes ____   No ____
Are you taking protein or amino acid supplements?   Yes ____   No ____
Does eating certain foods make you ill?   Yes ____   No ____
   If yes, which ones affect you the most? _____
                                          _____
                                          _____

Latha Balachandran, Angela Cacciatore, Julie Field, Ann Grediagin, Susan Hagood, Linda McMurray, Stephanie Perkins, Dept of Nutrition and Dietetics, Georgia State University, Atlanta.

Please respond to the following based on current intake. How often do you eat or drink the following?

Foods/Drinks	Never	Seldom (less than once per week)	Sometimes (2-4 times per week)	Often (5-7 times per week)	Frequently (more than once per day)
Red meat (beef, pork, lamb)					
Poultry					
Fish					
Processed meats (bacon, bologna, etc)					
Eggs					
Whole milk					
Low-fat milk					
Cheese					
Low-fat cheese					
Fruit juice					
Fresh fruits					
Vegetable juice					
Dark green vegetables					
Yellow, orange, or red vegetables					
Other vegetables					
Potatoes					
Whole-grain products					
Refined-grain products (white bread, etc)					
Dried beans, peas, lentils					
Margarine and/or butter					
Mayonnaise and/or salad dressing					
Fried foods					
Desserts					
Frozen desserts					
Frozen dinners					
At fast-food restaurants					
Add salt to your food					
Salty foods (chips, pretzels, pickles, etc)					
Water					
Regular sodas or sweetened drinks					
Diet sodas or drinks					
Sports drinks					
Alcohol					

How much control do you have over the selection of the foods you eat?   None _____   Some _____   Full _____

If you could, would you change your food selections?   Yes _____   No _____

How many meals do you eat per day?   2-4 _____   5-6 _____   6 or more _____

How many times per day do you snack?   2-4 _____   5-6 _____   6 or more _____

Sports Nutrition Questionnaire (Extensive)

Name: _____ Age: _____ y Date:_____

Sport: _____ Position:_____

Body Composition

Height: _____ cm   Weight:_____ kg

Waist circumference: _____cm   Hip circumference: _____ cm

Skinfolds

    Triceps:_____ mm   Chest: _____mm

    Suprailiac: _____ mm   Subscapular:_____ mm

    Abdomen:_____ mm   Thigh: _____mm

    Midaxillary:_____ mm

Blood Analysis

Triglycerides:_____   HDL:_____   LDL:_____

Cholesterol:_____   Sodium:_____   Potassium:_____

SGPT:_____   SGOT:_____   Ferritin:_____

Hemoglobin:_____   Hematocrit:_____   Glucose:_____

BUN:_____   Creatinine:_____   Alk phos:_____

General Medical History

1. Are you presently under the care of a physician or health practitioner for a medical problem?   Yes _____   No _____
   If yes, please explain:

   _____

2. Have you had any major illness or been hospitalized in the past 5 years?   Yes _____   No _____
   Past 10 years?   Yes _____   No _____
   If yes, please explain:

   _____

3. Are you presently taking any prescribed medication(s)?   Yes _____   No _____
   If yes, please provide name of medication and dosage:

   _____

4. Are you presently taking any nonprescribed medication(s)?   Yes _____   No _____
   If yes, please explain:

   _____

5. Have you had a supervised stress test in the past 5 years?   Yes _____   No _____
   If yes, what was the outcome of this test?

   _____

Latha Balachandran, Angela Cacciatore, Julie Field, Ann Grediagin, Susan Hagood, Linda McMurray, Stephanie Perkins, Dept of Nutrition and Dietetics, Georgia State University, Atlanta.

Please circle yes or no for the questions that follow. If you answer yes to any of these questions, please provide a brief explanation in the space provided below.

Have you been told by your physician that you have or have you experienced any of the following?

Explanation

1. Heart problems	Yes	No	_____
2. High blood pressure	Yes	No	_____
3. Low blood pressure	Yes	No	_____
4. Diabetes (high blood sugar)	Yes	No	_____
5. Hypoglycemia (low blood sugar)	Yes	No	_____
6. Asthma	Yes	No	_____
7. Shortness of breath with mild exertion	Yes	No	_____
8. Back discomfort or pain	Yes	No	_____
9. Broken bones or torn cartilage	Yes	No	_____
10. Muscle strains, ligament sprains	Yes	No	_____
11. Arthritis	Yes	No	_____
12. Gout	Yes	No	_____
13. High cholesterol	Yes	No	_____
14. High triglycerides	Yes	No	_____
15. Allergies	Yes	No	_____
16. Ulcers	Yes	No	_____

Family History

1. Has any member of your family (parents, siblings, grandparents) been diagnosed as having heart disease?   Yes _____ No _____
   If yes, please explain:

   _____

2. Has any member of your family had diabetes or hypoglycemia?   Yes _____ No _____
   If yes, please explain:

   _____

3. Has any member of your family died before the age of 65?   Yes _____ No _____
   If yes, please explain:

   _____

Special Eating Patterns

Are you following a special diet at this time?   Yes _____ No _____

If you are following a special diet, please check all that apply below. Diet prescribed by:_____

Diet	Physician	Dietitian	Coach or trainer	Other health care professional	Other nonlicensed person	Self
High calorie						
Low calorie						
Diabetic						
Low fat/low cholesterol						
Vegetarian						
High carbohydrate						
Low fiber						
High fiber						
Low sodium						
Diet for low blood sugar						
Liquid diet						
Diet for allergy						
Other						

Are you taking vitamin/mineral supplements?   Yes _____   No _____
Are you taking protein or amino acid supplements?   Yes _____   No _____
Does eating certain foods make you ill?   Yes _____   No _____
   If yes, which ones affect you the most? _____   _____   _____

Check the column that appropriately describes how you usually eat.

Then complete a 5-day food record. Follow the instructions on the forms provided (attached).

Food	Usual portion size	More than once per day	Daily	Weekly	Monthly	Rarely
Whole milk						
Skim milk						
Cheese						
Ice cream/pudding/yogurt						
Eggs						
Fish/shellfish						
Chicken/turkey						
Beef						
Liver						
Luncheon meats						
Sausage/hot dogs						
Dried beans/peas						
Peanut butter						
Pork/ham						
Bacon						
Butter						
Margarine						
Cooking oil						
Salad dressing						
Cream						
Mayonnaise						
Orange/grapefruit juice						
Raw fruit						
Canned fruit						
Cooked green vegetables						
Potatoes						
Green salad						
Carrots/yellow vegetables						
Cereal						
Rice/grits						
Pasta (spaghetti, noodles, macaroni)						
Bread						
Biscuit, roll, crackers						
Potato chips/snacks						
Cake/cookies						
Nuts						
Coffee						
Pie/pastry						
Sugar						
Sugar substitute						
Salt						
Salt substitute						
Pickles						
Syrup/honey						
Candy						
Regular soda						
Diet soda						

Food Record Data Collection Form

Please complete as accurately as possible, using the examples provided as a guide. Use only 1 form per day. Do not put information pertaining to more than 1 day on the same form. **Record everything you consume for accuracy.**

Day number (circle): 1   2   3   4   5

Name: _____   Date of recorded intake: _____

FOOD	TYPE	PREPARATION	AMOUNT	TIME CONSUMED
Chicken	Breast	Fried	Half breast	12:30 PM
Milk	Whole	–	12-oz glass	3:00 PM
Broccoli	Fresh	Steamed	1 stalk	6:30 PM

Appendix 6

Summary of the Recommended Dietary Allowances*

Age (y)	Weight (kg)	Weight (lb)	Height (cm)	Height (in)	Protein (g)	Vitamin A (µg RE)	Vitamin D (µg)	Vitamin E (mg α-TE)	Vitamin K (µg)	Vitamin C (mg)	Thiamin (mg)	Riboflavin (mg)	Niacin (mg NE)	Vitamin B6 (mg)	Folate (µg)	Vitamin B12 (µg)	Calcium (mg)	Phosphorus (mg)	Magnesium (mg)	Iron (mg)	Zinc (mg)	Iodine (µg)	Selenium (µg)
Infants																							
0.0-0.5	6	13	60	24	13	375	7.5	3	5	30	0.3	0.4	5	0.3	25	0.3	400	300	40	6	5	40	10
0.5-1.0	9	20	71	28	14	375	10	4	10	35	0.4	0.5	6	0.6	35	0.5	600	500	60	10	5	50	15
Children																							
1-3	13	29	90	35	16	400	10	6	15	40	0.7	0.8	9	1.0	50	0.7	800	800	80	10	10	70	20
4-6	20	44	112	44	24	500	10	7	20	45	0.9	1.1	12	1.1	75	1.0	800	800	120	10	10	90	20
7-10	28	62	132	52	28	700	10	7	30	45	1.0	1.2	13	1.4	100	1.4	800	800	170	10	10	120	30
Males																							
11-14	45	99	157	62	45	1000	10	10	45	50	1.3	1.5	17	1.7	150	2.0	1200	1200	270	12	15	150	40
15-18	66	145	176	69	59	1000	10	10	65	60	1.5	1.8	20	2.0	200	2.0	1200	1200	400	12	15	150	50
19-24	72	160	177	70	58	1000	10	10	70	60	1.5	1.7	19	2.0	200	2.0	1200	1200	350	10	15	150	70
25-50	79	174	176	70	63	1000	5	10	80	60	1.5	1.7	19	2.0	200	2.0	800	800	350	10	15	150	70
51 +	77	170	173	68	63	1000	5	10	80	60	1.2	1.4	15	2.0	200	2.0	800	800	350	10	15	150	70
Females																							
11-14	46	101	157	62	46	800	10	8	45	50	1.1	1.3	15	1.4	150	2.0	1200	1200	280	15	12	150	45
15-18	55	120	163	64	44	800	10	8	55	60	1.1	1.3	15	1.5	180	2.0	1200	1200	300	15	12	150	50
19-24	58	128	164	65	46	800	10	8	60	60	1.1	1.3	15	1.6	180	2.0	1200	1200	280	15	12	150	55
25-50	63	138	163	64	50	800	5	8	65	60	1.1	1.3	15	1.6	180	2.0	800	800	280	15	12	150	55
51 +	65	143	160	63	50	800	5	8	65	60	1.0	1.2	13	1.6	180	2.0	800	800	280	10	12	150	55
Pregnant					60	800	10	10	65	70	1.5	1.6	17	2.2	400	2.2	1200	1200	300	30	15	175	65
Lactating																							
1st 6 mo					65	1300	10	12	65	95	1.6	1.8	20	2.1	280	2.6	1200	1200	355	15	19	200	75
2nd 6 mo					62	1200	10	11	65	90	1.6	1.7	20	2.1	260	2.6	1200	1200	340	15	16	200	75

Note: The Committee on Dietary Allowances has published a separate table showing energy allowances in ranges for each age-sex group and another table of estimated safe and adequate daily dietary intakes for selected vitamins and minerals. The FDA has published a special table of selected RDA values for use on food labels.

*The allowances are intended to provide for individual variations among most normal, healthy people in the United States under usual environmental stresses. They were designed for the maintenance of good nutrition. Diets should be based on a variety of common foods in order to provide other nutrients for which human requirements have been less well defined. See the text for a more detailed discussion of the RDA and of nutrients not tabulated.

Reprinted with permission from *Recommended Dietary Allowances*. © 1989 by the National Academy of Sciences. Published by National Academy Press, Washington, DC

Appendix 7

Nutrients Significantly Affected by Selected Drugs

Nutrient	Drug Action	Drugs
Vitamin B_6	Function as vitamin B_6 antagonists or increase the turnover of B_6 in the body.	Isoniazid, cycloserine and other antituberculous drugs. Hydralazine. Penicillamine. L-Dopa. Oral contraceptives. Alcohol.
Folic acid	Function as folic acid antagonists; affect the absorption of folic acid or increase the turnover or loss of folate from the body.	Para-aminosalicylic acid. Methotrexate. Pyrimethamine. Isoniazid. Anticonvulsants. Triamterene. Trimethoprim. Oral contraceptives. Cycloserine. Salicylazosulfapyridine Acetylsalicylic acid. Pentamidine. Alcohol.
Vitamin B_{12}	Affect the absorption of vitamin B_{12}.	Neomycin. Biguanides. Para-aminosalicylic acid. Cholestyramine. Potassium choloride. Alcohol.
Niacin	By antagonizing vitamin B_6, cause depletion, because vitamin B_6 is a necessary coenzyme in the synthesis of niacin from tryptophan.	Isoniazid.
Riboflavin	Decreases riboflavin absorption by increasing GI motility.	Thyroxine.
	Displaces riboflavin from plasma binding site and causes hyperexcretion of riboflavin.	Boric acid.
Thiamin	Impairs absorption of thiamin or impairs the formation of the coenzyme form of the vitamin.	Alcohol.
	Increase requirements.	Digitalis alkaloids.
Ascorbic acid	Decrease the absorption or stimulate the metabolism of the vitamin.	Oral contraceptives.
	Deplete the tissues of the vitamin.	Acetylsalicylic acid. Alcohol. Anorectic agents. Anticonvulsants. Tetracycline.
	Depletes adrenal ascorbic acid.	Adrenal corticosteroids.

From Krause MV, Mahan LK. Food, Nutrition, and Diet Therapy. 7th ed. Philadelphia, Pa: WB Saunders Co; 1984. Used by permission.

Nutrient	Drug Action	Drugs
Vitamin A	Acts as a solvent for carotene and vitamin A and thus prevents absorption.	Mineral oil.
	Decrease absorption by damage to mucosa; inhibition of pancreatic lipase and inactivation of bile salts.	Cholestyramine. Neomycin. Alcohol. Colchicine (affects carotene).
Vitamin D	Affect absorption or metabolism of vitamin D.	Cholestyramine. Laxatives. Antacids. Mineral oil. Phenolphthalein.
	Accelerate the degradation of 25-OHD$_3$.	Anticonvulsants. Glutethimide.
	Block the production of 1,25-OH$_2$D$_3$ in the kidney.	Diphosphonates. Corticosteroids.
Vitamin E	Diminishes the carrier lipoprotein for vitamin E.	Clofibrate.
	Decreases absorption.	Mineral oil. Isoniazid.
Vitamin K	Decrease synthesis of vitamin K$_2$ by intestinal bacteria, but no effect on vitamin status unless vitamin K intake is inadequate.	Tetracyclines and other broad-spectrum antibiotics.
	Decrease absorption of vitamin K.	Mineral oil Neomycin. Cholestyramine.
	Cause vitamin K deficiency.	Coumarin aniticoagulants. Aspirin and other salicylates.
Iron	Depresses iron absorption.	Bicarbonate.
	Increases iron absorption.	Isoniazide
	Impairs the uptake of iron into protoporphyrin; capable of causing sideroblastic anemia.	Cholestyramine.
Zinc	Cause excessive urinary excretion of zinc.	Alcohol. D-Penicillamine. Corticosteroids. Estrogen component of oral contraceptives. Chlorthalidone. Thiazides. Furosemide.
Magnesium	Increase urinary excretion of magnesium.	Chlorothiazide. Hydrochlorothiazide. Ethacrynic acid. Ammonium chloride. Mercurial diuretics. Alcohol.
	Drug-induced steatorrhea causes formation of magnesium soaps and excessive fecal excretion of magnesium.	
Calcium	Cause malabsorption of calcium.	Prednisone and other glucocorticoids. Phenobarbital. Phenytion. Primidone. Glutethimide. Diphosphonates. Phenolphthalein. Neomycin.

Nutrient	Drug Action	Drugs
	Cause excessive urinary excretion of calcium.	Furosemide. Ethacrynic acid. Triamterene. Alcohol.
	Increase intestinal absorption of calcium.	Combination oral contraceptives.
Protein	Cause malabsorption of protein.	Neomycin.
	Inhibit protein synthesis.	Actinomycin D. Corticosteroids.
Fat	Cause malabsorption of fat.	Neomycin. Colchicine. Cholestyramine. Para-aminosalicyclic acid.
Carbohydrate	Cause malabsorption of lactose.	Neomycin. Colchicine.
	Cause malabsorption of sucrose.	Neomycin.
Sodium and potassium	Increase fecal excretion.	Neomycin. Colchicine.
Phosphate	Increase fecal excretion.	Aluminum hydroxide antacids.

Appendix 8

Exchange Lists for Meal Planning

Starch/Bread List

Each item in this list contains approximately 15 grams of carbohydrate, 3 grams of protein, a trace of fat, and 80 calories. Whole grain products average about 2 grams of fiber per exchange. Some foods are higher in fiber. Those foods that contain 3 or more grams of fiber per exchange are identified with an asterisk(*).

Cereals/Grains/Pasta

Bran cereals, concentrated* (such as Bran Buds, All Bran)	1/3 cup
Bran cereals, flaked*	1/2 cup
Bulgur (cooked)	1/2 cup
Cooked cereals	1/2 cup
Cornmeal (dry)	2 1/2 tbsp
Grape-Nuts	3 tbsp
Grits (cooked)	1/2 cup
Other ready-to-eat unsweetened cereals	3/4 cup
Pasta (cooked)	1/2 cup
Puffed cereal	1 1/2 cup
Rice, white or brown (cooked)	1/3 cup
Shredded wheat	1/2 cup
Wheat germ*	3 tbsp

Dried Beans/Peas/Lentils

Beans and peas (cooked)* (such as kidney, white, split, blackeye)	1/3 cup
Lentils (cooked)*	1/3 cup
Baked beans*	1/4 cup

Starchy Vegetables

Corn*	1/2 cup
Corn on cob, 6 in long*	1
Lima beans*	1/2 cup
Peas, green (canned or frozen)*	1/2 cup
Plantain*	1/2 cup
Potato, baked	1 small (3 oz)
Potato, mashed	1/2 cup
Squash, winter* (acorn, butternut)	1 cup
Yam, sweet potato, plain	1/3 cup

Bread

Bagel	1/2 (1 oz)
Bread sticks, crisp, 4 in long x 1/2 in	2 (2/3 oz)
Croutons, lowfat	1 cup
English muffin	1/2
Frankfurter or hamburger bun	1/2 (1 oz)
Pita, 6 in across	1/2
Plain roll, small	1 (1 oz)
Raisin, unfrosted	1 slice (1 oz)
Rye, pumpernickel	1 slice (1 oz)
Tortilla, 6 in across	1
White (including French, Italian)	1 slice (1oz)
Whole wheat	1 slice (1 oz)

Crackers/Snacks

Animal crackers	8
Graham crackers, 2 1/2 in square	3
Matzoh	3/4 oz
Melba toast	5 slices
Oyster crackers	24
Popcorn (popped, no fat added)	3 cups
Pretzels	3/4 oz
RyKrisp, 2 in X 3 1/2 in	4
Saltine-type crackers	6
Whole-wheat crackers, no fat added* (crisp breads, such as Finn, Kavli, Wasa)	2-4 slices (3/4 oz)

Starch Foods Prepared With Fat

(Count as 1 starch/bread exchange, plus 1 fat exchange.)

Biscuit, 2 1/2 in across	1
Chow mein noodles	1/2 cup
Corn bread, 2 in cube	1 (2 oz)
Cracker, round butter type	6
French fried potatoes, 2 in to 3 1/2 in long	10 (1 1/2 oz)
Muffin, plain, small	1
Pancake, 4 in across	2
Stuffing, bread (prepared)	1/4 cup
Taco shell, 6 in across	2
Waffle, 4 1/2 in square	1
Whole-wheat crackers fat added* (such as Triscuit)	4-6 (1 oz)

---

*3 grams or more of fiber per exchange.

Meat List
_____

Each serving of meat and substitutes on this list contains about 7 grams of protein. The amount of fat and number of calories varies, depending on what kind of meat or substitute you choose. The list is divided into three parts based on the amount of fat and calories: lean meat, medium-fat meat, and high-fat meat. One ounce (one meat exchange) of each of these includes:

	Carbohydrate (grams)	Protein (grams)	Fat (grams)	Calories (grams)
Lean	0	7	3	55
Medium-fat	0	7	5	75
High-fat	0	7	8	100

You are encouraged to use more lean and medium-fat meat, poultry, and fish in your meal plan. This will help decrease your fat intake, which may help decrease your risk for heart disease. The items from the high-fat group are high in saturated fat, cholesterol, and calories. You should limit your choices from the high-fat group to three (3) times per week. Meat and substitutes do not contribute any fiber to your meal plan. *Meats and meat substitutes that have 400 milligrams or more of sodium per exchange are indicated with a dagger (†). Meats and meat substitutes that have 400 mg or more of sodium if two or more exchanges are eaten are indicated with a double dagger (‡).*

Tips

1. Bake, roast, broil, grill, or boil these foods rather than frying them with added fat.
2. Use a nonstick pan spray or a nonstick pan to brown or fry these foods.
3. Trim off visible fat before and after cooking.
4. Do not add flour, bread crumbs, coating mixes, or fat to these foods when preparing them.
5. Weigh meat after removing bones and fat, and after cooking. Three ounces of cooked meat is about equal to 4 ounces of raw meat. Some examples of meat portions are:

   2 ounces meat (2 meat exchanges) = 1 small chicken leg or thigh
   $\frac{1}{2}$ cup cottage cheese or tuna

   3 ounces meat (3 meat exchanges) = 1 medium pork chop
   1 small hamburger
   $\frac{1}{2}$ of a whole chicken breast
   1 unbreaded fish fillet
   cooked meat, about the size of a deck of cards

6. Restaurants usually serve prime cuts of meat, which are high in fat and calories.

Lean Meat and Substitutes

(One exchange is equal to any one of the following items.)

Beef	USDA Select or Choice grades of lean beef, such as round, sirloin, and flank steak; tenderloin; and chipped beef†	1 oz
Pork	Lean pork, such as fresh ham; canned, cured or boiled ham†; Canadian bacon†, tenderloin.	1 oz
Veal	All cuts are lean except for veal cutlets (ground or cubed). Examples of lean veal are chops and roasts.	1 oz
Poultry	Chicken, turkey, Cornish hen (without skin)	1 oz
Fish	All fresh and frozen fish	1 oz
	Crab, lobster, scallops, shrimp, clams (fresh or canned in water)	2 oz
	Oysters	6 medium
	Tuna‡ (canned in water)	$\frac{1}{4}$ cup
	Herring‡ (uncreamed or smoked)	1 oz
	Sardines (canned)	2 medium
Wild Game	Venison, rabbit, squirrel	1 oz
	Pheasant, duck, goose (without skin)	1 oz
Cheese	Any cottage cheese‡	$\frac{1}{4}$ cup
	Grated parmesan	2 tbsp
	Diet cheeses† (with less than 55 calories per ounce)	1 oz
Other	95% fat-free luncheon meat†	1 $\frac{1}{2}$ oz
	Egg whites	3 whites
	Egg substitutes with less than 55 calories per $\frac{1}{2}$ cup	$\frac{1}{2}$ cup

Medium-Fat Meat and Substitutes

(One exchange is equal to any one of the following items.)

Beef	Most beef products fall into this category. Examples are: all ground beef, roast (rib, chuck, rump), steak (cubed, Porterhouse, T-bone), and meatloaf.	1 oz
Pork	Most pork products fall into this category. Examples are: chops, loin roast, Boston butt, cutlets.	1 oz
Lamb	Most lamb products fall into this category. Examples are: chops, leg, and roast.	1 oz
Veal	Cutlet (ground or cubed, unbreaded)	1 oz
Poultry	Chicken (with skin), domestic duck or goose (well drained of fat), ground turkey	1 oz
Fish	Tuna‡ (canned in oil and drained)	¹/₄ cup
	Salmon‡ (canned)	¹/₄ cup
Cheese	Skim or part-skim milk cheeses, such as:	
	Ricotta	¹/₄ cup
	Mozzarella	1 oz
	Diet cheeses† (with 56-80 calories per ounce)	1 oz
Other	86% fat-free luncheon meat‡	1 oz
	Egg (high in cholesterol, limit to 3 per week)	1
	Egg substitutes with 56-80 calories per ¹/₄ cup	¹/₄ cup
	Tofu (2¹/₂ in × 2³/₄ in × 1 in)	4 oz
	Liver, heart, kidney, sweetbreads (high in cholesterol)	1 oz

High-Fat Meat and Substitutes

Remember, these items are high in saturated fat, cholesterol, and calories,
and should be used only three (3) times per week.
(One exchange is equal to any one of the following items.)

Beef	Most USDA Prime cuts of beef, such as ribs, corned beef‡	1 oz
Pork	Spareribs, ground pork, pork sausage† (patty or link)	1 oz
Lamb	Patties (ground lamb)	1 oz
Fish	Any fried fish product	1 oz
Cheese	All regular cheeses, such as American,† Blue,† Cheddar,‡ Monterey Jack,‡ Swiss	1 oz
Other	Luncheon meat,† such as bologna, salami, pimento loaf	1 oz
	Sausage,† such as Polish, Italian smoked	1 oz
	Knockwurst†	1 oz
	Bratwurst‡	1 oz
	Frankfurter† (turkey or chicken)	1 frank (10/lb)
	Peanut butter (contains unsaturated fat)	1 tbsp

Count as One High-Fat Meat Plus One Fat Exchange

Frankfurter† (beef, pork, or combination)		1 frank (10/lb)

†400 mg or more of sodium per exchange.

‡400 mg or more of sodium if two or more exchanges are eaten.

Vegetable List

Each vegetable serving on this list contains about 5 grams of carbohydrate, 2 grams of protein, and 25 calories. Vegetables contain 2-3 grams of dietary fiber. Vegetables which contain 400 mg or more of sodium per exchange are identified with a dagger (†).

Vegetables are a good source of vitamins and minerals. Fresh and frozen vegetables have more vitamins and less added salt. Rinsing canned vegetables will remove much of the salt.

Unless otherwise noted, the serving size for vegetables (one vegetable exchange) is:

$1/2$ cup of cooked vegetables or vegetable juice
1 cup of raw vegetables

Artichoke ($1/2$ medium)

Asparagus

Beans (green, wax, Italian)

Bean sprouts

Beets

Broccoli

Brussels sprouts

Cabbage, cooked

Carrots

Cauliflower

Eggplant

Greens (collard, mustard, turnip)

Kohlrabi

Leeks

Mushrooms, cooked

Okra

Onions

Pea pods

Peppers (green)

Rutabaga

Sauerkraut†

Spinach, cooked

Summer squash (crookneck)

Tomato (one large)

Tomato/vegetable juice†

Turnips

Water chestnuts

Zucchini, cooked

Starchy vegetables such as corn, peas, and potatoes are found on the Starch/bread List.
For free vegetables, see Free Food List.

†400 mg or more of sodium per exchange.

Fruit List

Each item on this list contains about 15 grams of carbohydrate and 60 calories. Fresh, frozen, and dried fruits have about 2 grams of fiber per exchange. Fruits that have 3 or more grams of fiber per exchange have an asterisk (*) symbol. Fruit juices contain very little dietary fiber.

The carbohydrate and calorie content for a fruit exchange are based on the usual serving of the most commonly eaten fruits. Use fresh fruits or fruits frozen or canned without sugar added. Whole fruit is more filling than fruit juice and may be a better choice for those who are trying to lose weight. Unless otherwise noted, the serving size for one fruit exchange is:

$1/2$ cup of fresh fruit or fruit juice
$1/4$ cup of dried fruit

Fresh, Frozen, and Unsweetened Canned Fruit

Apple (raw, 2 in across)	1 apple
Applesauce (unsweetened)	$1/2$ cup
Apricots (medium, raw)	4 apricots
Apricots (canned)	$1/2$ cup, or 4 halves
Banana (9 in long)	$1/2$ banana
Blackberries (raw)*	$3/4$ cup
Blueberries (raw)*	$3/4$ cup
Cantaloupe (5 in across)	$1/3$ melon
(cubes)	1 cup
Cherries (large, raw)	12 cherries
Cherries (canned)	$1/2$ cup
Figs (raw, 2 in across)	2 figs
Fruit cocktail (canned)	$1/2$ cup
Grapefruit (medium)	$1/2$ grapefruit
Grapefruit (segments)	$3/4$ cup
Grapes (small)	15 grapes
Honeydew melon (medium)	$1/8$ melon
(cubes)	1 cup
Kiwi (large)	1 kiwi
Mandarin oranges	$3/4$ cup
Mango (small)	$1/2$ mango
Nectarine ($2^1/2$ in across)*	1 nectarine
Orange ($2^1/2$ in across)	1 orange
Papaya	1 cup
Peach ($2^3/4$ in across)	1 peach, or $3/4$ cup
Peaches (canned)	$1/2$ cup or 2 halves
Pear	$1/2$ large, or 1 small

Pears (canned)	$1/2$ cup, or 2 halves
Persimmon (medium, native)	2 persimmons
Pineapple (raw)	$3/4$ cup
Pineapple (canned)	$1/3$ cup
Plum (raw, 2 in across)	2 plums
Pomegranate*	$1/2$ pomegranate
Raspberries (raw)*	1 cup
Strawberries (raw, whole)*	$1^1/4$ cup
Tangerine ($2^1/2$ in across)*	2 tangerines
Watermelon (cubes)	$1^1/4$ cup

Dried Fruit

Apples*	4 rings
Apricots*	7 halves
Dates	$2^1/2$ medium
Figs*	$1^1/2$
Prunes*	3 medium
Raisins	2 tbsp

Fruit Juice

Apple juice/cider	$1/2$ cup
Cranberry juice cocktail	$1/3$ cup
Grapefruit juice	$1/2$ cup
Grape juice	$1/3$ cup
Orange juice	$1/2$ cup
Pineapple juice	$1/2$ cup
Prune juice	$1/3$ cup

*3 or more grams of fiber per exchange.

Milk List

Each serving of milk or milk products on this list contains about 12 grams of carbohydrate and 8 grams of protein. The amount of fat in milk is measured in percent (%) of butterfat. The calories vary, depending on what kind of milk you choose. The list is divided into three parts based on the amount of fat and calories: skim/very low-fat milk, low-fat milk, and whole milk. One serving (one milk exchange) of each of these includes:

	Carbohydrate (grams)	Protein (grams)	Fat (grams)	Calories (grams)
Skim/very low-fat	12	8	Trace	90
Low-fat	12	8	5	120
Whole	12	8	8	150

Milk is the body's main source of calcium, the mineral needed for growth and repair of bones. Yogurt is also a good source of calcium. Yogurt and many dry or powdered milk products have different amounts of fat. If you have questions about a particular item, read the label to find out the fat and calorie content.

Milk is good to drink, but it can also be added to cereal, and to other foods. Many tasty dishes such as sugar-free pudding are made with milk (see the Combination Foods list). Add life to plain yogurt by adding one of your fruit exchanges to it.

Skim and Very Low-fat Milk

Skim milk	1 cup
1/2% Milk	1 cup
1% Milk	1 cup
Low-fat buttermilk	1 cup
Evaporated skim milk	1/2 cup
Dry nonfat milk	1/3 cup
Plain nonfat yogurt	8 oz

Low-fat Milk

2% Milk	1 cup fluid
Plain low-fat yogurt (with added nonfat milk solids)	8 oz

Whole Milk

The whole milk group has much more fat per serving than the skim and low-fat groups. Whole milk has more than 3 1/4% butterfat. Try to limit your choices from the whole milk group as much as possible.

Whole milk	1 cup
Evaporated whole milk	1/2 cup
Whole plain yogurt	8 oz

Fat List

Each serving on the fat list contains about 5 grams of fat and 45 calories.

The foods on the fat list contain mostly fat, although some items may also contain a small amount of protein. All fats are high in calories and should be carefully measured. Everyone should modify fat intake by eating unsaturated fats instead of saturated fats. The sodium content of these foods varies widely. Check the label for sodium information.

Unsaturated Fats

Avocado	1/8 medium
Margarine	1 tsp
Margarine, diet‡	1 tbsp
Mayonnaise	1 tsp
Mayonnaise, reduced-calorie‡	1 tbsp
Nuts and seeds	
Almonds, dry roasted	6 whole
Cashews, dry roasted	1 tbsp
Pecans	2 whole
Peanuts	20 small or 10 large
Walnuts	2 whole
Other nuts	1 tbsp
Seeds, pine nuts, sunflower (without shells)	1 tbsp
Pumpkin seeds	2 tsp
Oil (corn, cottonseed, safflower, soybean, sunflower, olive, peanut)	1 tsp
Olives‡	10 small or 5 large

Salad dressing, mayonnaise-type	2 tsp
Salad dressing, mayonnaise-type, reduced-calorie	1 tbsp
Salad dressing (oil varieties)‡	1 tbsp
Salad dressing, reduced-calorie†	2 tbsp

(Two tablespoons of low-calorie salad dressing is a free food.)

Saturated Fats

Butter	1 tsp
Bacon‡	1 slice
Chitterlings	1/2 oz
Coconut, shredded	2 tbsp
Coffee whitener, liquid	2 tbsp
Coffee whitener, powder	4 tsp
Cream (light, coffee, table)	2 tbsp
Cream, sour	2 tbsp
Cream (heavy, whipping)	1 tbsp
Cream cheese	1 tbsp
Salt pork‡	1/4 oz

†400 mg or more of sodium per exchange.
‡400 mg or more of sodium if two or more exchanges are eaten.

Free Foods

A free food is any food or drink that contains less than 20 calories per serving. You can eat as much as you want of those items that have no serving size specified. You may eat two or three servings per day of those items that have a specific serving size. Be sure to spread them out through the day.

Drinks
Bouillon† or broth without fat
Bouillon, low-sodium
Carbonated drinks, sugar-free
Carbonated water
Club soda
Cocoa powder, unsweetened (1 tbsp)
Coffee/tea
Drink mixes, sugar-free
Tonic water, sugar-free

Nonstick pan spray

Fruit
Cranberries, unsweetened (1/2 cup)
Rhubarb, unsweetened (1/2 cup)

Vegetables
(raw, 1 cup)
Cabbage
Celery
Chinese cabbage*
Cucumber
Green onion
Hot peppers
Mushrooms
Radishes
Zucchini*

Salad greens
Endive
Escarole
Lettuce
Romaine
Spinach

Sweet substitutes
Candy, hard, sugar-free
Gelatin, sugar-free
Gum, sugar-free
Jam/jelly, sugar-free
  (less than 20 cal/2 tsp)
Pancake syrup, sugar-free (1-2 tbsp)
Sugar substitutes (saccharin, aspartame)
Whipped topping (2 tbsp)

Condiments
Catsup (1 tbsp)
Horseradish
Mustard
Pickles†, dill, unsweetened
Salad dressing, low-calorie (2 tbsp)
Taco sauce (3 tbsp)
Vinegar

Seasonings can be very helpful in making food taste better. Be careful of how much sodium you use. Read the label, and choose those seasonings that do not contain sodium or salt.

Basil (fresh)	Flavoring extracts	Hot pepper sauce	Onion powder	Soy sauce,† low-sodium
Celery seeds	(vanilla, almond,	Lemon	Oregano	("lite")
Chili powder	walnut, peppermint,	Lemon juice	Paprika	Wine, used in cooking
Chives	butter, lemon, etc)	Lemon pepper	Pepper	(1/4 cup)
Cinnamon	Garlic	Lime	Pimento	Worcestershire sauce
Curry	Garlic powder	Lime juice	Spices	
Dill	Herbs	Mint	Soy sauce†	

*3 grams or more of fiber per exchange.
†400 mg or more of sodium per exchange.

Combination Foods

Much of the food we eat is mixed together in various combinations. These combination foods do not fit into only one exchange list. It can be quite hard to tell what is in a certain casserole dish or baked food item. This is a list of average values for some typical combination foods.

Food	Amount	Exchanges
Casseroles, homemade	1 cup (8 oz)	2 starch, 2 medium-fat meat, 1 fat
Cheese pizza,† thin crust	1/4 of 15 oz or 1/4 of 10 in	2 starch, 1 medium-fat meat, 1 fat
Chili with beans*† (commercial)	1 cup (8 oz)	2 starch, 2 medium-fat meat, 2 fat
Chow mein† (without noodles or rice)	2 cups (16 oz)	1 starch, 2 vegetable, 2 lean meat
Macaroni and cheese†	1 cup (8 oz)	2 starch, 1 medium-fat meat, 2 fat
Soup		
Bean*†	1 cup (8 oz)	1 starch, 1 vegetable, 1 lean meat
Chunky, all varieties†	10 3/4 oz can	1 starch, 1 vegetable, 1 medium-fat meat
Cream† (made with water)	1 cup (8 oz)	1 starch, 1 fat
Vegetable† or broth-type†	1 cup (8 oz)	1 starch
Spaghetti and meatballs† (canned)	1 cup (8 oz)	2 starch, 1 medium-fat meat, 1 fat
Sugar-free pudding (made with skim milk)	1/2 cup	1 starch
If beans are used as a meat substitute		
Dried beans,* peas,* lentils*	1 cup (cooked)	2 starch, 1 lean meat

*3 grams or more of fiber per exchange.
†400 mg or more of sodium per exchange.

Foods for Occasional Use

Moderate amounts of some foods can be used in your meal plan, in spite of their sugar and fat content, as long as you maintain calorie and weight control. The following list includes average exchange values for some of these foods. Because they are concentrated sources of carbohydrate, and in some cases fat, you will notice that the portion sizes are very small.

Food	Amount	Exchanges
Angel food cake	1/12 cake	2 starch
Cake, no icing	1/12 cake, or a 3 in square	2 starch, 2 fat
Cookies	2 small (1 3/4 in across)	1 starch, 1 fat
Frozen fruit yogurt	1/3 cup	1 starch
Gingersnaps	3	1 starch
Granola	1/4 cup	1 starch, 1 fat
Granola bars	1 small	1 starch, 1 fat
Ice cream, any flavor	1/2 cup	1 starch, 2 fat
Ice milk, any flavor	1/2 cup	1 starch, 1 fat
Sherbet, any flavor	1/4 cup	1 starch
Snack chips,‡ all varieties	1 oz	1 starch, 2 fat
Vanilla wafers	6 small	1 starch

‡400 mg or more of sodium if two or more exchanges are eaten.

Appendix 9
24-Hour Recall Form

Directions:
1. Use this form to record ALL food and beverages, including snacks and alcoholic beverages, consumed within the last 24 hours.
2. Estimate portion sizes (3 oz of meat is about the size of a deck of cards) and include all liquids in cups or ounces. Be sure to include how the food was prepared (baked, fried, grilled) and any added condiments, fats (margarine, butter, oils, cream), salad dressings, sauces, or sweeteners.
3. Include all medications, food supplements, and vitamin and mineral supplements used.

Date: _____ Day of week: _____

Training routine: _____

Time	Location of Eating	Food/Beverage Item	How Prepared	Portion Size

Appendix 10
Food Frequency Questionnaire

I eat	Never	Seldom (once or less per week)	Sometimes (2-4 times per week)	Often (5-7 times per week)	Frequent (more than once per day)
Beef (3 oz portion size) Regular ground beef Lean ground beef Roast (sirloin, round, chuck) Steak (flank, sirloin, T-bone, porterhouse, tenderloin) Prime grades Corned beef					
Pork (3 oz portion size) Tenderloin Loin roast Center cut loin chops Commercial ground Spareribs Pork sausage					
Poultry (3 oz portion size) Chicken w/skin Chicken w/out skin Turkey Turkey, injected w/butter Chicken franks Goose, duck					
Veal (3 oz portion size) Chops Roast Breast					
Lamb (3 oz portion size) Roast Rib Breast Commercial ground					
Fish (3 oz portion size) Prebreaded, prefried Canned in oil Canned in water Shellfish Fresh or fresh frozen					
Processed meats Cold cuts, 1 oz Hot dogs, 1 medium					
Bread/starch Cold cereal, 1 cup Bran cereal, 1/3 cup Granola cereal, 1/2 cup Plain hot cereals, 1/2 cup Pasta, 1/2 cup Rice, 1/2 cup					

I eat	Never	Seldom (once or less per week)	Sometimes (2-4 times per week)	Often (5-7 times per week)	Frequent (more than once per day)
Pasta, rice in cream sauce, 1/2 cup					
Bread, wheat, rye, white, 1 slice					
English muffin, 1/2 whole					
Bagel, 1/2 whole					
Commercial biscuits, muffins, waffles, pancakes, French toast, 1 piece					
Plain crackers, bread sticks, pretzels, 4 pieces					
Snack crackers, serving varies for 1 oz					
Snack chips, serving varies for 1 oz					
Popcorn, 1 cup					
Fruits/vegetables					
Citrus fruit/juice 1 piece or 4 oz					
Fresh fruit, 1 piece					
Juice, 1/2 cup					
Canned/frozen fruit, 1/2 cup					
Dried fruit, 1/4 cup					
Canned vegetables, 1/2 cup					
Fresh/frozen vegetables, 1/2 cup					
Vegetables in sauce, 1/2 cup					
Raw vegetables, 1/2 cup to 1 cup					
Plain potatoes, 1/2 cup					
French fries, 1/2 cup					
Vegetable juice, 1/2 cup					
Vegetable soup, 1 cup					
Fats					
Butter, 1 tsp					
Margarine, 1 tsp					
Vegetable oil, 1 tsp					
Mayonnaise, 1 tsp					
Commercial salad dressing, 1 tbsp					
Diet salad dressing, 1 tbsp					
Sour cream, 1 tbsp					
Cream cheese, 1 tbsp					
Gravy, 1 tbsp					
Nuts, 12 whole					
Seeds, 1 tbsp					
Bacon, 1 slice					
Beverages					
Regular coffee, 1 cup					
Decaf coffee, 1 cup					
Regular soda, 12 oz					
Diet soda, 12 oz					
Beer, 12 oz					
Wine, 4 oz					
Liquor (whiskey, vodka, gin, brandy, liqueurs), 1 1/2 oz					
Dairy					
Nondairy creamer, 1 tbsp					
Cream, 1 tbsp					
Cheese (cheddar, Swiss, American), 1 oz					
Low-fat cheese product (part-skim), 1 oz					
Cottage cheese, 1/4 cup					
Whole milk, 8 oz					
Low-fat milk (1%-2%), 8 oz					
Skim milk (less than 1/2%), 8 oz					

I eat	Never	Seldom (once or less per week)	Sometimes (2-4 times per week)	Often (5-7 times per week)	Frequent (more than once per day)
Yogurt, low-fat, 8 oz					
Cream soup, 8 oz					
Desserts/sweets					
Pie/cake, 1 slice					
Candy, 1 oz					
Cookies, 2 medium					
Sweet rolls/Danish/doughnuts, 1 regular					
Candy bar, 1 medium					
Jam, jelly, syrup, 1 tbsp					
Chocolate, 1 oz					
Ice cream, 1/2 cup					
Pudding, 1/2 cup					
Ice milk, sherbet, 1/2 cup					
Frozen yogurt, 1/2 cup					
Other					
Frozen entrees, 8-9 oz serving					
Pizza, 1 slice					
Eggs, 1 medium					
Lentils, peas, beans, 1/2 cup					
Peanut butter, 1 tbsp					
Salt substitute, 1 tsp					
Sugar, 1 tsp					

How many times do you eat daily? _____

How many snacks do you eat daily? _____

Do you routinely eat breakfast? _____

lunch? _____

dinner? _____

Appendix 11
Food Diary

Directions:
1. Use this form to record ALL food and beverages, including snacks and alcoholic beverages, consumed on each day that the diary is kept. To assure the MOST accurate record, it is best to record items immediately after they are consumed.
2. Estimate portion sizes (3 oz of meat is about the size of a deck of cards) or measure items when possible. Record all liquids in cups or ounces. Be sure to include how the food is prepared (baked, fried, grilled) and any added condiments, fats (margarine, butter, oils, cream), salad dressings, sauces, or sweeteners. Where possible, save the label of unusual food items and/or convenience foods consumed.
3. Include all medications, food supplements, and vitamin and mineral supplements used each day and the amounts used.
4. Rate hunger on a scale of 1 to 5 (1 = low, 5 = high).

Date: _____ Day of week: _____

Training routine: _____

Time	Location of Eating	Food/Beverage Item	How Prepared	Portion Size	Hunger Rating (1-5)

Appendix 12

USDA Recommended Weight Standards

Height	Weight (lb)	
	Ages 19-34	Age 35+
5'0	97-128	108-138
5'1	101-132	111-143
5'2	104-137	115-148
5'3	107-141	119-152
5'4	111-146	122-157
5'5	114-150	126-162
5'6	118-155	130-167
5'7	121-160	134-172
5'8	125-164	138-178
5'9	129-169	142-183
5'10	132-174	146-188
5'11	136-179	151-194
6'0	140-184	155-199
6'1	144-189	159-205
6'2	148-195	164-210
6'3	152-200	168-216
6'4	156-205	173-222
6'5	160-211	177-228
6'6	164-216	182-234

From *Nutrition and Your Health: Dietary Guidelines for Americans.* Washington, DC: US Dept of Agriculture and US Dept of Health and Human Services; 1990. Home and Garden bulletin 232.

Appendix 13
Body-Composition Measurement Equipment

EQUIPMENT

Stadiometers, scales, miscellaneous
Holtain, Ltd
Pfister Import-Export, Inc

Harpenden stadiometer, portable, pocket
Raven Equipment, Ltd
Stanley-Mabo, Ltd
CMS Weighing Equipment, Ltd

Holtain electronic stadiometer
Holtain, Ltd

Blueprints for the production of stadiometers
Centers for Disease Control

Anthropometers
Harpenden anthropometer
Pfister Import-Export, Inc
Holtain, Ltd

GPM (Martin type) anthropometer
Pfister Import-Export, Inc
Owl Instruments, Inc

Recumbent length/sitting height measurement equipment
Infant heightometer
Hultafors AB
Infanitometer Instrumentation Corporation

Baby length measurer
Appropriate Health Resources and Technologies Action Group (AHRTAC)

Harpenden sitting height table
Harpenden neonatometer
Harpenden infantometer
Holtain electronic infantometer
Harpenden supine measuring table
Holtain, Ltd

Weighing scales
Designs for making scales locally
Hesperian Foundation
AHRTAC
Continental Scale Corporation
CMS Weighing Equipment, Ltd
Detecto Scales, Inc.
Salter International Measurement, Ltd
Marsden Weighing Machine Group, Ltd

Dial scales for field work
CMS Weighing Equipment, Ltd (model 235-PBW)
Salter International Measurement, Ltd (model 235)
John Chatillon and Sons
Rasmussen, Webb & Co

Electronic scales:
Toledo scale
Infant scale: "Baby weight" model 1365
Children/adult scales: "Weight plate"
a. Pediatric 12" × 12" plate, 150-lb capacity model 2300
b. Adult 18" × 18" plate, 300-lb capacity model 2300

Calipers
Sliding calipers (large)
Mediform sliding caliper (80 mm)

Sliding calipers (small)
Sliding caliper (Martin type)
Sliding caliper (Holtain, 14 cm)
Sliding caliper (Poech type)
Pfister Import-Export, Inc

Spreading calipers
Spreading caliper (Martin type) 0–300 mm
Spreading caliper (Martin type 0–600 mm
Pfister Import-Export, Inc

Adapted from *Anthropometric Standardization Reference Manual* (pp 161-164) by TG Lohman, AF Roche, and R Martorell, 1988, Champaign, IL: Human Kinetics. Copyright 1988 by Timothy G Lohman, Alex F Roche, and Reynoldo Martorell. Reprinted by permission.

Anthropometric tapes

Disposable paper tape for newly born infants
  Medline Industries

Retractable, fiberglass measuring tape
  Buffalo Medical Specialties (available through local distributors, eg, Burlingame Surgical Supply Co)

Retractable, flexible steel tape
  Keuffel and Esser Co. (200 cm no. 860358) (available through local distributors, eg, San Diego Blueprint)

Scoville-Dritz fiberglass measuring tape
  (available through local distributors, eg, Quinton Instruments)

Inser-Tape, Ross insertion tape
  Ross Laboratories

Linen measuring tape
  Pfister Import-Export, Inc

Gulick measuring tape
  Country Technology, Inc

Anthropometric tape measure (150 cm no. 67022)
  Country Technology, Inc

Skinfold calipers

Harpenden skinfold calipers
  H.E. Morse Co
  British Indicators, Ltd

Lange skinfold calipers
  Cambridge Scientific Industries
  Pfister Import-Export, Inc
  J.A. Preston Corp
  Owl Industries, Ltd

Lafayette skinfold calipers
  Lafayette Instrument Co

Slim Guide skinfold caliper
  Creative Health Products
  Rosscraft, Ltd
  Country Technology, Inc

Skyndex electronic body fat calculator—System I and II
  Cramer Products
  Human Performance Systems, Inc

Fat-O-Meter skinfold caliper
  Health & Education Services
  Miller & Sons Assoc, Inc

Fat Control caliper
  Fat Control, Inc

Adipometer skinfold caliper
  Ross Laboratories

McGaw skinfold caliper
  McGaw Laboratories

Holtain/Tanner/Whitehouse skinfold caliper and Holtain Slim-Kit caliper
  Holtain, Ltd
  Pfister Import-Export, Inc

Miscellaneous by Supplier

Pfister Import-Export, Inc
  Harpenden Vernier caliper
  Survey set—contains: anthropometer, skinfold caliper, 2 steel tapes, somatotype turntable, manual
  Base plate for anthropometer
  Curved cross bars
  Small instrument bag (Martin type) contains: sliding caliper, spreading caliper, steel measuring tape
  Large instrument bag (Martin type) contains: anthropometer, recurved measuring branches, sliding caliper, spreading caliper, steel measuring tape

SUPPLIERS

AHRTAC
85 Marlebone High St
London, W1M 3DE, UK

British Indicators, Ltd
Sutton Rd
St Albans, Herts UK

Burlingame Surgical Supply Co
1515 4th Ave
San Diego, CA 92101
Phone: 619/231-0187

Cambridge Scientific Industries
PO Box 265
Cambridge, MD 21613
Phone: 800/638-9566
301/228-5111

Centers for Disease Control
Division of Nutrition
1600 Clifton Rd
Atlanta, GA 30333

CMS Weighing Equipment, Ltd
18 Camden High St
London, NWI OJH, UK

Continental Scale Corp
7400 W 100th Pl
Bridgeview, IL 60455
Phone: 708/598-9100

Country Technology, Inc
PO Box 87
Gays Mills, WI 54631
Phone: 608/735-4718

Cramer Products
PO Box 1001
Gardner, KS 66030
Phone: 913/884-7511

Creative Health Products
5148 Saddle Ridge Rd
Plymouth, MI 48170
Phone: 313/453-5309
313/455-0177

Detecto Scales, Inc
Detecto International
103-00 Foster Ave
Brooklyn, NY 11236

Fat Control, Inc
PO Box 10117
Towson, MD 21204

H.E. Morse Co
455 Douglas Ave
Holland, MI 49423
Phone: 616/396-4604

Health & Education Services
Division of Novel Products
80 Fairbanks, Unit 12
Addison, IL 60101
Phone: 708/628-1787

Hesperian Foundation
PO Box 1692
Palo Alto, CA 94302

Holtain, Ltd
Crosswell, Crymmych, Dyfed
Wales

Hultafors AB
S-517 01 Bollebygd
Sweden

Human Performance Systems, Inc
PO Drawer 1324
Fayetteville, AR 72701
Phone: 501/521-3180

Infanitometer Instrumentation Corp
Elimeankatv-22-24
SF-00510
Helsinki, No. 51
Finland

J.A. Preston Corp
71 5th Ave
New York, NY 10003

John Chatillon and Sons
83-30 Kew Gardens Rd
Kew Gardens, NY 11415

Lafayette Instrument Co
PO Box 5729
Lafayette, IN 47903
Phone: 317/423-1505

McGaw Laboratories
Division of American Hospital Supply
Irvine, CA 92714

Marsden Weighing Machine Group, Ltd
388 Harrow Rd
London WG-2HV, UK

Mediform sliding caliper
5150 SW Griffith Dr
Beaverton, OR 97005
Phone: 800/633-3676
503/643-1670

Medline Industries
1825 Shermer Rd
Northbrook, IL 60062
Phone: 800/323-5886

Miller & Sons Assoc, Inc
New Rochelle, NY 10801

Owl Industries, Ltd
177 Idema Rd
Markham, Ontario L3R 1A9
Canada

Pfister Import-Export, Inc
450 Barell Ave
Carlstadt, NJ 07072
Phone: 201/939-4606

Quinton Instruments
2121 Terry Ave
Seattle, WA 98121
Phone: 800/426-0538
206/223-7373

Rasmussen, Webb & Co
1st Floor
12116 Laystall St
London ECIR-4UB, UK

Raven Equipment, Ltd
Little Easton
Dunmow, Essex, CM6 2ES, UK

Ross Laboratories
625 Cleveland Ave
Columbus, OH 43216

Rosscraft, Ltd
14732 16-A Ave
Surrey, BC V4A 5M7
Canada
Phone: 604/531-5049

Salter International Measurement, Ltd
George St
West Bromwich, Staffs, UK

San Diego Blueprint
4696 Ruffner Rd
San Diego, CA 92111
Phone: 619/565-4696

Toledo Scale
431 Ohio Pike
Suite 302, Way Cross Office Park
Toledo, OH
Phone: 513/528-2300

Appendix 14

Height/Wrist and Elbow Breadth

Estimating Frame Size From Height/Wrist Circumference Ratios

Frame Size	Men	Women
Small	>10.4	>11.0
Medium	9.6-10.4	10.1-11.0
Large	<9.6	<10.1

The wrist is measured where it bends (distal to the styloid process) on the right arm.

Adapted by permission from *Understanding Nutrition,* 2nd ed, by E.N. Whitney and M.N. Hamilton; copyright © 1984 by West Publishing Company. All rights reserved.

Measurement of wrist circumference

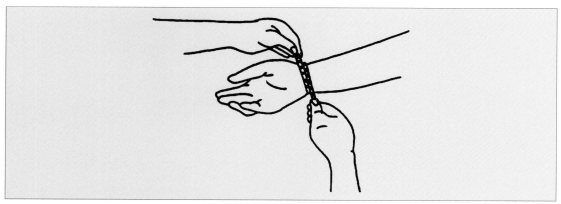

From Grant A, DeHoog S. *Nutritional Assessment and Support.* 4th ed. Seattle, Wash: Grant and DeHoog; 1991. Used by permission.

Frame Size by Elbow Breadth (cm) of US Male and Female Adults Derived From the Combined NHANES I and II Data Sets

Age, y	Frame Size		
	Small	Medium	Large
Males			
18-24	≤6.6	>6.6 and <7.7	≥7.7
25-34	≤6.7	>6.7 and <7.9	≥7.9
35-44	≤6.7	>6.7 and <8.0	≥8.0
45-54	≤6.7	>6.7 and <8.1	≥8.1
55-64	≤6.7	>6.7 and <8.1	≥8.1
65-74	≤6.7	>6.7 and <8.1	≥8.1
Females			
18-24	≤5.6	>5.6 and <6.5	≥6.5
25-34	≤5.7	>5.7 and <6.8	≥6.8
35-44	≤5.7	>5.7 and <7.1	≥7.1
45-54	≤5.7	>5.7 and <7.2	≥7.2
55-64	≤5.8	>5.8 and <7.2	≥7.2
65-74	≤5.8	>5.8 and <7.2	≥7.2

From Frisancho R. New standards of weight and body composition by frame size and height for assessment of nutritional status of adults and the elderly. © *Am J Clin Nutr.* 1984;40:806-819. American Society for Clinical Nutrition.

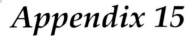

Appendix 15

Metropolitan Insurance Company Height and Weight Tables

Desirable Weight Ranges—Age 25 and Over*

Height (no shoes)		Men		Woment	
ft	in	Weight Range	Weight‡ MRW = 100	Weight Range	Weight MRW =100
4	9			90-118	100
4	10			92-121	103
4	11			95-124	106
5	0			98-127	109
5	1	105-134	117	101-130	112
5	2	108-137	120	104-134	116
5	3	111-141	123	107-138	120
5	4	114-145	126	110-142	124
5	5	117-149	129	114-146	128
5	6	121-154	133	118-150	132
5	7	125-159	138	122-154	136
5	8	129-163	142	126-159	140
5	9	133-167	146	130-164	144
5	10	137-172	150	134-169	148
5	11	141-177	155		
6	0	145-182	159		
6	1	149-187	164		
6	2	153-192	169		
6	3	157-197	174		

*Adapted from the 1959 Metropolitan Desirable Weight Table (weight in pounds, without clothing; height without shoes).

†For women between the ages of 18 and 25, subtract one pound for each year under 25.

‡Midpoint of medium frame range used to compute MRW: MRW = [(actual weight)/(midpoint of medium frame range)] x 100.

Adapted from Simopoulos AP. Dietary control of hypertension and obesity and body weight standards. Reprinted from *J Am Diet Assoc.* 1985;85:419.

1983 Metropolitan Height and Weight Tables

	Men				Women		
Height		Weight		Height		Weight	
	Small	Medium	Large		Small	Medium	Large
ft in	Frame	Frame	Frame	ft in	Frame	Frame	Frame
5 2	128-134	131-141	138-150	4 10	102-111	109-121	118-131
5 3	130-136	133-143	140-153	4 11	103-113	111-123	120-134
5 4	132-138	135-145	142-156	5 0	104-115	113-126	122-137
5 5	134-140	137-148	144-160	5 1	106-118	115-129	125-140
5 6	136-142	139-151	146-164	5 2	108-121	118-132	128-143
5 7	138-145	142-154	149-168	5 3	111-124	121-135	131-147
5 8	140-148	145-157	152-172	5 4	114-127	124-138	134-151
5 9	142-151	148-160	155-176	5 5	117-130	127-141	137-155
5 10	144-154	151-163	158-180	5 6	120-133	130-144	140-159
5 11	146-157	154-166	161-184	5 7	123-136	133-147	143-163
6 0	149-160	157-170	164-188	5 8	126-139	136-150	146-167
6 1	152-164	160-174	168-192	5 9	129-142	139-153	149-170
6 2	155-168	164-178	172-197	5 10	132-145	142-156	152-173
6 3	158-172	167-182	176-202	5 11	135-148	145-159	155-176
6 4	162-176	171-187	181-207	6 0	138-151	148-162	158-179

Weights at ages 25-29 based on lowest mortality. Weights in pounds according to frame (in indoor clothing weighing 5 lb for men or 3 lb for women, shoes with 1-in heels.)

Adapted from Metropolitan Life Insurance Company, 1 Madison Ave, New York, NY 10010. Reprinted with permission.

Appendix 16

Triceps Skinfold Percentiles, Arm Muscle Circumference Percentiles, Arm Muscle Area Percentiles

Triceps Skinfold Percentiles (mm), Males

Age	5th	10th	25th	50th	75th	90th	95th
1-2	6	7	8	10	12	14	16
2-3	6	7	8	10	12	14	15
3-4	6	7	8	10	11	14	15
4-5	6	7	8	10	11	14	15
5-6	6	6	8	9	11	12	14
6-7	6	6	8	9	11	14	15
7-8	5	6	7	8	10	13	16
8-9	5	6	7	9	12	15	17
9-10	5	6	7	8	10	13	16
10-11	6	6	7	10	13	17	18
11-12	6	6	8	10	14	18	21
12-13	6	6	8	11	16	20	24
13-14	6	6	8	11	14	22	28
14-15	5	5	7	10	14	22	26
15-16	4	5	7	9	14	21	24
16-17	4	5	6	8	11	18	24
17-18	4	5	6	8	12	16	22
18-19	5	5	6	8	12	16	19
19-25	4	5	6	9	13	20	24
25-35	4	5	7	10	15	20	22
35-45	5	6	8	12	16	20	24
45-55	5	6	8	12	16	20	23
55-65	6	6	8	12	15	20	25
65-75	5	6	8	11	14	19	22
75-80	4	6	8	11	15	19	22

Adapted from Frisancho A. New norms of upper limb fat and muscle areas for assessment of nutritional status. © *Am J Clin Nutr.* 1981;34:2540. American Society for Clinical Nutrition.

Triceps Skinfold Percentiles (mm), Females

Age	5th	10th	25th	50th	75th	90th	95th
1-2	6	7	8	10	12	14	16
2-3	6	8	9	10	12	15	16
3-4	7	8	9	11	12	14	15
4-5	7	8	8	10	12	14	16
5-6	6	7	8	10	12	15	18
6-7	6	6	8	10	12	14	16
7-8	6	7	9	11	13	16	18
8-9	6	8	9	12	15	18	24
9-10	8	8	10	13	16	20	22
10-11	7	8	10	12	17	23	27
11-12	7	8	10	13	18	24	28
12-13	8	9	11	14	18	23	27
13-14	8	8	12	15	21	26	30
14-15	9	10	13	16	21	26	28
15-16	8	10	12	17	21	25	32
16-17	10	12	15	18	22	26	31
17-18	10	12	13	19	24	30	37
18-19	10	12	15	18	22	26	30
19-25	10	11	14	18	24	30	34
25-35	10	12	16	21	27	34	37
35-45	12	14	18	23	29	35	38
45-55	12	16	20	25	30	36	40
55-65	12	16	20	25	31	36	38
65-75	12	14	18	24	29	34	36

Arm Muscle Circumference Percentiles (mm), Males

Age	5th	10th	25th	50th	75th	90th	95th
1-2	110	113	119	127	135	144	147
2-3	111	114	122	130	140	146	150
3-4	117	123	131	137	143	148	153
4-5	123	126	133	141	148	156	159
5-6	128	133	140	147	154	162	169
6-7	131	135	142	151	161	170	177
7-8	137	139	151	160	168	177	190
8-9	140	145	154	162	170	182	187
9-10	151	154	161	170	183	196	202
10-11	156	160	166	180	191	209	221
11-12	159	165	173	183	195	205	230
12-13	167	171	182	195	210	223	241
13-14	172	179	196	211	226	238	245
14-15	189	199	212	223	240	260	264
15-16	199	204	218	237	254	266	272
16-17	213	225	234	249	269	287	296
17-18	224	231	245	258	273	294	312
18-19	226	237	252	264	283	298	324
19-25	238	245	257	273	289	309	321
25-35	243	250	264	279	298	314	326
35-45	247	255	269	286	302	318	327
45-55	239	249	265	281	300	315	326
55-65	236	245	260	278	295	310	320
65-75	223	235	251	268	284	298	306

Arm Muscle Circumference Percentiles (mm), Females

Age	5th	10th	25th	50th	75th	90th	95th
1-2	105	111	117	124	132	139	143
2-3	111	114	119	126	133	142	147
3-4	113	119	124	132	140	146	152
4-5	115	121	128	136	144	152	157
5-6	125	128	134	142	151	159	165
6-7	130	133	138	145	154	166	171
7-8	129	135	142	151	160	171	176
8-9	138	140	151	160	171	183	194
9-10	147	150	158	167	180	194	198
10-11	148	150	159	170	180	190	197
11-12	150	158	171	181	196	217	223
12-13	162	166	180	191	201	214	220
13-14	169	175	183	198	211	226	240
14-15	174	179	190	201	216	232	247
15-16	175	178	189	202	215	228	244
16-17	170	180	190	202	216	234	249
17-18	175	183	194	205	221	239	257
18-19	174	179	191	202	215	237	245
19-25	179	185	195	207	221	236	249
25-35	183	188	199	212	228	246	264
35-45	186	192	205	218	236	257	272
45-55	187	193	206	220	238	260	274
55-65	187	196	209	225	244	266	280
65-75	185	195	208	225	244	264	279

Arm Muscle Area Percentiles (mm²), Males

Age	5th	10th	25th	50th	75th	90th	95th
1-2	956	1014	1133	1278	1447	1644	1720
2-3	973	1040	1190	1345	1557	1690	1787
3-4	1095	1201	1357	1484	1618	1750	1853
4-5	1207	1264	1408	1579	1747	1926	2008
5-6	1298	1411	1550	1720	1884	2089	2285
6-7	1360	1447	1605	1815	2056	2297	2493
7-8	1497	1548	1808	2027	2246	2494	2886
8-9	1550	1664	1895	2089	2296	2628	2788
9-10	1811	1884	2067	2288	2657	3053	3257
10-11	1930	2027	2182	2575	2903	3486	3882
11-12	2016	2156	2382	2670	3022	3359	4226
12-13	2216	2339	2649	3022	3496	3968	4640
13-14	2363	2546	3044	3553	4081	4502	4794
14-15	2830	3147	3586	3963	4575	5368	5530
15-16	3138	3317	3788	4481	5134	5631	5900
16-17	3625	4044	4352	4951	5753	6576	6980
17-18	3998	4252	4777	5286	5950	6886	7726
18-19	4070	4481	5066	5552	6374	7067	8355
19-25	4508	4777	5274	5913	6660	7606	8200
25-35	4694	4963	5541	6214	7067	7847	8436
35-45	4844	5181	5740	6490	7265	8034	8488
45-55	4546	4946	5589	6297	7142	7918	8458
55-65	4422	4783	5381	6144	6919	7670	8149
65-75	3973	4411	5031	5716	6432	7074	7458

Arm Muscle Area Percentiles (mm²), Females

Age	5th	10th	25th	50th	75th	90th	95th
1-2	885	973	1084	1221	1378	1535	1621
2-3	973	1029	1119	1269	1405	1595	1727
3-4	1014	1133	1227	1396	1563	1690	1846
4-5	1058	1171	1313	1475	1644	1832	1958
5-6	1238	1301	1423	1598	1825	2012	2159
6-7	1354	1414	1513	1683	1877	2182	2323
7-8	1330	1441	1602	1815	2045	2332	2469
8-9	1513	1566	1808	2034	2327	2657	2996
9-10	1723	1788	1976	2227	2571	2987	3112
10-11	1740	1784	2019	2296	2583	2873	3093
11-12	1784	1987	2316	2612	3071	3739	3953
12-13	2092	2182	2579	2904	3225	3655	3847
13-14	2269	2426	2657	3130	3529	4081	4568
14-15	2418	2562	2874	3220	3704	4294	4850
15-16	2426	2518	2847	3248	3689	4123	4756
16-17	2308	2567	2865	3248	3718	4353	4946
17-18	2442	2674	2996	3336	3883	4552	5251
18-19	2398	2538	2917	3243	3694	4461	4767
19-25	2538	2728	3026	3406	3877	4439	4940
25-35	2661	2826	3148	3573	4138	4806	5541
35-45	2750	2946	3359	3783	4428	5240	5877
45-55	2784	2956	3378	3858	4520	5375	5964
55-65	2784	3063	3477	4045	4750	5632	6247
65-75	2737	3018	3444	4019	4739	5566	6214

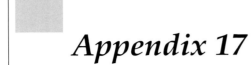

Appendix 17

Skinfold Measurement Data Collection Form and Prediction Tables

Skinfold Measurements

Name_____Date_____Age_____Sex_____Height_____Weight_____

Measurements:

_____ Chest

_____ Abdominal

_____ Thigh

_____ Triceps

_____ Suprailium

_____ Axilla

_____ Subscapular

_____ Total

Calculations: (Use appropriate formula)

_____ Body fat %

_____ Pounds of fat

_____ Pounds of LBW

_____ Classification

_____ Ideal body weight

Percentage Body Fat—Classifications*

Classification	Male	Female
Lean	Less than 8%	Less than 15%
Healthy	8-15%	15-22%
Plump	16-19%	23-27%
Fat	20-24%	28-33%
Obese (overfat)	Above 24%	Above 33%

Note: Average college male = 15%   Average college female = 25%

Average middle-aged American male = 23%   Average middle-aged American female = 32%

Athletic Norms

Long distance runners (elite)	4- 9%	6-15%
Wrestlers	4-10%	—
Gymnasts	4-10%	10-17%
Competitive body builders	6-10%	10-17%
Swimmers (elite)	5-11%	14-24%
Basketball athletes	7-11%	18-27%
Tennis players	14-17%	19-22%

*Body fat ranges vary depending on type of equipment and regression equation used for calculation.

From Nieman DC. *The Sports Medicine Fitness Course.* Palo Alto, Calif: Bull Publishing Co; 1986. Used by permission.

Percentage of Body Fat Based on Four Skinfold Measurements*

Skinfolds	Males (age in y)				Females (age in y)			
(mm)	17-29	30-39	40-49	50+	16-29	30-39	40-49	50+
15	4.8	—	—	—	10.5	—	—	—
20	8.1	12.2	12.2	12.6	14.1	17.0	19.8	21.4
25	10.5	14.2	15.0	15.6	16.8	19.4	22.2	24.0
30	12.9	16.2	17.7	18.6	19.5	21.8	24.5	26.6
35	14.7	17.7	19.6	20.8	21.5	23.7	26.4	28.5
40	16.4	19.2	21.4	22.9	23.4	25.5	28.2	30.3
45	17.7	20.4	23.0	24.7	25.0	26.9	29.6	31.9
50	19.0	21.5	24.6	26.5	26.5	28.2	31.0	33.4

Skinfolds	Males (age in y)				Females (age in y)			
(mm)	17-29	30-39	40-49	50+	16-29	30-39	40-49	50+
55	20.1	22.5	25.9	27.9	27.8	29.4	32.1	34.6
60	21.2	23.5	27.1	29.2	29.1	30.6	33.2	35.7
65	22.2	24.3	28.2	30.4	30.2	31.6	34.1	36.7
70	23.1	25.1	28.3	31.6	31.2	32.5	35.0	37.7
75	24.0	25.9	30.3	32.7	32.2	33.4	35.9	38.7
80	24.8	26.6	31.2	33.8	33.1	34.3	36.7	39.6
85	25.5	27.2	32.1	34.8	34.0	35.1	37.5	40.4
90	26.2	27.8	33.0	35.8	34.8	35.8	38.3	41.2
95	26.9	28.4	33.7	36.6	35.6	36.5	39.0	41.9
100	27.6	29.0	34.4	37.4	36.4	37.2	39.7	42.6
105	28.2	29.6	35.1	38.2	37.1	37.9	40.4	43.3
110	28.8	30.1	35.8	39.0	37.8	38.6	41.0	43.9
115	29.4	30.6	36.4	39.7	38.4	39.1	41.5	44.5
120	30.0	31.1	37.0	40.4	39.0	39.6	42.0	45.1
125	30.5	31.5	37.6	41.1	39.6	40.1	42.5	45.7
130	31.0	31.9	38.2	41.8	40.2	40.6	43.0	46.2
135	31.5	32.3	38.7	42.4	40.8	41.1	43.5	46.7
140	32.0	32.7	39.2	43.0	41.3	41.6	44.0	47.2
145	32.5	33.1	39.7	43.6	41.8	42.1	44.5	47.7
150	32.9	33.5	40.2	44.1	42.3	42.6	45.0	48.2
155	33.3	33.9	40.7	44.6	42.8	43.1	45.4	48.7
160	33.7	34.3	41.2	45.1	43.3	43.6	45.8	49.2
165	34.1	34.6	41.6	45.6	43.7	44.0	46.2	49.6
170	34.5	34.8	42.0	46.1	44.1	44.4	46.6	50.0
175	34.9	—	—	—	—	44.8	47.0	50.4
180	35.3	—	—	—	—	45.2	47.4	50.8
185	35.6	—	—	—	—	45.6	47.8	51.2
190	35.9	—	—	—	—	45.9	48.2	51.6
195	—	—	—	—	—	46.2	48.5	52.0
200	—	—	—	—	—	46.5	48.8	52.4
205	—	—	—	—	—	—	49.1	52.7
210	—	—	—	—	—	—	49.4	53.0

From Durnin JVGA, Wormersley J. Body fat assessed from total body density and its estimation from skinfold thickness: measurements on 481 men and women aged from 16-72 years. *Br J Nutr.* 1974;32:77. Used by permission

*Measurements made on the right side of the body using biceps, triceps, subscapular, and suprailiac skinfolds.

Percentage Fat Estimate for Men: Sum of Chest, Abdomen, and Thigh Skinfolds

Sum of Skinfolds (mm)	Age to Last Year								
	Under 22	23-27	28-32	33-37	38-42	43-47	48-52	53-57	Over 57
8-10	1.3	1.8	2.3	2.9	3.4	3.9	4.5	5.0	5.5
11-13	2.2	2.8	3.3	3.9	4.4	4.9	5.5	6.0	6.5
14-16	3.2	3.8	4.3	4.8	5.4	5.9	6.4	7.0	7.5
17-19	4.2	4.7	5.3	5.8	6.3	6.9	7.4	8.0	8.5
20-22	5.1	5.7	6.2	6.8	7.3	7.9	8.4	8.9	9.5
23-25	6.1	6.6	7.2	7.7	8.3	8.8	9.4	9.9	10.5
26-28	7.0	7.6	8.1	8.7	9.0	9.8	10.3	10.9	11.4
29-31	8.0	8.5	9.1	9.6	10.2	40.7	11.3	11.8	12.4
32-34	8.9	9.4	10.0	10.5	11.1	11.6	12.2	12.8	13.3
35-37	9.8	10.4	10.9	11.5	12.0	12.6	13.1	13.7	14.3
38-40	10.7	11.3	11.8	12.4	12.9	13.5	14.1	14.6	15.2
41-43	11.6	12.2	12.7	13.3	13.8	14.4	15.0	15.5	16.1
44-46	12.5	13.1	13.6	14.2	14.7	15.3	15.9	16.4	17.0
47-49	13.4	13.9	14.5	15.1	15.6	16.2	16.8	17.3	17.9
50-52	14.3	14.8	15.4	15.9	16.5	17.1	17.6	18.2	18.8
53-55	15.1	15.7	16.2	16.8	17.4	17.9	18.5	19.1	19.7
56-58	16.0	16.5	17.1	17.7	18.2	18.8	19.4	20.0	20.5
59-61	16.9	17.4	17.9	18.5	19.1	19.7	20.2	20.8	21.4
62-64	17.6	18.2	18.8	19.4	19.9	20.5	21.1	21.7	22.2

Sum of Skinfolds (mm)	Age to Last Year Under 22	23-27	28-32	33-37	38-42	43-47	48-52	53-57	Over 57
65-67	18.5	19.0	19.6	20.2	20.8	21.3	21.9	22.5	23.1
68-70	19.3	19.9	20.4	21.0	21.6	22.2	22.7	23.3	23.9
71-73	20.1	20.7	21.2	21.8	22.4	23.0	23.6	24.1	24.7
74-76	20.9	21.5	22.0	22.6	23.2	23.8	24.4	25.0	25.5
77-79	21.7	23.2	22.8	23.4	24.0	24.6	25.2	25.8	26.3
80-82	22.4	23.0	23.6	24.2	24.8	25.4	25.9	26.5	27.1
83-85	23.2	23.8	24.4	25.0	25.5	26.1	26.7	27.3	27.9
86-88	24.0	24.5	25.1	25.7	26.3	26.9	27.5	28.1	28.7
89-91	24.7	25.3	25.9	26.5	27.1	27.6	28.2	28.8	29.4
92-94	25.4	26.0	26.6	27.2	27.8	28.4	29.0	29.6	30.2
95-97	26.1	26.7	27.3	27.9	28.5	29.1	29.7	30.3	30.9
98-100	26.9	27.4	28.0	28.6	29.2	29.8	30.4	31.0	31.6
101-103	27.5	28.1	28.7	29.3	29.9	30.5	31.1	31.7	32.3
104-106	28.2	28.8	29.4	30.0	30.6	31.2	31.8	32.4	33.0
107-109	28.9	29.5	30.1	30.7	31.3	31.9	32.5	33.1	33.7
110-112	29.6	30.2	30.8	31.4	32.0	32.6	33.2	33.8	34.4
113-115	30.2	30.8	31.4	32.0	32.6	33.2	33.8	34.5	35.1
116-118	30.9	31.5	32.1	32.7	33.3	33.9	34.5	35.1	35.7
119-121	31.5	32.1	32.7	33.3	33.9	34.5	35.1	35.7	36.4
122-124	32.1	32.7	33.3	33.9	34.5	35.1	35.8	36.4	37.0
125-127	32.7	33.3	33.9	34.5	35.1	35.8	36.4	37.0	37.6

From Jackson AS, Pollock ML. Practical assessment of body composition. *Phys Sports Med*. 1985;13:76-89. Used by permission.

Percentage Fat Estimate for Women: Sum of Triceps, Suprailium, and Thigh Skinfolds

Sum of Skinfolds (mm)	Age to Last Year Under 22	23-27	28-32	33-37	38-42	43-47	48-52	53-57	Over 57
23-25	9.7	9.9	10.2	10.4	10.7	10.9	11.2	11.4	11.7
26-28	11.0	11.2	11.5	11.7	12.0	12.3	12.5	12.7	13.0
29-31	12.3	12.5	12.8	13.0	13.3	13.5	13.8	14.0	14.3
32-34	13.6	13.8	14.0	14.3	14.5	14.8	15.0	15.3	15.5
35-37	14.8	15.0	15.3	15.5	15.8	16.0	16.3	16.5	16.8
38-40	16.0	16.3	16.5	16.7	17.0	17.2	17.5	17.7	18.0
41-43	17.2	17.4	17.7	17.9	18.2	18.4	18.7	18.9	19.2
44-46	18.3	18.6	18.8	19.1	19.3	19.8	19.8	20.1	20.3
47-49	19.5	19.7	20.0	20.2	20.5	20.7	21.0	21.2	21.5
50-52	20.6	20.8	21.1	21.3	21.6	21.8	22.1	22.3	22.6
53-55	21.7	21.9	22.1	22.4	22.6	22.9	23.1	23.4	23.6
56-58	22.7	23.0	23.2	23.4	23.7	23.9	24.2	24.4	24.7
59-61	23.7	24.0	24.2	24.5	24.7	25.0	25.2	25.5	25.7
62-64	24.7	25.0	25.2	25.5	25.7	26.0	26.7	26.4	26.7
65-67	25.7	25.9	26.2	26.4	26.7	26.9	27.2	27.4	27.7
68-70	26.6	26.9	27.1	27.4	27.6	27.9	28.1	28.4	28.6
71-73	27.5	27.8	28.0	28.3	28.5	28.8	29.0	29.3	29.5
74-76	28.4	28.7	28.9	29.2	29.4	29.7	29.9	30.2	30.4
77-79	29.3	29.5	29.8	30.0	30.3	30.5	30.8	31.0	31.3
80-82	30.1	30.4	30.6	30.9	31.1	31.4	31.6	31.9	32.1
83-85	30.9	31.2	31.4	31.7	31.9	32.2	32.4	32.7	32.9
86-88	31.7	32.0	32.2	32.5	32.7	32.9	33.2	33.4	33.7
89-91	32.5	32.7	33.0	33.2	33.5	33.7	33.9	34.2	34.4
92-94	33.2	33.4	33.7	33.9	34.2	34.4	34.7	34.9	35.2
95-97	33.9	34.1	34.4	34.6	34.9	35.1	35.4	35.6	35.9
98-100	34.6	34.8	35.1	35.3	35.5	35.8	36.0	36.3	36.5
101-103	35.3	35.4	35.7	35.9	36.2	36.4	36.7	36.9	37.2
104-106	35.8	36.1	36.3	36.6	36.8	37.1	37.3	37.5	37.8
107-109	36.4	36.7	36.9	37.1	37.4	37.6	37.9	38.1	38.4
110-112	37.0	37.2	37.5	37.7	38.0	38.2	38.5	38.7	38.9
113-115	37.5	37.8	38.0	38.2	38.5	38.7	39.0	39.2	39.5
116-118	38.0	38.3	38.5	38.8	39.0	39.3	39.5	39.7	40.0

Sum of Skinfolds (mm)	Age to Last Year								
	Under 22	23-27	28-32	33-37	38-42	43-47	48-52	53-57	Over 57
119-121	38.5	38.7	39.0	39.2	39.5	39.7	40.0	40.2	40.5
122-124	39.0	39.2	39.4	39.7	39.9	40.2	40.4	40.7	40.9
125-127	39.4	39.6	39.9	40.1	40.4	40.6	40.9	41.4	41.4
128-130	39.8	40.0	40.3	40.5	40.8	41.0	41.3	41.5	41.8

From Jackson AS, Pollock ML. Practical assessment of body composition. *Phys Sports Med.* 1985;13:76-89. Used by permission.

Percentage Fat Estimate for Men: Sum of Triceps, Chest, and Subscapula Skinfolds

Sum of Skinfolds (mm)	Age to Last Year								
	Under 22	23-27	28-32	33-37	38-42	43-47	4835 2	53-57	Over 57
8-10	1.5	2.0	2.5	3.1	3.6	4.1	4.6	5.1	5.6
11-13	3.0	3.5	4.0	4.5	5.1	5.6	6.1	6.6	7.1
14-16	4.5	5.0	5.5	6.0	6.5	7.0	7.6	8.1	8.6
17-19	5.9	6.4	6.9	7.4	8.0	8.5	9.0	9.5	10.0
20-22	7.3	7.8	8.3	8.8	9.4	9.9	10.4	10.9	11.4
23-25	8.6	9.2	9.7	10.2	10.7	11.2	11.8	12.3	12.8
26-28	10.0	10.5	11.0	11.5	12.1	12.6	13.1	13.6	14.2
29-31	11.2	11.8	12.3	12.8	13.4	13.9	14.4	14.9	15.5
32-34	12.5	13.0	13.5	14.1	14.6	15.1	15.7	16.2	16.7
35-37	13.7	14.2	14.6	15.3	15.8	16.4	16.9	17.4	18.0
38-40	14.9	15.4	15.9	16.5	17.0	17.6	18.1	18.6	19.2
41-43	16.0	16.6	17.1	17.6	18.2	18.7	19.3	19.8	20.3
44-46	17.1	17.7	18.2	18.7	19.3	19.8	20.4	20.9	21.5
47-49	18.2	18.7	19.3	19.8	20.4	20.9	21.4	22.0	22.5
50-52	19.2	19.7	20.3	20.8	21.4	21.9	22.5	23.0	23.6
53-55	20.2	20.7	21.3	21.8	22.4	22.9	23.5	24.0	24.6
56-58	21.1	21.7	22.2	22.8	23.3	23.9	24.4	25.0	25.5
59-61	22.0	22.6	23.1	23.7	24.2	24.8	25.3	25.9	26.5
62-64	22.9	23.4	24.0	24.5	25.1	25.7	26.2	26.8	27.3
65-67	23.7	24.3	24.8	25.4	25.9	26.5	27.1	27.6	28.2
68-70	24.5	25.0	25.6	26.2	26.7	27.3	27.8	28.4	29.0
71-73	25.2	25.8	26.3	26.9	27.5	28.0	28.6	29.1	29.7
74-76	25.9	26.5	27.0	27.6	28.2	28.7	29.3	29.9	30.4
77-79	26.6	27.1	27.7	28.2	28.8	29.4	29.9	30.5	31.1
80-82	27.2	27.7	28.3	28.9	29.4	30.0	30.6	31.1	31.7
83-85	27.7	28.3	28.8	29.4	30.0	30.5	31.1	31.7	32.3
86-88	28.2	28.8	29.4	29.9	30.5	31.1	31.6	32.2	32.8
89-91	28.7	29.3	29.8	30.4	31.0	31.5	32.1	32.7	33.3
92-94	29.1	29.7	30.3	30.8	31.4	32.0	32.6	33.1	33.4
95-97	29.5	30.1	30.6	31.2	31.8	32.4	32.9	33.5	34.1
98-100	29.8	30.4	31.0	31.6	32.1	32.7	33.3	33.9	34.4
101-103	30.1	30.7	31.3	31.8	32.4	33.0	33.6	34.1	34.7
104-106	30.4	30.9	31.5	32.1	32.7	33.2	33.8	34.4	35.0
107-109	30.6	31.1	31.7	32.3	32.9	33.4	34.0	34.6	35.2
110-112	30.7	31.3	31.9	32.4	33.0	33.6	34.2	34.7	35.3
113-115	30.8	31.4	32.0	32.5	33.1	33.7	34.3	34.9	35.4
116-118	30.9	31.5	32.0	32.6	33.2	33.8	34.3	34.9	35.5

From Jackson AS, Pollock ML. Practical assessment of body composition. *Phys Sports Med.* 1985;13:76-89. Used by permission.

Percentage Fat Estimate for Women: Sum of Triceps, Abdomen, and Suprailium Skinfolds

Sum of Skinfolds (mm)	Age to Last Year								
	18-22	23-27	28-32	33-37	38-42	43-47	48-52	53-57	Over 57
8-12	8.8	9.0	9.2	9.4	9.5	9.7	9.9	10.1	10.3
13-17	10.8	10.9	11.1	11.3	11.5	11.7	11.8	12.0	12.2
18-22	12.6	12.8	13.0	13.2	13.4	13.5	13.7	13.9	14.1

Sum of Skinfolds (mm)	Age to Last Year								
	18-22	23-27	28-32	33-37	38-42	43-47	48-52	53-57	Over 57
23-27	14.5	14.6	14.8	15.0	15.2	15.4	15.6	15.7	15.9
28-32	16.2	16.4	16.6	16.8	17.0	17.1	17.3	17.5	17.7
33-37	17.9	18.1	18.3	18.5	18.7	18.9	19.0	19.2	19.4
38-42	19.6	19.8	20.0	20.2	20.3	20.5	20.7	20.9	21.1
43-47	21.2	21.4	21.6	21.8	21.9	22.1	22.3	22.5	22.7
48-52	22.8	22.9	23.1	23.3	23.5	23.7	23.8	24.0	24.2
53-57	24.2	24.4	24.6	24.8	25.0	25.2	25.3	25.5	25.7
58-62	25.7	25.9	26.0	26.2	26.4	26.6	26.8	27.0	27.1
63-67	27.1	27.2	27.4	27.6	27.8	28.0	28.2	28.3	28.5
68-72	28.4	28.6	28.7	28.9	29.1	29.3	29.5	29.7	29.8
73-77	29.6	29.8	30.0	30.2	30.4	30.6	30.7	30.9	31.1
78-82	30.9	31.0	31.2	31.4	31.6	31.8	31.9	32.1	32.3
83-87	32.0	32.2	32.4	32.6	32.7	32.9	33.1	33.3	33.5
88-92	33.1	33.3	33.5	33.7	33.8	34.0	34.2	34.4	34.6
93-97	34.1	34.3	34.5	34.7	34.9	35.1	35.2	35.4	35.6
98-102	35.1	35.3	35.5	35.7	35.9	36.0	36.2	36.4	36.6
103-107	36.1	36.2	36.4	36.6	36.8	37.0	37.2	37.3	37.5
108-112	36.9	37.1	37.3	37.5	37.7	37.9	38.0	38.2	38.4
113-117	37.8	37.9	38.1	38.3	39.2	39.4	39.6	39.8	39.2
118-122	38.5	38.7	38.9	39.1	39.4	39.6	39.8	40.0	40.0
123-127	39.2	39.4	39.6	39.8	40.0	40.1	40.3	40.5	40.7
128-132	39.9	40.1	40.2	40.4	40.6	40.8	41.0	41.2	41.3
133-137	40.5	40.7	40.8	41.0	41.2	41.4	41.6	41.7	41.9
138-142	41.0	41.2	41.4	41.6	41.7	41.9	42.1	42.3	42.5
143-147	41.5	41.7	41.9	42.0	42.2	42.4	42.6	42.8	43.0
148-152	41.9	42.1	42.3	42.3	42.6	42.8	43.0	43.2	43.4
153-157	42.3	42.5	42.6	42.8	43.0	43.2	43.4	43.6	43.7
158-162	42.6	42.8	43.0	43.1	43.3	43.5	43.7	43.9	44.1
163-167	42.9	43.0	43.2	43.4	43.6	43.8	44.0	44.1	44.3
168-172	43.1	43.2	43.4	43.6	43.8	44.0	44.2	44.3	44.5
173-177	43.2	43.4	43.6	43.8	43.9	44.1	44.3	44.5	44.7
178-182	43.3	43.5	43.7	43.8	44.0	44.2	44.4	44.6	44.8

From Jackson AS, Pollock ML. Practical assessment of body composition. *Phys Sports Med.* 1985;13:76-89. Used by permission.

Appendix 18

Body-Composition Measurements for Various Sports

Body-Composition Values for Male and Female Athletes

Athletic Group or Sport	Sex	Age (y)	Height (cm)	Weight (kg)	Relative Fat %	Reference
Baseball	Male	20.8	182.7	83.3	14.2	Novak
	Male	—	—	—	11.8	Forsyth
	Male	26.0	185.4	87.5	16.2	Gurry
	Male	27.3	185.8	86.4	12.6	Coleman
	Male	27.4	183.1	88.0	12.6	Wilmore
Pitchers	Male	26.7	188.1	89.8	14.7	Coleman
Infielders	Male	27.4	183.1	83.2	12.0	Coleman
Outfielders	Male	28.3	185.9	85.6	9.9	Coleman
Basketball	Female	19.1	169.1	62.6	20.8	Sinning
	Female	19.4	173.0	68.3	20.8	Vaccaro
	Female	19.4	167.0	63.9	26.9	Conger
Centers	Male	27.7	214.0	109.2	7.1	Parr
Forwards	Male	25.3	200.6	96.9	9.0	Parr
Guards	Male	25.2	188.0	83.6	10.6	Parr
Bicycling	Male	—	180.3	67.1	8.8	Burke
	Female	—	167.7	61.3	15.4	Burke
Canoeing/	Male	23.7	182.0	79.6	12.4	Rusko
Paddlers	Male	20.1	179.9	76.3	10.4	Vaccaro
Dancing, Ballet	Female	15.0	161.1	48.4	16.4	Clarkson
General	Female	21.2	162.7	51.2	20.5	Novak
Fencers	Male	20.4	174.9	68.0	12.2	Vander
Football	Male	19.3	186.8	93.1	13.7	Smith
	Male	20.3	184.9	96.4	13.8	Novak
	Male	—	—	—	13.9	Forsyth
Defensive backs	Male	17-23	178.3	77.3	11.5	Wickkiser
	Male	24.5	182.5	84.8	9.6	Wilmore
Offensive backs	Male	17-23	179.7	79.8	12.4	Wickkiser
	Male	24.7	183.8	90.7	9.4	Wilmore
Linebackers	Male	17-23	180.1	87.2	13.4	Wickkiser
	Male	24.2	188.6	102.2	14.0	Wilmore
Offensive linemen	Male	17-23	186.0	99.2	19.1	Wickkiser
	Male	24.7	193.0	112.6	15.6	Wilmore
Defensive linemen	Male	17-23	186.6	97.8	18.5	Wickkiser
	Male	25.7	192.4	117.1	18.2	Wilmore
Quarterbacks/kickers	Male	24.1	185.0	90.1	14.4	Wilmore
Golf	Female	33.3	168.9	61.8	24.0	Crews
Gymnastics	Male	20.3	178.5	69.2	4.6	Novak
	Female	14.0	—	—	17.0	Parizkova
	Female	15.2	161.1	50.4	13.1	Moffatt
	Female	19.4	163.0	57.9	23.8	Conger
	Female	20.0	158.5	51.5	15.5	Sinning
	Female	23.0	—	—	11.0	Parizkova
	Female	23.0	—	—	9.6	Parizkova
Ice hockey	Male	22.5	179.0	77.3	13.0	Rusko
	Male	26.3	180.3	86.7	15.1	Wilmore
Jockeys	Male	30.9	158.2	50.3	14.1	Wilmore
Orienteering	Male	31.2	—	72.2	16.3	Knowlton
	Female	29.0	—	58.1	18.7	Knowlton

Athletic Group or Sport	Sex	Age (y)	Height (cm)	Weight (kg)	Relative Fat %	Reference
Pentathlon	Female	21.5	175.4	65.4	11.0	Krahenbuhl
Racquetball	Male	25.0	181.7	80.3	8.1	Pipes
Lightweight	Male	21.0	186.0	71.0	8.5	Hagerman
	Female	23.0	173.0	68.0	14.0	Hagerman
Rowing	Male	25.6	192.0	93.0	6.5	Secher
Rugby	Male	28.1	181.6	86.3	9.1	Maud
Skating, Speed	Male	21.0	181.0	76.5	11.4	Kusko
	Male	—	181.0	73.6	9.0	Vanlugen
Figure	Male	21.3	166.9	59.6	9.1	Niinimaa
	Female	16.5	158.8	48.6	12.5	Niinimaa
Skiing	Male	25.9	176.6	74.8	7.4	Sprynarova
Alpine	Male	16.5	173.1	65.5	11.0	Song
	Male	21.0	178.0	78.0	9.9	Veicsteinas
	Male	21.2	176.0	70.1	14.1	Rusko
	Male	21.8	177.8	75.5	10.2	Haymes
	Female	19.5	165.1	58.8	20.6	Haymes
Cross-country	Male	21.2	176.0	66.6	12.5	Niinimaa
	Male	22.7	176.2	73.2	7.9	Haymes
	Male	25.6	174.0	69.3	10.2	Rusko
	Female	20.2	163.4	55.9	15.7	Haymes
	Female	24.3	163.0	59.1	21.8	Rusko
Nordic	Male	21.7	181.7	70.4	8.9	Haymes
Combination	Male	22.9	176.0	70.4	11.2	Rusko
Ski jumping	Male	22.2	174.0	69.9	14.3	Rusko
Soccer	Male	26.0	176.0	75.5	9.6	Raven
US junior	Male	17.5	178.3	72.3	9.4	Kirkendahl
US Olympic	Male	20.6	179.3	72.5	9.1	Kirkendahl
US collegiate	Male	20.0	175.3	72.4	10.9	Kirkendahl
US national	Male	22.5	178.6	76.2	9.9	Kirkendahl
M I S L	Male	26.9	177.3	74.5	10.5	Kirkendahl
Swimming	Male	15.1	166.8	59.1	10.8	Vaccaro
	Male	20.6	182.9	78.9	5.0	Novak
	Male	21.8	182.3	79.1	8.5	Sprynarova
	Female	19.4	168.0	63.8	26.3	Conger
Sprint	Female	—	165.1	57.1	14.6	Wilmore
Middle distance	Female	—	166.6	66.8	24.1	Wilmore
Distance	Female	—	166.3	60.9	17.1	Wilmore
Synchronized swimming	Female	20.1	166.2	55.8	24.0	Roby
Tennis	Male	—	—	—	15.2	Forsyth
	Male	42.0	179.6	77.1	16.3	Vodak
	Female	39.0	163.3	55.7	20.3	Vokak
Track and field	Male	21.3	180.6	71.6	3.7	Novak
	Male	—	—	—	8.8	Forsyth
Runners	Male	22.5	177.4	64.5	6.3	Sprynarova
Distance	Male	26.1	175.7	64.2	7.5	Costill
	Male	26.2	177.0	66.2	8.4	Rusko
	Male	26.2	177.1	63.1	4.7	Pollock
	Male	40-49	180.7	71.6	11.2	Pollock
	Male	47.2	176.5	70.7	13.2	Lewis
	Male	55.3	174.5	63.4	18.0	Barnard
	Male	50-59	174.7	67.2	10.9	Pollock
	Male	60-69	175.7	67.1	11.3	Pollock
	Male	70-75	175.6	66.8	13.6	Pollock
	Female	19.9	161.3	52.9	19.2	Malina
	Female	32.4	169.4	57.2	15.2	Wilmore
	Female	37.8	165.1	54.1	15.5	Upton
	Female	43.8	161.5	53.8	18.3	Vaccaro
Middle distance	Male	20.1	178.1	71.9	6.9	Wilmore
	Male	24.6	179.0	72.3	12.4	Rusko
Sprint	Female	20.1	164.9	56.7	19.3	Malina
	Male	20.1	178.2	72.8	5.4	Wilmore
	Male	46.5	177.0	74.1	16.5	Barnard

Athletic Group or Sport	Sex	Age (y)	Height (cm)	Weight (kg)	Relative Fat %	Reference
Cross-country	Female	15.6	164.2	51.1	15.3	Butts
	Female	15.6	163.3	50.9	15.4	Butts
Race walking	Male	26.7	178.7	68.5	7.8	Franklin
Discus	Male	26.4	190.8	110.5	16.3	Wilmore
	Male	28.3	186.1	104.7	16.4	Fahey
	Female	21.1	168.1	71.0	25.0	Malina
Jumpers and hurdlers	Female	20.3	165.9	59.0	20.7	Malina
Shot put	Male	22.0	191.6	126.2	19.6	Behnke
	Male	27.0	188.2	112.5	16.5	Fahey
	Female	21.5	167.6	78.1	28.0	Malina
Triathlon	Male	—	—	—	7.1	Holly
	Female	—	—	—	12.6	Holly
Volleyball	Male	26.1	192.7	85.5	12.0	Puhl
	Female	19.4	166.0	59.8	25.3	Conger
	Female	19.9	172.2	64.1	21.3	Kovaleski
	Female	21.6	178.3	70.5	17.9	Puhl
Weight lifting	Male	24.9	166.4	77.2	9.8	Sprynarova
Power	Male	25.5	173.6	89.4	19.9	Hakkinen
	Male	26.3	176.1	92.0	15.6	Fahey
Olympic	Male	25.3	177.1	88.2	12.2	Fahey
Body builders	Male	25.6	176.9	87.6	13.4	Hakkinen
	Male	27.6	178.8	88.1	8.3	Pipes
	Male	29.0	172.4	83.1	8.4	Fahey
	Female	27.0	160.8	53.8	13.2	Freedson
Wrestling	Male	11.3	141.2	34.2	12.7	Sady
	Male	15-18	172.3	66.3	6.9	Katch
	Male	19.6	174.6	74.8	8.8	Sinning
	Male	20.6	174.8	67.3	4.0	Stine
	Male	22.0	—	—	5.0	Parizkova
	Male	23.0	—	79.3	14.3	Taylor
	Male	24.0	173.3	77.5	12.7	Hakkinen
	Male	26.0	177.8	81.8	9.8	Fahey
	Male	27.0	176.0	75.7	10.7	Gale

Maximal Oxygen Uptake (mL $\bullet$ kg^{-1} $\bullet$ min^{-1}) of Male and Female Athletes

Athletic Group or Sport	Sex	Age (y)	Height (cm)	Weight (kg)	$\dot{V}O_2$max	Reference
Baseball/	Male	21	182.7	83.3	52.3	Novak
Softball	Male	26	185.4	87.5	41.6	Gurry
	Male	28	183.6	88.1	52.0	Wilmore
	Female	19-23	—	—	55.3	Rubal
Basketball	Female	19	167.0	63.9	42.3	Conger
	Female	19	169.1	62.6	42.9	Sinning
	Female	19	173.0	68.3	49.6	Vaccaro
Centers	Male	28	214.0	109.2	41.9	Parr
Forwards	Male	25	200.6	96.9	45.9	Parr
Guards	Male	25	188.0	83.6	50.0	Parr
Bicycling	Male	24	182.0	74.5	68.2	Gollnick
(competitive)	Male	24	180.4	79.2	70.3	Hermansen
	Male	25	180.0	72.8	67.1	Burke
	Male	—	180.3	67.1	74.0	Burke
	Male	—	—	—	74.0	Saltin
	Male	—	—	—	69.1	Strømme
	Female	20	165.0	55.0	50.2	Burke
	Female	—	167.7	61.3	57.4	Burke
Canoeing/	Male	18	—	66.5	71.2	Tesch
Paddlers	Male	19	173.0	64.0	60.0	Sidney
	Male	20	179.9	76.3	60.1	Vaccaro
	Male	22	190.5	80.7	67.7	Hermansen
	Male	24	182.0	79.6	66.1	Rusko
	Male	25	—	78.0	69.2	Tesch
	Male	26	181.0	74.0	56.8	Gollnick

Athletic Group or Sport	Sex	Age (y)	Height (cm)	Weight (kg)	V̇o₂max	Reference
	Female	18	166.0	57.3	49.2	Sidney
Dancing, Ballet	Male	24	177.5	68.0	48.2	Cohen
	Male	28	175.0	64.0	59.3	Mostardi
	Male	29	177.0	69.0	56.0	Schantz
	Female	15	161.1	48.4	48.9	Clarkson
	Female	24	165.6	49.5	43.7	Cohen
	Female	25	165.0	50.0	48.6	Mostardi
	Female	28	164.0	51.0	51.0	Schantz
General	Female	21	162.7	51.2	41.5	Novak
Fencing	Male	20	174.9	68.0	50.2	Vander
Football	Male	19	186.8	93.1	56.5	Smith
	Male	20	184.9	96.4	51.3	Novak
Defensive backs	Male	25	182.5	84.8	53.1	Wilmore
Offensive backs	Male	25	183.8	90.7	52.2	Wilmore
Linebackers	Male	24	188.6	102.2	52.1	Wilmore
Offensive line	Male	25	193.0	112.6	49.9	Wilmore
Defensive line	Male	26	192.4	117.1	44.9	Wilmore
Quarterbacks/kickers	Male	24	185.0	90.1	49.0	Wilmore
Golf	Female	33	168.9	61.8	34.2	Crews
Gymnastics	Male	20	178.5	69.2	55.5	Novak
	Female	15	161.1	50.4	45.2	Moffatt
	Female	15	159.7	48.8	49.8	Hermansen
	Female	19	163.0	57.9	36.3	Conger
Ice hockey	Male	11	140.5	35.5	56.6	Cunningham
	Male	22	179.0	77.3	61.5	Rusko
	Male	24	179.3	81.8	54.6	Seliger
	Male	26	180.1	86.4	53.6	Wilmore
Jockey	Male	31	158.2	50.3	53.8	Wilmore
Orienteering	Male	25	179.7	70.3	71.1	Hermansen
	Male	31	—	72.2	61.6	Knowlton
	Male	52	176.0	72.7	50.7	Gollnick
	Female	23	165.8	60.0	60.7	Hermansen
	Female	29	—	58.1	46.1	Knowlton
Pentathlon	Female	21	175.4	65.4	45.9	Krahenbuhl
Racquetball/	Male	24	183.7	81.3	60.0	Hermansen
Handball	Male	25	181.7	80.3	58.3	Pipes
Rowing	Male	—	—	—	65.7	Strømme
	Male	23	192.7	89.9	62.7	Mickelson
	Male	24	180.0	71.8	72.0	Secher
	Male	25	189.9	86.9	66.9	Hermansen
	Male	26	192.0	93.0	63.0	Secher
Heavyweight	Male	23	192.0	88.0	68.9	Hagerman
Lightweight	Male	21	186.0	71.0	71.1	Hagerman
	Female	23	173.0	68.0	60.3	Hagerman
Rugby	Male	28	181.6	86.3	45.9	Maud
Skating, Speed	Male	—	181.0	73.6	64.4	van Ingen Schenau
	Male	20	175.5	73.9	56.1	Maksud
	Male	21	181.0	76.5	72.9	Rusko
	Male	25	183.1	82.4	64.6	Hermansen
	Female	20	168.1	65.4	52.0	Hermansen
	Female	21	164.5	60.8	46.1	Maksud
Figure	Male	21	166.9	59.6	58.5	Niinimaa
	Female	17	158.8	48.6	48.9	Niinimaa
Skiing, Alpine	Male	16	173.1	65.5	65.6	Song
	Male	21	176.0	70.1	63.8	Rusko
	Male	21	178.0	78.0	52.4	Veicsteinas
	Male	22	178.5	77.6	63.1	Brown
	Male	22	177.8	75.5	66.6	Haymes
	Male	26	176.6	74.8	62.3	Sprynarova
	Female	19	165.1	58.8	52.7	Haymes
Cross-country	Male	21	176.0	66.6	63.9	Niinimaa
	Male	23	176.2	73.2	73.0	Haymes
	Male	25	180.4	73.2	73.9	Hermansen

Athletic Group or Sport	Sex	Age (y)	Height (cm)	Weight (kg)	V̇o₂max	Reference
	Male	26	174.0	69.3	78.3	Rusko
	Male	—	—	—	72.8	Strømme
	Female	20	163.4	55.9	61.5	Haymes
	Female	24	163.0	59.1	68.2	Rusko
	Female	25	165.7	60.5	56.9	Hermansen
	Female	—	—	—	58.1	Strømme
Nordic	Male	23	176.0	70.4	72.8	Rusko
	Male	22	181.7	70.4	67.4	Haymes
Ski jumping	Male	22	174.0	69.9	61.3	Rusko
Soccer	Male	26	176.0	75.5	58.4	Raven
US junior	Male	18	178.3	72.3	61.8	Kirkendahl
Swimming	Male	12	150.4	41.2	52.5	Cunningham
	Male	13	164.8	52.1	52.9	Cunningham
	Male	15	169.6	59.8	56.6	Cunningham
	Male	15	166.8	59.1	56.8	Vaccaro
	Male	20	181.4	76.7	55.7	Magel
	Male	20	181.0	73.0	50.4	Charbonnier
	Male	21	182.9	78.9	62.1	Novak
	Male	21	181.0	78.3	69.9	Gollnick
	Male	22	182.3	79.1	56.9	Sprynarova
	Male	22	182.3	79.7	55.9	Cunningham
	Female	12	154.8	43.3	46.2	Cunningham
	Female	13	160.0	52.1	43.4	Cunningham
	Female	15	164.8	53.7	40.5	Cunningham
Sprint	Male	19	181.1	75.0	58.3	Shephard
Mid-distance	Male	22	178.0	74.6	55.4	Shephard
Long-distance	Male	21	179.0	74.9	65.4	Shephard
	Female	19	168.0	63.8	37.6	Conger
Synchronized	Female	20	166.2	55.8	43.2	Roby
Tennis	Male	12	147.9	38.5	56.3	Buti
	Male	42	179.6	77.1	50.2	Vodak
	Female	12	150.9	42.9	52.6	Buti
	Female	39	163.3	55.7	44.2	Vodak
Track and field	Male	21	180.6	71.6	66.1	Novak
Runners	Male	22	177.4	64.5	64.0	Sprynarova
	Male	23	177.0	69.5	72.4	Gollnick
Sprint	Male	17-22	—	—	51.0	Thomas
	Male	46	177.0	74.1	47.2	Barnard
Mid-distance	Male	20	178.1	71.9	55.8	Wilmore
	Male	25	180.1	67.8	70.1	Costill
	Male	25	179.0	72.3	69.8	Rusko
Distance	Male	10	144.3	31.9	56.6	Mayers
	Male	17-22	—	—	65.5	Thomas
	Male	26	177.1	63.1	76.9	Pollock
	Male	26	176.1	64.5	72.2	Hermansen
	Male	26	178.9	63.9	77.4	Costill
	Male	26	177.0	66.2	78.1	Rusko
	Male	27	178.7	64.9	73.2	Costill
	Male	32	177.3	64.3	70.3	Costill
	Male	35	174.0	63.1	66.6	Costill
	Male	36	177.3	69.6	65.1	Hagan
	Male	40-49	180.7	71.6	57.5	Pollock
	Male	55	174.5	63.4	54.4	Barnard
	Male	50-59	174.7	67.2	54.4	Pollock
	Male	60-69	175.7	67.1	51.4	Pollock
	Male	70-75	175.6	66.8	40.0	Pollock
	Male	—	—	—	72.5	Davies
	Female	16	162.2	48.6	63.2	Burke
	Female	16	163.3	50.9	50.8	Butts
	Female	21	170.2	58.6	57.5	Hermansen
	Female	25	165.7	52.3	59.8	Upton
	Female	32	169.4	57.2	59.1	Wilmore
	Female	38	165.1	54.1	55.5	Upton

Athletic Group or Sport	Sex	Age (y)	Height (cm)	Weight (kg)	$\dot{V}O_2max$	Reference
	Female	38	165.5	54.7	55.5	Upton
	Female	44	161.5	53.8	43.4	Vaccaro
	Female	—	—	—	58.2	Davies
Cross-country	Female	16	163.3	50.9	50.8	Butts
Race walking	Male	27	178.7	68.5	62.9	Franklin
Jumpers	Male	17-22	—	—	55.0	Thomas
Shot/discus	Male	17-22	—	—	49.5	Thomas
	Male	26	190.8	110.5	42.8	Wilmore
	Male	27	188.2	112.5	42.6	Fahey
	Male	28	186.1	104.7	47.5	Fahey
Triathlon	Male	—	—	—	72.0	Holly
	Female	—	—	—	58.7	Holly
Volleyball	Male	25	187.0	84.5	56.4	Conlee
	Male	26	192.7	85.5	56.1	Puhl
	Female	19	166.0	59.8	43.5	Conger
	Female	20	172.2	64.1	56.0	Kovaleski
	Female	22	183.7	73.4	41.7	Spence
	Female	22	178.3	70.5	50.6	Puhl
Weight lifting	Male	25	171.0	81.3	40.1	Gollnick
	Male	25	166.4	77.2	42.6	Sprynarova
Power	Male	26	173.6	89.4	41.9	Hakkinen
	Male	26	176.1	92.0	49.5	Fahey
Olympic	Male	25	177.1	88.2	50.7	Fahey
Body builder	Male	26	176.9	87.6	50.8	Hakkinen
	Male	27	178.8	88.1	46.3	Pipes
	Male	29	172.4	83.1	41.5	Fahey
Wrestling	Male	11	141.2	34.2	54.0	Sady
	Male	21	174.8	67.3	58.3	Stine
	Male	23	—	79.2	50.4	Taylor
	Male	24	173.3	77.5	57.8	Hakkinen
	Male	24	175.6	77.7	60.9	Nagel
	Male	26	177.0	81.8	64.0	Fahey
	Male	27	176.0	75.7	54.3	Gale

REFERENCES

Adams, J., Mottola, M., Bagnall, K.M., & McFadden, K.D. (1982). Total body fat content in a group of professional football players. *Canadian Journal of Applied Sports and Science, 7,* 36-40.

Astrand, P.O., & Rodahl, K. (1986). *Textbook of work physiology* (3rd ed.). New York: McGraw-Hill Publishing Co.

Barnard, R.J., Grimditch, G.K., & Wilmore, J.H. (1979). Physiological characteristics of sprint and endurance Masters runners. *Medicine and Science in Sports, 11,* 167-171.

Bar-Or, O. (1975). Predicting athletic performance. *Physician and Sportsmedicine, 3* (#2), 80-85.

Behnke, A.R., & Wilmore, J.H. (1974). *Evaluation and regulation of body build and composition.* Englewood Cliffs, NJ: Prentice-Hall.

Bergh, U., Thorstensson. A., Sjodin, B., Hulten, B., Piehl, K., & Karlsson, J. (1978). Maximal oxygen uptake and muscle fiber types in trained and untrained humans. *Medicine and Science in Sports, 10,* 151-154.

Brown, C.H., & Wilmore, J.H. (1974). The effects of maximal resistance training on the strength and body composition of women athletes. *Medicine and Science in Sports, 6,* 174-177.

Brown, S.L., & Wilkinson, J.G. (1983). Characteristics of national, divisional, and club male alpine ski racers. *Medicine and Science in Sports and Exercise, 15,* 491-495.

Burke, E.J., & Brush, F.C. (1979). Physiological and anthropometric assessment of successful teenage female distance runners. *Research Quarterly, 50,* 180-187.

Burke, E.R. (1980). Physiological characteristics of competitive cyclists. *Physician and Sportsmedicine, 8* (#7), 78-84.

Burke, E.R., Cerny, F., Costill, D., & Fink, W. (1977). Characteristics of skeletal muscle in competitive cyclists. *Medicine and Science in Sports, 9,* 109-112.

Buti, T., Elliott, B., & Morton, A. (1984). Physiological and anthropometric profiles of elite prepubescent tennis players. *Physician and Sportsmedicine, 12* (#1), 111-116.

Butts, N.K. (1982). Physiological profile of high school female cross-country runners. *Physician and Sportsmedicine, 10,* 103-111.

Butts, N.K. (1982). Physiological profiles of high school female cross country runners. *Research Quarterly for Exercise and Sport, 53,* 8-14.

Charbonnier, J.P., Lacour, J.R., Riffat, J., & Flandrois, R. (1975). Experimental study of the performance of competition swimmers. *European Journal of Applied Physiology, 34,* 157-167.

Clarkson, P.M., Freedson, P.S., Keller, B., Carney, D., & Skrinar, M. (1985). Maximal oxygen uptake, nutritional patterns and body composition of adolescent female ballet dancers. *Research Quarterly for Exercise and Sport, 56,* 180-184.

Clement, D.B., Asmundson, C., Taunton, C., Taunton, J.E., Ridley, D., & Banister, E.W. (1979). The sport scientist's role in identification of performance criteria for distance runners. *Canadian Journal of Applied Sports Science, 4,* 143-148.

Coleman. A.E. (1981). Skinfold estimates of body fat in major league baseball players. *Physician and Sportsmedicine, 9* (#10), 77-82.

Conger, P.R., & Macnab, R.B.J. (1967). Strength, body composition, and work capacity of participants and nonparticipants in women's intercollegiate sports. *Research Quarterly, 38,* 184-192.

Conlee, R.K., McGown, C.M., Fisher, A.G., Dalsky, G.P., & Robinson, K.C. (1982). Physiological effects of power volleyball. *Physician and Sportsmedicine, 10* (#2), 93-97.

Costill, D.L. (1967). The relationship between selected physiological variables and distance running performance. *Journal of Sports Medicine, 7,* 61-66.

Costill, D.L. (1970). Metabolic responses during distance running. *Journal of Applied Physiology, 28,* 251-255.

Costill, D.L., Bowers, R., & Kammer, W.F. (1970). Skinfold estimates of body fat among marathon runners. *Medicine and Science in Sports, 2,* 93-95.

Costill, D.L., Daniels, J., Evans, W., Fink, W., Krahenbuhl, G., & Saltin, B. (1976). Skeletal muscle enzymes and fiber composition in male and female track athletes. *Journal of Applied Physiology, 40,* 149-154.

Costill, D.L., Fink, W.J., & Pollock, M.L. (1976). Muscle fiber composition and enzyme activities of elite distance runners. *Medicine and Science in Sports, 8,* 96-100.

Costill, D.L., Thomason, H., & Roberts, E. (1973). Fractional utilization of the aerobic capacity during distance running. *Medicine and Science in Sports, 5,* 248-252.

Costill, D.L., & Winrow, E. (1970). Maximal oxygen intake among marathon runners. *Archives of Physical and Medical Rehabilitation, 51,* 317-320.

Crews, D., Thomas, G., Shirreffs, J.H., & Helfrich, H.M. (1984). A physiological profile of ladies professional golf association tour players. *Physician and Sportsmedicine, 12* (#5), 69-76.

Cunningham, D.A., & Eynon, R.B. (1973). The working capacity of young competitive swimmers, 10-16 years of age. *Medicine and Science in Sports, 5,* 227-231.

Cunningham, D.A., Telford, P., & Swart, G.T. (1976). The cardiopulmonary capacities of young hockey players: Age 10. *Medicine and Science in Sports, 8,* 23-25.

Cureton, T.K. (1951). *Physical fitness of champion athletes.* Urbana, IL; University of Illinois Press.

Davies, C.T.M. (1971). Body composition in children: A reference standard for maximum aerobic power output on a stationary bicycle ergometer. In, Proceedings of the III International Symposium on Pediatric Work Physiology. *Acta Paediatrica Scandinavica* (Suppl) *217,* 136-137.

Davies, C.T.M., & Thompson, M.W. (1979). Aerobic performance of female marathon and male ultramarathon athletes. *European Journal of Applied Physiology, 41,* 233-245.

deGaray, A.L., Levine, L., & Carter, J.E.L. (Eds). (1974). *Genetic and anthropological studies of Olympic athletes.* New York: Academic Press.

Drinkwater, B.L. (1973). Physiological responses of women to exercise. *Exercise and Sport Sciences Reviews, 1,* 125-153.

Drinkwater, B.L. (1984). Women and exercise: Physiological aspects. *Exercise and Sport Sciences Reviews, 12,* 21-51.

Edstrom, L., & Ekblom, B. (1972). Differences in sizes of red and white muscle fibers in vastus lateralis of musculus quadriceps femoris of normal individuals and athletes: Relation to physical performance. *Scandinavian Journal of Clinical Laboratory Investigation, 30,* 175-181.

Ekblom, B. (1986). Applied physiology of soccer. *Sports Medicine, 3,* 50-60.

Fahey, T.D., Akka, L., & Rolph, R. (1975). Body composition and $\dot{V}O_2$ max of exceptional weight-trained athletes. *Journal of Applied Physiology, 39,* 559-561.

Forsyth, H.L., & Sinning, W.E. (1973). The anthropometric estimation of body density and lean body weight of male athletes. *Medicine and Science in Sports, 5,* 174-180.

Franklin, B.A., Kaimal, K.P., Moir, T.W., & Hellerstein, H.K. (1981). Characteristics of national-class race walkers. *Physician and Sportsmedicine, 9,* (#9), 101-108.

Freedson, P.S., Mihevic, P.M., Loucks, A.B., & Girandola, R.N. (1983). Physique, body composition, and psychological characteristics of competitive female body builders. *Physician and Sportsmedicine, 11,* (#5), 85-93.

Gale, J.B., & Flynn, K.W. (1974). Maximal oxygen consumption and relative body fat of high-ability wrestlers. *Medicine and Science in Sports, 6,* 232-234.

Gollnick, P.D., Armstrong, R.B., Saubert, IV, C.W., Piehl, K., & Saltin, B. (1972). Enzyme activity and fiber composition in skeletal muscle of untrained and trained men. *Journal of Applied Physiology, 33,* 312-319.

Gurry, M., Pappas, A., Michaels, J., Maher, P., Shakman, A., Goldberg, R., & Rippe, J. (1985). A comprehensive preseason fitness evaluation for professional baseball players. *Physician and Sportsmedicine, 13* (#6), 63-74.

Hagan, R.D., Smith, M.G., & Gettman, L.R. (1981). Marathon performance in relation to maximal aerobic power and training indices. *Medicine and Science in Sports and Exercise, 13,* 185-189.

Hagberg, J.M., & Coyle, E.F. (1983). Physiological determinants of endurance performance as studied in competitive racewalkers. *Medicine and Science in Sports and Exercise, 15,* 287-289.

Hagerman, F.C., Hagerman, G.R., & Mickelson, T.C. (1979). Physiological profiles of elite rowers. *Physician and Sportsmedicine, 7* (#7), 74-83.

Hakkinen, K., Alen, M., & Komi, P.V. (1984). Neuromuscular, anaerobic, and aerobic performance characteristics of elite power athletes. *European Journal of Applied Physiology, 53,* 97-105.

Haymes, E.M., & Dickinson, A.L. (1980). Characteristics of elite male and female ski racers. *Medicine and Science in Sports and Exercise, 12,* 153-158.

Hermansen, L. (1973). Oxygen transport during exercise in human subjects. *Acta Physiologica Scandinavica,* (Suppl) 399, 1-104.

Hermansen, L., & Andersen, K.L. (1965). Aerobic work capacity in young Norwegian men and women. *Journal of Applied Physiology, 20,* 425-431.

Holly, R.G., Barnard, R.J., Rosenthal, M., Applegate, E., & Pritikin, N. (1986). Triathlete characterization and response to prolonged strenuous competition. *Medicine and Science in Sports and Exercise, 18,* 123-127.

Katch, F.I., & Michael, E.D. (1971). Body composition of high school wrestlers according to age and wrestling weight category. *Medicine and Science in Sports, 3,* 190-194.

Kirkendahl, D.T. (1985). The applied sport science of soccer. *Physician and Sportsmedicine, 13,* (#4), 53-59.

Knowlton, R.G., Ackerman, K.J., Fitzgerald, P.I., Wilde, S.W., & Tahamont, M.V. (1980). Physiological and performance characteristics of United States championship class orienteers. *Medicine and Science in Sports and Exercise, 12,* 164-169.

Kovaleski, J.E., Parr, R.B., Hornak, J.E., & Roitman, J.L. (1980). Athletic profile of women college volleyball players. *Physician and Sportsmedicine, 8* (#2), 112-118.

Krahenbuhl, G.S., Wells, C.L., Brown, C.H., & Ward, P.E. (1979). Characteristics of national and world class female pentathletes. *Medicine and Science in Sports, 11,* 20-23.

Lewis, S., Haskell, W.L., Klein, H., Halpern, J., & Wood, P.D. (1975). Prediction of body composition in habitually active middle-aged men. *Journal of Applied Physiology, 39,* 221-225.

Magal, J.R., & Faulkner, J.A. (1967). Maximum oxygen uptakes of college swimmers. *Journal of Applied Physiology, 22,* 929-933.

Maksud, M.G., Wiley, R.L., Hamilton, L.H., & Lockhart, B. (1970). Maximal $\dot{V}O_2$, ventilation, and heart rate of Olympic speed skating candidates. *Journal of Applied Physiology, 29,* 186-190.

Malina, R.M., Harper, A.B., Avent, H.H., & Campbell, D.E. (1971). Physique of female track and field athletes. *Medicine and Science in Sports, 3,* 32-38.

Malina, R.M., & Rarick, G.L. (1973). Growth, Physique and motor performance. In G.L. Rarick (Ed). *Physical activity, human growth and development* (pp. 125-153). New York: Academic Press.

Maud, P.J., & Schultz, B.B. (1984). The U.S. national rugby team: A physiological and anthropometric assessment. *Physician and Sportsmedicine, 12,* (#9), 86-99.

Mayers, N., & Gutin, B. (1979). Physiological characteristics of elite prepubertal cross-country runners. *Medicine and Science in Sports, 11,* 172-176.

Mickelson, T.C., & Hagerman, F.C. (1982). Anaerobic threshold measurements of elite oarsmen. *Medicine and Science in Sports and Exercise, 14,* 440-444.

Moffatt, R.J., Surina, B., Golden, B., & Ayres, N. (1984). Body composition and physiological characteristics of female high school gymnasts. *Research Quarterly for Exercise and Sport, 55,* 80-84.

Mostardi, R.A., Porterfield, J.A., Greenberg, B., Goldberg, D., & Lea, M. (1983). Musculoskeletal and cardiopulmonary characteristics of the professional ballet dancer. *Physician and Sportsmedicine, 11,* (#12), 53-61.

Nagle, F.J., Morgan, W.P., Hellickson, R.O., Serfass, R.C., & Alexander, J.F. (1975). Spotting success traits in Olympic contenders. *Physician and Sportsmedicine, 3,* 31-36.

Nicholas, J.A., & Hershman, E.B. (Eds). (1984). *Profiling.* (Clinics in Sports Medicine, Volume 3, #1) Philadelphia: W.B. Saunders Company.

Niinimaa, V. (1982). Figure skating: What do we know about it? *Physician and Sportsmedicine, 10* (#1), 51-56.

Niinimaa, V., Dyon, M., & Shephard, R.J. (1978). Performance and efficiency of intercollegiate cross-country skiers. *Medicine and Science in Sports, 10,* 91-93.

Novak, L.P., Hyatt, R.E., & Alexander, J.F. (1968). Body composition and physiologic function of athletes. *Journal of the American Medical Association, 205,* 764-770.

Novak, L.P., Magill, L.A., & Schutte, J.E. (1978). Maximal oxygen intake and body composition of female dancers. *European Journal of Applied Physiology, 39,* 277-282.

Parizkova, J. (1973). Body composition and exercise during growth and development. In G.I. Rarick (Ed.) *Physical activity, human growth and development.* New York: Academic Press. (pp. 97-124).

Parizkova, J., & Poupa, D. (1963). Some metabolic consequences of adaptation to muscular work. *British Journal of Nutrition, 17,* 341-345.

Parr, R.B., Wilmore, J.H., Hoover, R., Bachman, D., & Kerlan, R.K. (1978). Professional basketball players: Athletic profiles. *Physician and Sportsmedicine, 6* (#4), 77-84.

Pipes, T.V. (1979). Physiological characteristics of elite body builders. *Physician and Sportsmedicine, 7* (#3), 116-122.

Pipes, T.V. (1979). The racquetball pro: A physiological profile. *Physician and Sportsmedicine, 7* (#10), 91-94.

Pollock, M.L. (1973). The quantification of endurance training programs. *Exercise and SportsSciences Reviews, 1,* 155-188.

Pollock, M.L. (1977). Submaximal and maximal working capacity of elite distance runners. Part I. Cardiorespiratory aspects. *New York Academy of Science, 301,* 310-322.

Pollock, M.L., Miller, H.S., & Wilmore, J. (1974). Physiological characteristics of champion American track athletes 40 to 75 years of age. *Journal of Gerontology, 29,* 645-649.

Prince, F.P., Hikida, R.S., & Hagerman, F.C. (1977). Muscle fiber types in women athletes and non-athletes. *Pflugers Archives, 371,* 161-165.

Puhl, J., Case, S., Fleck, S., & Van Handel, P. (1982). Physical and physiological characteristics of elite volleyball players. *Research Quarterly for Exercise and Sports, 53,* 257-262.

Raven, P.B., Gettman, L.R., Pollock, M.L., & Cooper, K.H. (1976). A physiological evaluation of professional soccer players. *British Journal of Sports Medicine, 10,* 209-216.

Roby, F.B., Buono, M.J., Constable, S.H., Lowdon, B.J., & Tsao, W.Y. (1983). Physiological characteristics of champion synchronized swimmers. *Physician and Sportsmedicine, 11* (#4), 136-147.

Rusko, H., Havu, M., & Karvinen, E. (1978). Aerobic performance capacity in athletes. *European Journal of Applied Physiology, 38,* 151-159.

Sady, S.P., Thomson, W.H., Berg, K., & Savage, M. (1984). Physiological characteristics of high-ability prepubescent wrestlers. *Medicine and Science in Sports and Exercise, 16,* 72-76.

Saltin, B., & Astrand, P.O. (1967). Maximal oxygen uptake in athletes. *Journal of Applied Physiology, 23,* 353-358.

Schantz, P.G., & Astrand, P.O. (1984). Physiological characteristics of classical ballet. *Medicine and Science in Sports and Exercise, 16,* 472-476.

Secher, N.H. (1983). The physiology of rowing. *Journal of Sports Science, 1,* 23-53.

Secher, N.H., Vaage, O., Jensen, K. & Jackson, R.C. (1983). Maximal aerobic power in oarsmen. *European Journal of Applied Physiology, 51,* 155-162.

Seliger, V., Kostka, V., Grusova, D., Kovak, J., Machovcova, J., Pauer, M., Pribylova, A., & Urbankova, R. (1972). Energy expenditure and physical fitness of ice-hockey players. *Internationale Zeitschrift für Angewandte Physiologie, 30,* 283-291.

Shephard, R.J., Godin, G., & Campbell, R. (1974). Characteristics of sprint, medium, and long-distance swimmers. *European Journal of Applied Physiology, 32,* 99-103.

Sidney, K., & Shephard, R.J. (1973). Physiological characteristics and performance of the white-water paddler. *European Journal of Applied Physiology, 32,* 55-70.

Sinning, W.E. (1973). Body composition, cardiorespiratory function, and rule changes in women's basketball. *Research Quarterly, 44,* 313-321.

Sinning, W.E. (1974). Body composition assessment of college wrestlers. *Medicine and Science in Sports, 6,* 139-145.

Sinning, W.E., & Lindberg, G.D. (1972). Physical characteristics of college-age women gymnasts. *Research Quarterly, 43,* 226-234.

Smith, D.P., & Byrd, R.J. (1976). Body composition, pulmonary function and maximal oxygen consumption of college football players. *Journal of Sports Medicine, 16,* 301-308.

Song, T.M.K. (1982). Relationship of physiological characteristics to skiing performance. *Physician and Sportsmedicine, 10,* (#12), 96-102.

Spence, D.W., Disch, J.G., Fred, H.L., & Coleman, A.E. (1980). Descriptive profiles of highly skilled women volleyball players. *Medicine and Science in Sports and Exercise, 12,* 299-302.

Sprynarova, S., & Parizkova, J. (1971). Functional capacity and body composition in top weightlifters, swimmers, runners and skiers. *International Zeitschrift für Angewandte Physiologie, 29,* 184-194.

Stine, G., Ratliff, R., Shierman, G., & Grana, W.A. (1979). Physical profile of the wrestlers at the 1977 NCAA championships. *Physician and Sportsmedicine, 7* (#11), 98-105.

Strømme, S.B., Ingjer, F., & Meen, H.D. (1977). Assessment of maximal aerobic power in specifically trained athletes. *Journal of Applied Physiology, 42,* 833-837.

Tanner, J.M. (1964). *The physique of the Olympic athlete.* London: George Allen and Unwin Ltd.

Taylor, A.W., Brassard, L., Proteau, L., & Robin, D. (1979). A physiological profile of Canadian Greco-Roman wrestlers. *Canadian Journal of Applied Sport Sciences, 4,* 131-134.

Tesch, P., Piehl, K., Wilson, G., & Karlsson, J. (1976). Physiological investigations of Swedish elite canoe competitors. *Medicine and Science in Sports, 8,* 214-218.

Thorstensson, A., Larsson, L., Tesch, P., & Karlsson, J. (1977). Muscle strength and fiber composition in athletes and sedentary men. *Medicine and Science in Sports, 9,* 26-30.

Upton, S.J., Hagan, R.D., Lease, B., Rosentswieg, J., Gettman, L.R., & Duncan, J.J. (1984). Comparative physiological profiles among young and middle-aged female distance runners. *Medicine and Science in Sports and Exercise, 16,* 67-71.

Upton, S.J., Hagan, R.D., Rosentswieg, J., & Gettman, L.R. (1983). Comparison of the physiological profiles of middle-aged women distance runners and sedentary women. *Research Quarterly for Exercise and Sport, 54,* 83-87.

Vaccaro, P., Clarke, D.H., & Morris, A.F. (1980). Physiological characteristics of young well-trained swimmers. *European Journal of Applied Physiology, 44,* 61-66.

Vaccaro, P., Clarke, D.H., & Wrenn, J.P. (1979). Physiological profiles of elite women basketball players. *Journal of Sports Medicine, 19,* 45-54.

Vaccaro, P., Dummer, G.M., & Clarke, D.H. (1981). Physiological characteristics of female masters swimmers. *Physician and Sportsmedicine, 9* (#12), 75-78.

Vaccaro, P., Gray, P.R., Clarke, D.H., & Morris, A.F. (1984). Physiological characteristics of world class white-water slalom paddlers. *Research Quarterly for Exercise and Sport, 55,* 206-210.

Vaccaro, P., Morris, A.F., & Clarke, D.H. (1981). Physiological characteristics of masters female distance runners. *Physician and Sportsmedicine, 9* (#7), 105-108.

Vander, L.B., Franklin, B.A., Wrisley, D., Scherf, J., Kogler, A.A., & Rubenfire, M. (1984). Physiological profile of national-class national collegiate athletic association fencers. *Journal of American Medical Association, 252,* 500-503.

van Ingen Schenau, G.J., deGroot, G., & Hollander, A.P. (1983). Some technical, physiological and anthropometrical aspects of speed skating. *European Journal of Applied Physiology, 50,* 343-354.

Veicsteinas, A., Ferretti, G., Margonato, V., Rosa, G., & Tagliabue, D. (1984). Energy cost of and energy sources for alpine skiing in top athletes. *Journal of Applied Physiology, 56,* 1187-1190.

Vodak, P.A., Savin, W.M., Haskell, W.L., & Wood, P.D. (1980). Physiological profile of middle-aged male and female tennis players. *Medicine and Science in Sports and Exercise, 12,* 159-163.

Wickkiser, J.D., & Kelly, J.M. (1975). The body composition of a college football team. *Medicine and Science in Sports, 7,* 199-202.

Wilmore, J.H. (1974). Alterations in strength, body composition and anthropometric measurements consequent to a 10-week weight training program. *Medicine and Science in Sports, 6,* 133-138.

Wilmore, J.H. (1983). Body composition in sport and exercise: Directions for future research. *Medicine and Science in Sports and Exercise, 15,* 21-31.

Wilmore, J.H. (1984). The assessment of and variation in aerobic power in world class athletes as related to specific sports. *American Journal of Sports Medicine, 12,* 120-127.

Wilmore, J.H., & Bergfeld, J.A. (1979). A comparison of sports: Physiological and medical aspects. In R.H. Strauss (Ed.) *Sports medicine and physiology.* Philadelphia: W.B. Saunders.

Wilmore, J.H., & Brown, C.H. (1974). Physiological profiles of women distance runners. *Medicine and Science in Sports, 6,* 178-181.

Wilmore, J.H., Brown, C.H., & Davies, J.A. (1977). Body physique and composition of the female distance runner. *Annals of the New York Academy of Science, 301,* 764-776.

Wilmore, J.H., Parr, R.B., Haskell, W.L., Costill, D.L., Milburn, I.J., & Kerlan, R.K. (1976). Football pros' strengths—and CV weakness—charted. *Physician and Sportsmedicine, 4* (#10), 45-54.

Appendix 19

Nutrition and the NFL: Experiences of a Registered Dietitian

Susan Kleiner

Elite athletes have long been aware that nutrition can play a critical role in their performance. But myths and misconceptions were their usual basis for planning diets. Only recently have those athletes discovered the science of sports nutrition, and nutritionists and dietitians have played a leading role in getting the information to the consumer.

Endurance athletes have gained the most benefit from new discoveries that can enhance performance. Very little work was focused on strength-training athletes. As drug use in sports becomes less tolerated by the sports governing bodies, strength-training athletes in particular have begun to look for alternative methods of performance enhancement. The research base is also beginning to expand.

This change in atmosphere, from drug-tolerance to drug-abhorrence, has opened one door to sports nutritionists that was previously tightly closed: the National Football League.

My path to the door of an NFL organization was unplanned, but completely natural. All of my research and much of my consulting focused on strength-training and bodybuilding athletes. When the new head coach for the team arrived, he had been well trained in the importance of good nutrition by the team nutritionist of his former team. The coach requested that the team physician recommend a nutritionist for the team. Because the team physician and I were well acquainted, I was quickly interviewed for the job.

This was a critical meeting. With an excellent understanding of nutrition, the coach was aware of where nutrition fits into an entire training program for professional football players. My job was to show him that I understood that place, as well.

As with all athletes, nutrition is only one part of football players' entire training regimen. A great athlete requires, first and foremost, a great genetic potential to perform. At these elite heights, those who try hard but lack the genetic makeup just can't make it. Second, proper training and coaching will make a great difference, especially during the rookie year in the pros. All alone, these two factors can definitely create a great athlete. But how long will this athlete be able to keep up the pace? Nutrition is the third important factor in the training regimen of athletes, but, especially with strength and power athletes, its impact is felt more over the long term, rather than the short term.

One of the main jobs of a team nutritionist is weight-control counseling. Weight control is a major concern of pro football players, and the nutritionist's impact may be both short and long term. Depending on the coach, players may be asked to gain weight any way they can, gain only muscle weight, lose weight slowly, or lose by next week. A dietitian plays a major role in educating these athletes on healthful yet practical ways to gain and lose weight.

321

But making weight is the issue, not health. Regardless of our own desires to create healthy football players, we must remember that health is not *their* goal. Their sole goal is performance. If we don't help them achieve that because our own goals get in the way, then we are of no service to the team.

This may seem as if we, as health professionals and sports nutritionists, must serve two masters. Not exactly. With so many nutrition misconceptions floating around the locker rooms, our input is extremely valuable, both to help the athlete achieve his goals, as well as to achieve our own. The athlete who starves and dehydrates himself to make weight is a perfect injury target for Sunday afternoon, if not during practice or weigh-in day. Suggesting realistic weight-loss goals based on percentage-body-fat measures (to coaches) and alternatives to extreme dieting practices (to athletes) can make a great difference to the entire team.

Football players, like most Americans, eat too much fat. Since many can handle the calories, they don't feel the body weight impact of a high-fat diet as much as an average individual. Generally, however, athletes will perform better on a high-carbohydrate, rather than a high-fat, diet. Therefore, offering basic nutrition education that follows the general guidelines of a high-carbohydrate, low-fat diet is another very important part of a team nutritionist's job.

Learning by example is just as important in the NFL as in a clinical setting. If the dietitian cannot review and suggest the menus for minicamps, training camp, pregame meals, and other meals that the organization feeds the team, then much of the work of nutrition education will be lost. It is critical for a team nutritionist to offer this input, so that diet information remains consistent and obviously has the support of the coaches and management.

The most important time for nutrition counseling and intervention is during the preseason, especially just before and during training camp. Once the season begins, there are so many issues involved in learning and practicing the weekly strategies that too much nutrition information is distracting, rather than supportive.

Some kind of contact with the team as a whole should be maintained during the season to reinforce nutrition basics. Weekly nutrition tips and nutrition sessions with wives and companions are good ways to maintain that contact. Specific players may need individual counseling. Some may begin to gain weight because they are less active now than during preseason. Injured players may need special attention.

The overall impact of nutritional changes may not be obvious the first season, and they may never be measurably obvious. There are too many factors to truly separate the unique effect that nutrition may have on the performance of individual players or on the team as a whole.

After considering superior genetic potential and training, high-performance nutrition practices have the potential to influence the athletic performance of these elite athletes at a level of 2% to 3%. At this level of athletic endeavor, this seemingly small amount may make the difference of 1 or 2 yards at the end of an exhausting game; the difference between a lost opportunity and a winning touchdown.

If a nutritionist is successful in modifying the diets and nutrition practices of pro football players, one would hope that the ultimate influences would be athletes who might stay healthier during the season, heal more readily after injuries, maintain a higher level of performance year after year, and possibly extend their professional athletic lifetimes.

In fact, our greatest influence may come at the end of their professional playing careers. Former professional football players are notorious for continuing to indulge in high-fat diets, even though their exercise routines have been significantly reduced since retirement. This life-style usually leads to obesity and places these players at a very high risk for chronic diseases. If what we teach football players during their careers helps them alter their dietary patterns during retirement, we may have made the most important impact on their health status long after we have helped them achieve their athletic goals.

It is certain that the NFL did well before sports nutritionists and it could continue to do well without us. Without drugs to enhance performance, coaches and trainers have begun to look to nutrition as a legal alternative. Although nutrition will never create the physical changes in athletes that drugs might support, following the principles of sports nutrition science can certainly help athletes achieve realistic goals naturally—and legally.

Appendix 20

Joint Position of The American Dietetic Association and The Canadian Dietetic Association: Nutrition for Physical Fitness and Athletic Performance for Adults

The American Dietetic Association and The Canadian Dietetic Association support access to accurate and appropriate information that explains the interrelationships between exercise and nutrition, reinforces the important role of nutrition, and encourages appropriate food choices to achieve optimal physical fitness and athletic performance.

Weight/area (lbs)
On 150-pound room Percent utilization   Effect

1.5

wt/area (lbs)   On 200-pound room   150-pound room

Percent situation   1.0   1.5

Effect   ↑ B temp   1.0

$\dfrac{1 \cdot 5}{10 \cdot 5}$

Appendix 21
Suggested Reading List

► **SECTION I**

Books

Gollnick P. Energy metabolism and prolonged exercise. In: Lamb D, Murray R, eds. *Prolonged Exercise.* Indianapolis, Ind: Benchmark Press; 1988.

Goodhart RS, Shils ME, eds. *Modern Nutrition in Health and Disease.* 6th ed. Philadelphia, Pa: Lea & Febiger; 1980.

Hunt S, Groff J. *Advanced Nutrition and Human Metabolism.* St Paul, Minn: West Publishing Co; 1990.

McArdle WD, Katch FI, Katch VL. *Exercise Physiology: Energy, Nutrition, and Human Performance.* 2nd ed. Philadelphia, Pa: Lea & Febiger; 1986.

National Research Council. *Recommended Dietary Allowances.* 10th ed. Washington, DC: National Academy Press; 1989.

Powers S, Howley E. *Exercise Physiology: Theory and Application to Fitness and Performance.* Dubuque, Iowa: Wm C Brown; 1990.

Williams MH. *Nutrition for Fitness and Sport.* 3rd ed. Dubuque, Iowa: Wm C Brown Publishers; 1992.

Articles

Bergstrom J, Hultman E. Nutrition for maximal sports performance. *JAMA.* 1972;221:999.

Bouchard C, Lortie J. Heredity and human performance. *Sports Med.* 1984;1:38.

Brehm B, Gutin B. Recovery energy expenditure for steady state exercise in runners and nonexercisers. *Med Sci Sports Exerc.* 1986;18:205-210.

Costill D. Energy supply in endurance activities. *Int J Sports Med.* 1984;5(suppl):19-20.

Costill DL, Miller J. Nutrition for endurance sports: carbohydrate and fluid balance. *Int J Sports Med.* 1980;1:2.

Coyle EF, Coggan AR. Effectiveness of carbohydrate feeding in delaying fatigue during prolonged exercise. *Sports Med.* 1984;1:446.

Durnin J. The energy cost of exercise. *Proc Nutr Soc.* 1985;44:273-282.

Forbes G, Brown M. Energy need for weight maintenance in human beings: effects of body size and composition. *J Am Diet Assoc.* 1989;89:499-502.

Holloszy JO, Coyle EF. Adaptations of skeletal muscle to endurance exercise and their metabolic consequences. *J Appl Physiol.* 1984;56:831.

Horton E. Metabolic fuels, utilization, and exercise. *Am J Clin Nutr.* 1989;49:931-932.

Howley E, Glover M. The caloric costs of running and walking one mile for men and women. *Med Sci Sports Exerc.* 1974;6:235-237.

Karlsson J. Saltin B. Lactate, ATP, and CP in working muscles during exhaustive exercise in man. *J Appl Physiol.* 1970;29:598.

Krahenbuhl GS, Pangrasi R. Characteristics associated with running performance in young boys. *Med Sci Sports Exerc.* 1983;15:488.

Schwartz R, Ravussin E, Massari M, et al. The thermic effect of carbohydrates versus fat feeding in man. *Metabolism.* 1985;34:285-293.

Sedlick D, Cohen B. The effect of acute nutritional status on postexercise energy expenditure. *Med Sci Sports Exerc.* 1990;22:S49.

Sherman WM, Costill DL. The marathon: dietary manipulation to optimize performance. *Am J Sports Med.* 1984;12:44.

Stainsby W, Brooks G. Control of lactic acid metabolism in contracting muscles and during exercise. *Exerc Sports Sci Rev.* 1990;18:29-63.

Thomas T, Londeree B. Energy cost during prolonged walking vs jogging exercise. *Phys Sports Med.* 1989;17:93-102.

Werblow JA. Nutritional knowledge, attitudes, and food patterns of women athletes. *J Am Diet Assoc.* 1978;73:242.

► SECTION II

Books

American College of Sports Medicine. *Guidelines for Graded Exercise Testing Prescription.* 4th ed. Philadelphia, Pa: Lea & Febiger; 1991.

American Heart Association. *Dietary Guidelines for Healthy American Adults.* Dallas, Tex: 1986. American Heart Association, AHA publication 21-0030.

Astrand PO, Rodahl K. *Textbook of Work Physiology.* 3rd ed. New York, NY: McGraw-Hill; 1986.

Berning JR, Steen SN, eds. *Sports Nutrition for the 90s: The Health Professional's Handbook.* Gaithersburg, Md: Aspen Publishers Inc; 1991.

Bouchard C, Johnston F, eds. *Fat Distribution During Growth and Later Outcomes.* New York, NY: Alan R. Liss; 1988.

Gibson RS. *Principles of Nutritional Assessment.* New York, NY: Oxford University Press; 1990.

Goodhart RS, Shils ME, eds. *Modern Nutrition in Health and Disease.* 6th ed. Philadelphia, Pa: Lea & Febiger; 1980.

Lohman TG, Roche AF, Martorell R, eds. *Anthropometric Standardization Reference Manual.* Champaign, Ill: Human Kinetics Publishers; 1988.

McArdle WD, Katch FI, Katch VL. *Exercise Physiology: Energy, Nutrition, and Human Performance.* 2nd ed. Philadelphia, Pa: Lea & Febiger; 1986.

Nieman DC. *The Sports Medicine Fitness Course.* Palo Alto, Calif: Bull Publishing Co; 1990.

Nutrition and Your Health: Dietary Guidelines for Americans. 3rd ed. Washington, DC: US Dept of Agriculture, US Dept of Health and Human Services; 1990. Home and Garden bulletin 232.

Roche A, ed. *Body Composition Assessments in Youth and Adults.* Columbus, Ohio: Ross Laboratories; 1985.

Shils M, Young V. *Modern Nutrition in Health and Disease.* 7th ed. Philadelphia, Pa: Lea & Febiger; 1988.

Articles

Acheson KJ, Campbell IT, Edholm OG, Miller DS, Stock MJ. The measurement of food and energy intake in man—an evaluation of some techniques. *Am J Clin Nutr.* 1980;33:1147-1154.

Benardot D, Czerwinski C. Selected body composition and growth measures of junior elite gymnasts. *J Am Diet Assoc.* 1991;91:209-216.

Clarys JP, Martin AD, Drinkwater DT. Gross tissue weights in the human body by cadaver dissection. *Hum Biol.* 1984;56:459-473.

Conway JM, Norris KH, Bodwell CE. A new approach for the estimation of body composition: infrared interactance. *Am J Clin Nutr.* 1984;40:1123-1130.

Frisancho AR. New standard of weight and body composition by frame size and height for assessment of nutritional status of adults and the elderly. *Am J Clin Nutr.* 1984;40:808-819.

Jackson AS. Research design and analysis of data procedures for predicting body density. *Med Sci Sports Exerc.* 1984;16:616-620.

Jackson B, Dujovne CA, DeCoursey S, Beyer P, Brown EF, Hassanein K. Methods to assess relative reliability of diet records: minimum records for monitoring lipid and calorie intake. *J Am Diet Assoc.* 1986;86:1531-1535.

Katch F, Michael ED, Horvath SM. Estimation of body volume by underwater weighing: description of a simple method. *J Appl Physiol.* 1967;23:811-813.

Katch VL, Freedson PS, Katch FI, Smith L. Body frame size: validity of self-appraisal. *Am J Clin Nutr.* 1982;36:676-679.

Krall EA, Dwyer JT. Validity of a food frequency questionnaire and a food diary in a short-term recall situation. *J Am Diet Assoc.* 1987;87:1374-1376.

Lohman TG. Assessment of body composition in children *Pediatr Exerc Sci.* 1989;1:19-30.

Lohman TG, Pollock ML, Slaughter MH, Brandon LJ, Boileau RA. Methodological factors and the prediction of body fat in female athletes. *Med Sci Sports Exerc.* 1984;16:92-96.

Lohman TG. Skinfolds and body density and their relation to body fatness: a review. *Hum Biol.* 1981;53:181-225.

Roche AF. The bioelectrical estimation of body composition. *Hum Biol.* 1987;59:213.

Steen SN, Brownell K. Patterns of weight loss and regain in wrestlers: has the pattern changed? *Med Sci Sports Exerc.* 1990;22:762-768.

▶ **SECTION III**

Books

American College of Obstetricians and Gynecologists. *Exercise During Pregnancy and the Postnatal Period.* Washington, DC: American College of Obstetricians and Gynecologists; 1985.

Graef JW, Cone TE, eds. *Manual of Pediatric Therapeutics.* Boston, Mass: Little, Brown and Co; 1980.

McArdle WD, Katch FI, Katch VL. *Exercise Physiology: Energy, Nutrition, and Human Performance.* 2nd ed. Philadelphia, Pa: Lea & Febiger; 1986.

Report of the Ross Symposium: The Theory and Practice of Athletic Nutrition: Bridging the Gap. Columbus, Ohio: Ross Laboratories; 1990.

Shils M, Young V. *Modern Nutrition in Health and Disease.* Philadelphia, Pa: Lea & Febiger; 1988.

US Dept of Health and Human Services, Public Health Service. *The Surgeon General's Report on Nutrition and Health.* Washington DC: US Government Printing Office; 1988. DHHS (PHS) publication 88-50210.

US Dept of Health and Human Services, Joint National Committee on Detection, Evaluation, and Treatment of High Blood Pressure: The 1988 Report. Bethesda, Md: National Heart, Lung, and Blood Institute; 1988. NIH publication 88-1088.

Wilmore JH. *Sports Medicine for Children and Youth: Report of 10th Ross Roundtable on Approaches to Common Pediatric Problems.* Columbus, Ohio: Ross Laboratories; 1979.

Articles

Borgen JS, Corbin C. Eating disorders among female athletes. *Phys Sports Med.* 1987;15:89-95.

Clapp JF. The course of labor after endurance exercise during pregnancy. *Am J Obstet Gynecol.* 1990;163:1799-1805.

Fishbein EG, Phillips M. How safe is exercise during pregnancy? *J Obstet Gynecol Neonatal Nurs.* 1990;19:45-49.

Goldberg L, Elliot DL. The effect of physical activity on lipid and lipoprotein levels. *Med Clin North Am.* 1985;69:41.

Huch R, Erkkola R. Pregnancy and exercise—exercise and pregnancy: a short review. *Br J Obstet Gynaecol.* 1990;97:208-14.

Loucks AB. Effects of exercise training on the menstrual cycle: existence and mechanisms. *Med Sci Sports Exerc.* 1990;22:275-280.

Rosen L, McKeag D, Hough D, Curley V. Pathogenic weight control behavior in female athletes. *Phys Sports Med.* 1986;14:79-86.

Sedlet K, Ireton-Jones C. Energy expenditure and the abnormal eating pattern of a bulimic: a case report. *J Am Diet Assoc.* 1989;89:74-77.

Tzankoff SP, Norris AH. Effect of muscle mass decrease on age-related BMR changes. *J Appl Physiol.* 1977;32:1001.

Van Swearingen J. Iron deficiency in athletes: consequences or adaptation in strenuous activity. *J Orthoped Sports Phys Ther.* 1986;7:192.

Wolfe LA, Hall P, Webb KA, Goodman L, Monga M, McGrath MJ. Prescription of aerobic exercise during pregnancy. *Sports Med.* 1989;8:273-301.

▶ SECTION IV
Books

American College of Sports Medicine. *Guidelines for Graded Exercise Testing Prescription.* 4th ed. Philadelphia, Pa: Lea & Febiger; 1991.

American Heart Association. *Dietary Guidelines for Healthy American Adults.* Dallas, Tex: American Heart Association; 1986. AHA publication 21-0030.

Berning JR, Steen SN, eds. *Sports Nutrition for the 90s: The Health Professional's Handbook.* Gaithersburg, Md: Aspen Publishers, Inc; 1991.

Clark N. *Nancy Clark's Sports Nutrition Guidebook: Eating to Fuel Your Active Lifestyle.* Champaign, Ill: Leisure Press; 1990.

Coleman E. *Eating for Endurance.* Palo Alto, Calif: Bull Publishing; 1988.

Combs GF Jr. *The Vitamins: Fundamental Aspects in Nutrition and Health.* San Diego, Calif: Academic Press Inc; 1992.

Goodhart RS, Shils ME, eds. *Modern Nutrition in Health and Disease.* 6th ed. Philadelphia, Pa: Lea & Febiger; 1980.

McArdle WD, Katch FI, Katch VL. *Exercise Physiology: Energy, Nutrition, and Human Performance.* 2nd ed. Philadelphia, Pa: Lea & Febiger; 1986.

National Research Council. *Recommended Dietary Allowances.* 10th Ed. Washington, DC: National Academy Press; 1989.

Powers S, Howley E. *Exercise Physiology: Theory and Application to Fitness and Performance.* Dubuque, Iowa: Wm C Brown; 1990.

Smith N, Worthington-Roberts B. *Food for Sport.* Palo Alto, Calif: Bull Publishing; 1989.

Williams MH. *Nutrition for Fitness and Sport.* 3rd ed. Dubuque, Iowa: Wm C Brown Publishers; 1992.

Articles

Boyer SJ, Blume FD. Weight loss and changes in body composition at high altitude. *J Appl Physiol.* 1984;57:1580-1585.

Costill DL, Saltin B. Factors limiting gastric emptying during rest and exercise. *J Appl Physiol.* 1974;37:679.

Ivy J. Muscle glycogen synthesis after exercise and effect of time of carbohydrate ingestion. *J Appl Physiol.* 1988;64:1480-1485.

Jandrain B, Krentowski G, Pirnay F, et al. Metabolic availability of glucose ingested three hours before prolonged exercise in emptying. *Med Sci Sports Exerc.* 1986;18:658-662.

Loat ER, Rhodes EC. Jet-lag and human performance. *Sports Med.* 1989;8:226-238.

Nadel ER. Control of sweating rate while exercising in the heat. *Med Sci Sports Exerc.* 1979;11:31-35.

Sawka MN, Francesconi RP, Young AJ, Pandolf KB. Influence of hydration level and body fluids on exercise performance in the heat. *JAMA.* 1984;252:1165-1169.

Sherman WM, Costill DL, Fink WJ, Miller JM. The effect of exercise and diet manipulation on muscle glycogen and its subsequent use during performance. *Int J Sports Med.* 1981;2:114-119.

▶ SECTION V

Books

Barrett S, ed. *The Health Robbers.* Philadelphia, Pa: Stickley Co; 1980.

Berning JR, Steen SN, eds. *Sports Nutrition for the 90s: The Health Professional's Handbook.* Gaithersburg, Md: Aspen Publishers Inc; 1991.

Hickson J, Wolinsky I. *Nutrition in Exercise and Sport.* Boca Raton, Fla: CRC Press; 1989.

Williams MH. *Nutrition for Fitness and Sport.* 3rd ed. Dubuque, Iowa: Wm C Brown Publishers; 1992.

Articles

Applegate L. Fad diets and supplement use in athletes. *Sports Sci Exch.* 1988;1:1-4.

Douglas P, Douglas J. Nutrition knowledge and food practices of high school athletes. *J Am Diet Assoc.* 1984;84:1198-1202.

Kleiner S. Beware of nutrition quackery. *Phys Sports Med.* 1990;18:46-49.

Kris-Etherton PM. The facts and fallacies of nutritional supplements for athletes. *National Coach.* Spring 1990;25:6-9.

Position of The American Dietetic Association. Identifying food and nutrition misinformation. *J Am Diet Assoc.* 1988;88:1589-1591.

Yesalis C. Winning and performance-enhancing drugs—our dual addiction. *Phys Sports Med.* 1990;18:161-167.

Index